GERIATRICS, GERONTOLOGY AND ELDERLY ISSUES

CURRENT CHALLENGES AND MANAGEMENT OF DISEASES IN THE ELDERLY POPULATION

Geriatrics, Gerontology and Elderly Issues

Additional books and e-books in this series can be found on Nova's website under the Series tab.

GERIATRICS, GERONTOLOGY AND ELDERLY ISSUES

CURRENT CHALLENGES AND MANAGEMENT OF DISEASES IN THE ELDERLY POPULATION

ABHAI KUMAR
EDITOR

nova
Medicine & Health
New York

Library of Congress Cataloging-in-Publication Data

Names: Kumar, Abhai, editor.
Title: Current challenges and management of diseases in the elderly population / [edited by Abhai Kumar].
Description: New York: Nova Science Publishers, Inc., [2019] | Series: Geriatrics, gerontology and elderly issues | Includes bibliographical references and index. |
Identifiers: LCCN 2020000024 (print) | LCCN 2020000025 (ebook) | ISBN 9781536173048 (hardcover) | ISBN 9781536173055 (adobe pdf)
Subjects: LCSH: Older people--Diseases. | Older people--Diseases--Treatment. | Geriatrics.
Classification: LCC RC952.5 .C87 2019 (print) | LCC RC952.5 (ebook) | DDC 618.97--dc23
LC record available at https://lccn.loc.gov/2020000024
LC ebook record available at https://lccn.loc.gov/2020000025

Published by Nova Science Publishers, Inc. † New York

CONTENTS

FOREWORD

Debasis Bagchi, PhD, MACN, CNS, MAIChE
Director of Scientific Affairs, Victory Nutrition International Inc., Concord, CA
Department of Pharmacological and Pharmaceutical Sciences, University of Houston College of Pharmacy, Houston, TX
Adjunct Faculty, Texas Southern University, Houston, TX
Past President of American College of Nutrition, Clearwater, FL
Past Chairman of International Society of Nutraceuticals and Functional Foods (ISNFF)
Dr. Bagchi received the Master of American College of Nutrition Award in October 2010. Past Chair, Nutraceuticals and Functional Foods Division, Institute of Food Technologists (IFT), Chicago, IL.
Distinguished Advisor, Japanese Institute for Health Food Standards (JIHFS), Tokyo, Japan
Email: debasisbagchi@gmail.com.

In 2017, a survey was conducted by the United Nations in Ageing Population and it was reported that the number of people who are 60 years old will double and the number of 80 years old people will triple over the next 30 years, respectively [1]. The Department of Economic and Social Affairs Population Division of the United Nations further reported that the population in lower age groups will be reduced [1]. US Census Bureau also reported in 2017 that according to the current statistics 15% of the population are older adults and the Bureau estimated that this number will increase to 23.5% in 2060 [2,3]. A similar report by the European Commission in 2017 stated that 19% of the total population is currently 65-year old or older, which is estimated to increase to 25% of total population in 2080 [4]. Same trend has been reported for the other sub-continents.

Furthermore, ageing population suffer from diverse chronic diseases including diverse cardiovascular problems, diabetes, metabolic disorders, gastrointestinal diseases, ocular problems, cancer, respiratory distress and several others [5,6]. World Health Organization estimated 41 million deaths per year in the world from these diverse diseases and the number is increasing [5,6]. CDC (Centers for Disease Control and Prevention) estimated that in USA, about 50% of all ageing adults suffer from more than one chronic disease, while 25% have two or more chronic diseases [7]. Rijken et al. reported in 2013 [8] that in Europe, approximately 50 million adults suffer from multiple chronic diseases, while the Swedish Agency for Health and Care Services Analysis reported [9] in 2014 that 44% of the older population in Sweden suffer from one chronic disease, while 25% suffer from two or more chronic diseases.

The timing of the forthcoming book "Current Challenges and Management of Diseases of Elderly Population" edited by Dr. Abhai Kumar, PhD, from the Interdisciplinary School of Life Sciences, Banaras Hindu University, Varanasi, India, is perfectly appropriate. It is important to emphasize that Dr. Kumar gathered significant experience and expertise in neurodegeneration research in the top-notch institutions in India and USA. Dr. Kumar published numerous cutting-edge peer-reviewed publications and book chapters. The book comprises of ten leading chapters by leading researchers and academicians demonstrating the critical and salient features of diverse advancing age related diseases including diabetes, neurodegenerative disorders, bone health and two dedicated chapters emphasizing osteoporosis problems in women, ocular health and intricate aspects of metabolic syndrome. In addition, this book comprises of detailed chapters on cutting edge technologies including the applications of metabolomics, rejuvenation and activation of aged T cells, critical aspects of epigenetic elements and stem cell aging, as well as utilization of sophisticated analytical techniques in the detection of diverse aging related health maladies. Finally, several chapters focused on how appropriate diet, functional foods, micronutrients, polyphenols and other phytonutrients may he utilized to reverse or slow down the diverse detrimental health problems.

This book will immensely help the researchers, health professionals and medical professionals, especially involved in neurological and neurodegeneration research studies.

REFERENCES

[1] Department of Economic and Social Affairs Population Division. United Nations. (2017). *World Population Ageing 2017*. New York, NY. https://www.un.org/en/development/desa/population/publications/pdf/ageing/WPA2017_Report.pdf (accessed Oct 10, 2019).

[2] *United States Census Bureau.* (2017). Older Population and Aging. https://www.census.gov/topics/population/older-aging.html (accessed Oct 10, 2019).

[3] *The U.S. Census Bureau (2017) National Population Projections.* https://www.census.gov/programs-surveys/popproj.html (accessed Oct 10, 2019).

[4] *European Commission. (2017).* Eurostat regional yearbook 2017. Luxembourg: Publications Office of the European Union. https://ec.europa.eu/regional_policy/en/newsroom/news/2017/09/14-09-2017-eurostat-regional-yearbook-2017 (accessed Oct 10, 2019).

[5] *World Health Organization (WHO).* (2013). A universal truth: No health without a workforce. Third Global Forum on Human Resources for Health Report. Geneva: World Health Organization (WHO).https://www.who.int/workforcealliance/knowledge/resources/hrhreport2013/en/ (accessed Oct 10, 2019).

[6] World Health Organization (WHO). *Noncommunicable diseases fact sheet.* http://www.who.int/en/news-room/fact-sheets/detail/noncommunicable-diseases/ (accessed Oct 10, 2019).

[7] Centers for Disease Control and Prevention. (2017). *Chronic diseases: The leading causes of death and disability in the United States.* https://www.cdc.gov/chronicdisease/overview/index.htm (accessed Oct 10, 2019).

[8] Rijken M, Struckmann V, Dyakova M, Melchiorre MG, Rissanen S, van Ginneken E. (2013). *ICARE4EU: Improving care for people with multiple chronic conditions in Europe*. http://www.icare4eu.org/pdf/icare4eu-improving.pdf (accessed Oct 10, 2019).

[9] The Swedish Agency for Health and Care Services Analysis. (2014). VIPs in health care? *About challenges in health care for persons with chronic illness. Stockholm: The Swedish Agency for Health and Care Services Analysis*. https://www.vardanalys.se/in-english/reports/vips-in-health-care/ (accessed Oct 10, 2019)

PREFACE

The shift in epidemiological transition due to decrease in mortality and high fertility is characterized by waning of infectious and acute diseases and emerging importance of chronic and degenerative diseases1. The major epidemiologic trend of current century is rise in chronic and degenerative diseases in countries throughout the world regardless of income level [1,2].

By 2030, non communicable diseases are projected to account for more than one-half of the disease burden in low-income countries and more than three-fourths in middle-income countries. Infectious and parasitic diseases will account for 30 percent and 10 percent, respectively, in low- and middle-income countries. Among the 60-and-over population, non communicable diseases already account for more than 87 percent of the burden in low-, middle-, and high-income countries [1,2]. The health problem in adulthood and later stage of life is linked with infection and health conditions early in life. The aged people suffering from one chronic disease or infectious disease are more vulnerable for multiple diseases, for example type 2 diabetes and immunosuppression are well known comorbid risk factors that have serious health consequences for older people [3].

Population Aging is likely to influence pattern of health care spending in both developed and developing countries in the decades to come. In developed countries, where acute care and institutional long-term care services are widely available, the use of medical care services by adults rises with age, and per capita expenditures on health care are relatively high among older age groups [4,5]. Accordingly, the rising proportion of older people is placing upward pressure on overall health care spending in the developed world, although other factors such as income growth and advances in the technological capabilities of medicine generally play a much larger role [6].

The two most populous countries of world India and China will challenge national infrastructure mainly health system. The increase in old age population above 65 years will swell up by 330 and 228 million in China and India by 2050 as compared with current 110 and 68 million. The constitution of older people at age above 85 years or older are around 12%and 6% in developed and developing countries respectively [3,7,8] . In various part of the world the oldest are the fastest growing part of total population, on the global level the 85 and over population is projected to increase 351 percent between 2010 and 2050, compared to 188 percent increase for the population aged 65 or older and 22 percent increase for the population under age 65 [9,10,11]

The current book emphasizes various diseases challenges and management in the elderly population during aging. Chapter 1 deals with the importance of stem cell based regulation of cell homeostasis during ageing, mainly methylation/demethylation of DNA encoding different proteins responsible for cell maintenance and regeneration during ageing. Chapter 2 discuss about the compromised immune-responsiveness during old age by failure in activation of T-cell. Chapter 3 emphasized about the most prevalent problem around the globe Type-2 Diabetes Mellitus which leads to diabetic neuropathy, pathogenesis and management of disease. Chapter 4 encompass information on bone diseases which are very common in elderly population, different type of bone disease like osteoporosis, Paget disease, osteoarthritis, osteomalacia their pathogenesis and management. Chapter 5 highlights the role of Vitamin D in bone formation and metabolic activity mainly after menopause in elderly women's in Asian population. Chapter 6. Provide insight about different type of eye disease that occurs during old age and their management through preventive measures. Chapter 7. Changes in body metabolite is result of paradigm changes in physiology during ageing, biomarker identification through metabolomics can provide specific marker for disease identification, the chapter provide complete information on tools and techniques for biomarker identification through metabolomics. Chapter 8. The complete information on changes in DNA, RNA and proteins inside cells at particular time line could tag specific changes as signature of disease manifestation; these changes are elucidated through omics and imaging techniques for identification of neurodegeneration in this part Chapter 9. It focus on various neurodegenerative diseases, their pathogenesis and prevention through plant flavonoids Chapter 10. The information related to brain health on basis of nutraceuticals and dietary factor, their role in brain physiology and different types of diets to improve brain functioning and treating brain diseases in older population

In summary, this book covers a broad range of topics related to elderly population related major diseases and their management, and various treatment options, rendering it an invaluable resource for professionals interested in gerontology and geriatric care. Our sincere thanks to all our eminent contributors and Dr. Smita Singh for his continued support, cooperation, and assistance.

REFERENCES

[1] Abegunde, D. O., Mathers, C. D., Adam, T., Ortegon, M., Strong, K. *The burden and costs of chronic diseases in low-income and middle-income countries*. The Lancet 2007 (December 8); 370:1929-1938

[2] Avendano, M., Glymour, M. M., Banks, J., Mackenbach, J. P. *Health disadvantage in US adults aged 50 to 74 years: A comparison of the health of rich and poor Americans with that of Europeans*. American Journal of Public Health 2009: 99/3:540-548.

[3] Chatterji S., Kowal P., Mathers C., Naidoo N., Verdes E., Smith J. P., Suzman R. *The health of aging populations in China and India*. Health Affairs 2008; 27/4:1052-1063.

[4] Christensen K., Doblhammer G., Rau R., Vaupel J. W. *Ageing populations: The challenges ahead.* The Lancet 2009; 374/9696: 1196-1208.

[5] Crimmins EM, Preston SH, Cohen B., eds. International Differences in Mortality at Older Ages. Dimensions and Sources. Washington, DC: The National Academies Press, 2010. European Commission. 2009 Ageing Report: Economic and Budgetary Projections for the EU-27 Member States (2008-2060). Brussels: European Communities, 2009. Available at: http://www.da.dk/bilag/publication14992_ageing_report.pdf.

[6] Kinsella K, He, W. An Aging World: 2008. Washington, DC: National Institute on Aging and U.S. Census Bureau, 2009. Lafortune, G., Balestat, G. *Trends in Severe Disability Among Elderly People. Assessing the Evidence in 12 OECD Countries and the Future Implications*. OECD Health Working Papers 26. Paris: Organization for Economic Cooperation and Development, 2007.

[7] Lopez, A. D., Mathers, C. D., Ezzati, M., Jamison, D. T., Murray, C. J. L., eds. Global Burden of Disease and Risk Factors. Washington, D. C.: *The World Bank Group*, 2006.

[8] National Institute on Aging. Growing Older in America: The Health and Retirement Study. Washington, DC: U.S. *Department of Health and Human Services, 2007.*

[9] Oxley, H. Policies for Healthy Ageing: An. Overview. *OECD Health Working Papers 42. Paris: Organization for Economic Cooperation and Development*, 2009.

[10] Plassman, B. L., Langa, K. M., Fisher, G. G., Heeringa, S. G., Weir, D. R., Ofstedal, MB, Burke, JR, Hurd, MD, Potter, GG, Rodgers, WL, Steffens, DC, Willis, R. J., and Wallace, R. B. *Prevalence of dementia in the United States: The aging, demographics, and memory study.* Neuroepidemiology 2007; 29:125-132.

[11] Rohwedder, S., Willis, R. J. Mental retirement. Journal of Economic Perspectives 2010 Winter; 24/1: 119-138. Zeng, Y., G Danan, Land KC. *The association of childhood socioeconomic conditions with healthy longevity at the oldest old ages in China*. Demography, 2007; 44/3:497-518.

In: Current Challenges and Management … ISBN: 978-1-53617-304-8
Editor: Abhai Kumar

Chapter 1

STEM CELL AGING: AN EPIGENETIC PERSPECTIVE

Kulwant Singh*, PhD
and Chandra Prakash Chaturvedi†, PhD
Stem Cell Research Center, Department of Hematology,
Sanjay Gandhi Post Graduate Institute of Medical Sciences,
Lucknow, UP, India

ABSTRACT

Adult stem cells are indispensable for long-term maintenance of various tissues of an organism. Loss of adult stem cell functions has been associated with aging, leading to compromised tissue repair and regeneration. As epigenetic mechanisms are instrumental for stem cell lineage progression, their deregulation has been emerging as an important driver of stem cell dysfunctions during aging stem. Here we have highlighted the way epigenetic regulators control the stem cell function under normal homeostatic conditions and how deregulation of these mechanisms results in alterations of their functions and emergence of

* Corresponding Author's Email: ksinghcdri@gmail.com.
† Corresponding Author's Email: chaturvedicp75@rediffmail.com.

age-associated human diseases. As epigenetic signatures are mostly reversible, precise understanding of these mechanisms are crucial for slowing down or preventing the process of stem cell aging and also provide opportunities to design novel epigenetic based therapeutic regimens for treatment of age-associated human disorders.

Keywords: stem cell, aging, epigenetics, DNA methylation, histone modifications, microRNA

1. Introduction

In the developing embryo, stem cells mediate organogenesis, whereas postnatal, are responsible for fitness of various tissues throughout the life of the organism as adult stem cells (Goodell and Rando 2015). The lineage of adult stem cells is determined during embryonic development from specialized population of progenitor cells therefore, key developmental pathways operated during embryogenesis are recapitulated in these cells to ensure postnatal regeneration and organ homeostasis. Adult stem cells are tissue-specific rare populations of cells located in specialized micro-environment termed as 'stem cell niche', where stem cells regulate the cellular turnover by replacing cells lost or damaged to the normal biological activities and repair tissues in response to injury. Tissue-specific stem cells must self-renew to maintain a stem cell pool for long-term tissue regeneration. Adult stem cells such as muscle stem cells (satellite cell), hematopoietic stem cell, hair follicle stem cells, etc. exist in dormant phase of quiescence (G^0 phase of cell cycle), which facilitate their identification in somatic tissues through specific biomarkers. In response to natural activation signals or after tissue damage, quiescent stem cells become activated, enter in cell cycle and undergoes first round of cell division to give rise to two progenitor cells. One progenitor cell repopulates the stem cell niche (self-renewal) whereas the other progenitor cell differentiate into the cell types to repair the damaged tissue of the organ in which they reside (Figure 1).

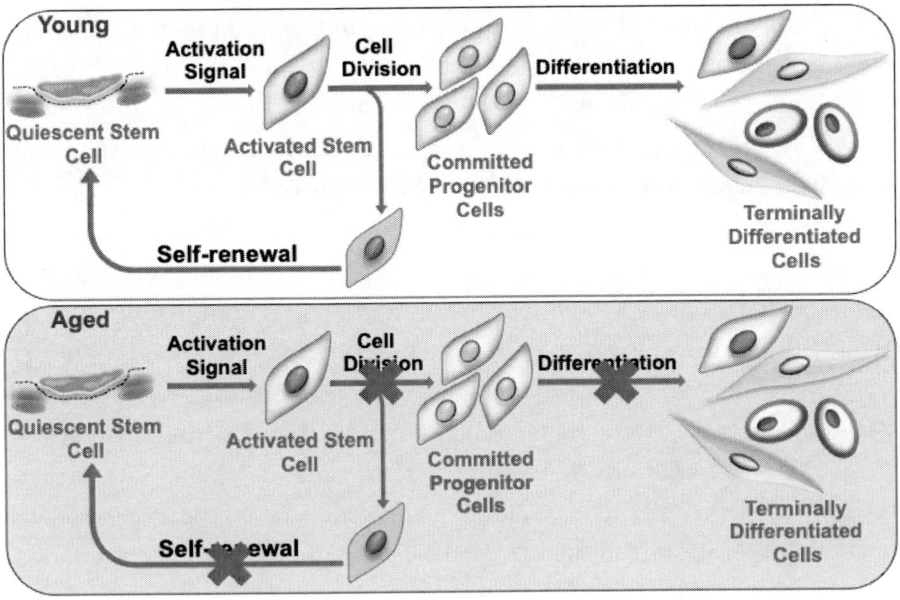

Figure 1. Tissue specific adult stem cells reside in a specialized microenvironment (stem cell niche) in a quiescent state. Upon activation through extrinsic signals, stem cells can self-renew or differentiate to produce committed progenitor cells that proliferate and terminally differentiate into tissue-specific effector cell types. During aging, stem cell self-renewal, proliferation, and differentiation are deregulated.

The regeneration capacity of adult stem cells declines during the aging of the organisms leading to defective tissue regeneration and homeostasis (Oh, Lee, and Wagers 2014; L. Liu and Rando 2011; Behrens et al. 2014; Rossi, Jamieson, and Weissman 2008). Aging can alter stem cell fitness at almost all levels including self-renewal, activation, proliferation and capability to differentiate into effector cell types (Figure 1) (Table 1) (Keyes and Fuchs 2018). For example aged hematopoietic stem cells (HSCs) show increased self-renewal and proliferation potential along with higher propensity to differentiate towards the myeloid lineage (Rossi et al. 2005). In addition, aging HSCs also display reduced engraftment capacity and impairment in long-term reconstitution of immune system (Rossi et al. 2005; Sudo et al. 2000; Dykstra et al. 2011; Cho, Sieburg, and Muller-Sieburg 2008). Similar to HSCs, aged muscle stem cells (MuSCs) display impaired regeneration after injury because of reduced self-renewal and proliferation potential along with increased fibrosis (Conboy et al. 2003; Carlson and Conboy 2007). MuSCs also tend to take alternative lineage from myogenic to fibrogenic and adipogenic lineage during aging (Taylor-Jones et al. 2002; Brack et al. 2007). Such decline in stem cell functions results in changes in the pathophysiology of tissues and emergence of age-related degenerative diseases. Although the mechanistic basis of decline in stem cell function during aging is not completely understood however numerous studies have shown that loss of stem cell polarity (Florian et al. 2012), telomere attrition (Armanios 2013), changes in proteostasis (Warr et al. 2013), replicative stress (Flach et al. 2014), DNA damage (Rossi et al. 2007; Yahata et al. 2011; Jiapeng Wang et al. 2014; Beerman and Rossi 2014), mitochondrial dysfunctions (Bratic and Larsson 2013) and alterations in stem cell niche (Gopinath and Rando 2008) etc. contribute to stem cell aging. A shift in the epigenetic landscape has also been reported as an important mechanistic driver of stem cell aging (Beerman and Rossi 2015; Ermolaeva et al. 2018). As epigenetic marks are mostly reversible, precise understanding of the mechanisms is instrumental for slowing down or preventing the process of stem cell aging.

Table 1. Alterations in stem cell characteristics with age (Modified from Keyes and Fuchs, 2018)

Stem Cell type	Self-renewal	Proliferation	Differentiation	Regeneration and repair capacity
HSCs	Increased	Increased	Increased propensity towards myeloid lineage	Decreased engraftment potential, immune response
HFSCs	Not affected	Reduced	Not affected	Decreased hair cycling and delayed wound healing
ISCs	Not affected	Reduced	Increased propensity towards secretory lineage cells	Reduced generation after UV exposure, delayed response
MuSCs	Decreased	Reduced	Increased fibrosis after injury	Decreased engraftment potential and myofiber regeneration
NSCs	Decreased	Reduced	Not affected	Unknown

Epigenetic regulation refers to heritable changes in gene expression that are not attributed to the change in the gene sequence (Waddington 2012) (Goldberg, Allis, and Bernstein 2007; Bird 2007). Epigenetic signatures such as DNA methylation, histone modification, microRNAs, etc. allow lineage specification of stem cells into defined set of functionally different cell types despite having same genetic sequence. Stem cells imbued with epigenetic memory, which is heritably transmitted to their daughter cells, thus the chromatin marks set at specific loci in stem cells during embryogenesis can prime transcriptional activation or repression of the loci in downstream progeny (Brand et al. 2019). For example, progeny cells derived from stem cells either remember their chromatin signatures as stem cells (self-renewal) or partially erase their chromatin signatures to take a new identity (differentiation). In differentiated cells, epigenetic mechanisms also co-ordinate the cellular activity and inhibit access to lineage inappropriate gene expression program (Hodges et al. 2011). Thus, chromatin architecture of stem cells is instrumental in preserving stem cell identity and functions.

This chapter describes how the epigenetic mechanisms regulate adult stem cell functions and how deregulation of these mechanisms in aging stem cells leads to defective tissue regeneration and homeostasis. The epigenetic signatures discussed in the context of stem cell aging are as follows.

2. Epigenetic Regulation of Stem Cell Fate Decision and Aging

2.1. DNA Methylation/Demethylation in Stem Cell Fate Decision and Aging

DNA methylation refers to the addition of methyl group at the 5th carbon atom of cytosine nucleotide in DNA to give rise to 5-methyl cytosine. DNA methylation predominantly occurs at CpG dinucleotides, which represent about 28 million sites, unevenly distributed throughout mammalian genome (Field et al. 2018). At regulatory regions of housekeeping and developmentally regulated genes, CpG dinucleotides are clustered to constitute so-called CpG Island (Schubeler 2015). DNA methylation at CpG dinucleotide constitutes most abundant DNA modification in mammalian cells. Generally most of the CpGs exist in methylated state, however methylation patterns of genes and regulatory sequences determine the level of gene expressions. For example, DNA methylation at gene body promotes gene expression and suppresses transcription initiation at internal cryptic sites (Neri et al. 2017)(X. Yang et al. 2014). Distal regulatory sequences like enhancers contain intermediate level of CpG methylation (Elliott et al. 2015; Stadler et al. 2011), which sometimes promotes gene silencing (Deaton and Bird 2011; Hon et al. 2014). In general, CpG Islands exist in unmethylated state under normal conditions, however upon methylation they promote gene silencing (Deaton and Bird 2011). Mechanistically, DNA methylation controls gene expression either by affecting transcription factors binding or patterning the histone modifications (Reddington, Pennings and Meehan 2013; Rose and Klose 2014; Yin et al. 2017).

DNA methylation is a dynamic process. The 'writers' for 5-methyl cytosine are DNA methyltransferases (Dnmts) namely Dnmt1, Dnmt3A, Dnmt3B and 'erasers' are ten-eleven translocation (TET) family of proteins. Dnmt1 recognizes the hemimethylated sites generated after DNA replication and adds methylation mark to cytosine on the newly synthesized daughter strand thereby responsible for maintenance of methylation mark (Schubeler 2015). In contrast, Dnmt3A, Dnmt3B, and Dnmt3L catalyze de novo DNA methylation in non-proliferating cells. Mammalian cells express three different TET enzymes namely TET1, TET2, and TET3 that mediate demethylation (X. Wu and Zhang 2017). Genetic ablation of Dnmts and TET family of proteins causes loss and gain of DNA methylation respectively suggesting that cellular levels of these enzymes regulate methylation and demethylation dynamics of DNA. The altered lineage progression of multiple Dnmt1 knock out stem cells (Table 2) suggests that at least a subset of methylation marks present in the stem cells are critical for the fate decision of downstream lineages. Of note many of the phenotypes observed for loss of Dnmt1 resembles those associated with aging phenotypes like myeloid lineage skewing of the aged HSCs, age-related increment in astrocytes and abnormal bulge cell differentiation (Keyes and Fuchs 2018). De novo DNA methylation has also been reported to be critical for adult stem cell differentiation (Hodges et al. 2011; Bock et al. 2012; Kaaij et al. 2013; Ji et al. 2010). Genetic ablation of Dnmt3A in several tissues reveals that de novo DNA methylation is crucial for stem cell differentiation (Table 2). Based on importance of DNA methylation in stem cell functions and correlation between aging phenotypes and phenotypes observed for Dnmts knockouts, it is plausible to predict that DNA methylation may play critical roles in decline of tissue-specific stem cell functions during aging.

In aging stem cells, the basal DNA methylation level progressively diverges and the phenomenon is referred as 'epigenetic drift', which is also observed in individuals with identical genetic backgrounds like monozygotic twins (Fraga et al. 2005). In fact DNA methylome of the different tissues and organs can be precisely used to predict the biological age of the mouse and human (Field et al. 2018). Global DNA methylation profile of purified HSCs isolated from young and old mice shows that HSCs display global hypermethylation during aging (D. Sun et al. 2014). However in somatic and other stem cells, global decrement in DNA methylation level but hypermethylation of CpG islands at specific loci have also been documented (Hahn et al. 2017; Petkovich et al. 2017; Stubbs et al. 2017; Fernandez et al. 2015; Cole et al. 2017; Maegawa et al. 2017). Surprisingly, the altered DNA methylation pattern in HSCs does not correlate with transcriptional outcomes on these loci. In other words, increased DNA methylation did not correspond to decreased gene expression or vice versa (Hodges et al. 2011; Ji et al. 2010; Bock et al. 2012; Kaaij et al. 2013; Beerman et al. 2013; D. Sun et al. 2014). Surprisingly, many of these hypermethylated genes are not expressed in HSCs but exclusively transcribed in the progenitor cells of downstream lineages with altered expression patterns (Beerman et al. 2013). These findings establish that the methylation memory acquired by HSCs during embryonic development get altered in aging stem cells, which eventually leads to alterations in differentiation potential of the downstream progenitor cells. This led to the alterations in frequency of distribution of blood cell types in the peripheral blood of aged individuals (Beerman and Rossi 2014) (Figure 2).

Table 2. Changes in stem cell properties upon genetic ablation of Dnmts and TETs

Gene	Gene ablation method	Stem Cell	Phenotype	Reference
Dnmt1	Knockdown	Skin	Diminished self-renewal and premature differentiation of epidermal progenitor cells	(Sen et al. 2010)
Dnmt1	Conditional knockout	Bulge stem cell	Compromised self-renewal, Decreased proliferation, abnormal differentiation	(J. Li et al. 2012)
Dnmt1	Conditional knockout	NSCs	Premature differentiation towards astroglia	(G Fan et al. 2001; Guoping Fan et al. 2005)
Dnmt1	Conditional knockout	ISCs	Delayed differentiation	(Sheaffer et al. 2014)
Dnmt1	Conditional knockout	HSCs	Defect in self-renewal and differentiation leading to skewed lineage output biased to myelopoiesis	(Trowbridge et al. 2009; Broske et al. 2009)
Dnmt3A	Knockout	NSCs	Impaired differentiation	(H. Wu et al. 2010)
Dnmt3A	Conditional knockout	HSCs	Increased self-renewal and decreased differentiation	(Challen et al. 2011)
TET1	Conditional knockout	NPCs	Decreased NPCs proliferation and no effect on differentiation	(R.-R. Zhang et al. 2013)
TET1	Knockout	HSCs	Increased self-renewal, Promotes B-cell lineage differentiation and develop B-cell lymphoma at old age	(Cimmino et al. 2015)
TET2	Conditional knockout	HSCs	Increased self-renewal, high level of myeloid lineage output and myeloid transformation	(Ko et al. 2011; Moran-Crusio et al. 2011)(Shide et al. 2012)
TET3	Knockout	NPCs derived from TET3 knockout ESCs	Dysregulation of maintenance of the NPCs with increased apoptosis.	(T. Li et al. 2015)

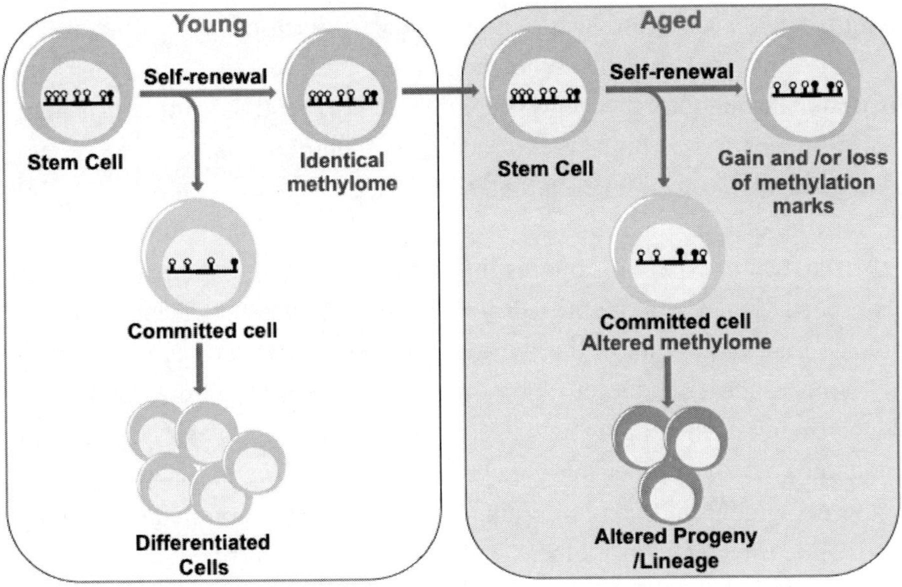

Figure 2. Aging-associated alterations in DNA methylation in stem cells can influence the gene expression programs in downstream progeny. DNA methylation signatures established in adult stem cells during embryonic development are maintained in young stem cells via self-renewal and passes in down progeny in regulated manner. In aging stem cells, DNA methylome is altered, which is amplified within stem cell pool and propagated to downstream progenies results emergence of functionally altered differentiated cells.

Clonal dominance is a hallmark of aging stem cells (Ermolaeva et al. 2018). A single aged stem cell with genetic and epigenetic alterations can perpetuate and amplified within the stem cell pool via self-renewal, which can alter the clonal composition of stem cell pool. Clones inculcated with proliferative and metabolic advantages are amplified because of strong benefits in cell-to-cell competition and compartment colonization. Additional genetic or epigenetic mutations in these clones could eventually transform them into malignant cells (Figure 3) (McKerrell et al. 2015; Okuchi et al. 2016; Shlush et al. 2014). The frequency of such somatic mutations is extremely rare in blood of young individuals i.e., less than 1% in person of <50 years age and exponentially increases up to 30-50% in 70 years old person (McKerrell et al. 2015). The presence of these mutations is associated with a significant increase in the risk of hematological malignancies and age-related cardiovascular diseases and all-cause of mortality. Although most of the mutations identified in these clones are dispersed throughout the genome but three frequently disrupted protein-coding genes with high recurrence are identified as key epigenetic regulators, Dnmt3A, TET2 and ASXL1 (Additional sex comb-like 1) and considered as functional drivers of clonal hematopoiesis (Genovese et al. 2014; Jaiswal et al. 2014). Interestingly, these mutated epigenetic enzymes have been frequently identified within leukemic cells. These findings indicate that alterations in the epigenome of the stem cells are crucial for the emergence of clonal dominance in hematopoietic stem cell compartment during aging and also support the hypothesis that altered epigenome of the clones provoke them to transform in leukemic cells. Aging dependent and somatic mutation-driven clonal dominance has also been documented in other stem cell compartments including physiologically normal eyelid epidermal cells and spermatogonial cells indicating that clonal dominance may or may not result in tumorigenesis (Martincorena et al. 2015; Goriely and Wilkie 2012).

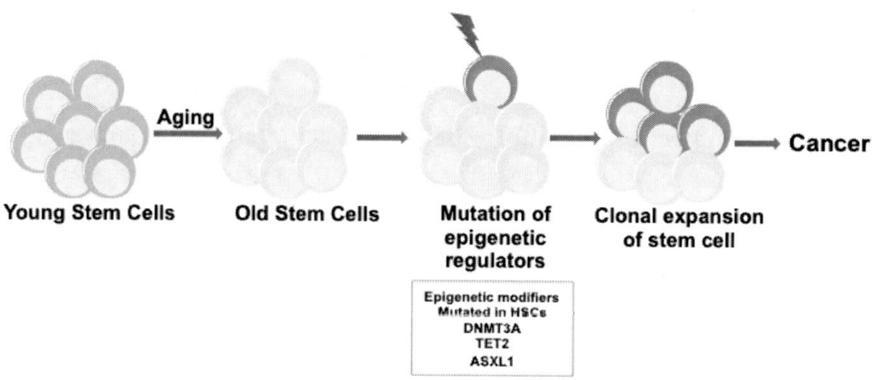

Figure 3. Aging adult stem cell epigenome undergoes an epigenetic drift driven by several extrinsic and intrinsic factors. Epigenetic drift increases self-renewal and impairs the differentiation of adult stem cells. Within these aged stem cells somatic mutations in key epigenetic regulators can lead to selection of mutant stem cells (Dark gray) that gains clonal dominance leading to impairment of stem cell differentiation and onset of malignancy.

The mechanistic basis for epigenome mediated clonal dominance of mutant stem and/or progenitor cells in aged organisms remains poorly understood but one hypothesis suggests that the epigenetic programmes established and maintained in adult stem cells may slowly evolve away from concise regulation of developmental pathways during aging leading to alterations in developmental programmes. This may result in hyper-activation of self-renewal genes and/or skewing in gene expression programmes regulating differentiation thus imbalance between self-renewal and differentiation resulting in selection of mutant stem cell clones (Ermolaeva et al. 2018).

2.2. Histone Modifications in Stem Cell Fate Decision

Posttranslational modifications of histones have been shown to play vital roles in the regulation of gene expression during stem cell fate decisions (Bannister and Kouzarides 2011; Rinaldi and Benitah 2015). The core histone proteins that package the DNA and constitute nucleosomes are subject of variety of post translational modifications including lysine acetylation, lysine and arginine methylation, serine and threonine phosphorylation, lysine ubiquitylation, sumoylation and ADP ribosylation, etc. (Bannister and Kouzarides 2011; Sadakierska-Chudy and Filip 2015). Among these posttranslational modifications, acetylation and methylation are the most extensively studied histone modifications in context of stem cell functions. Like DNA methylation, histone modifications are also highly dynamic processes and are mediated through action of specific set of ‘readers’ ‘writers’ and ‘erasers’. The writers for histone acetylation are referred as Histone acetyltransferases (HATs) and erasers are histone deacetylases (HDACs). More than 20 types of HATs have been identified and classified into five families: GNAT1, MYST, TAFII250, P300/CBP, and nuclear receptor coactivators such as ACTR (Trisciuoglio, Di Martile, and Del Bufalo 2018). Similarly, HDACs are also classified in to four classes; Class I HDACs include HDAC 1, 2, 3, and 8; Class II HDACs are comprised of HDAC 4, 5, 6, 7, 9, and 10; Enzymes belong to Class III are known as sirtuins and include SIRTs 1-7; HDAC11 constitutes Class IV enzyme, which retains features of both Class I and II enzymes (Huynh, Everts, and Ampornaramveth 2017). Similarly writers for histone methylation marks are called histone methyltransferases (HMTs) and erasers are referred as histone demethylases (HDMs). HMTs including SET1, SET7/9, Ash1, ALL-1, MLL, ALR, Trx, and SMYD3 catalyze methylation of histone H3 at lysine 4 (H3-K4) whereas ESET, G9a, SUV39-h1, SUV39-h2, SETDB1, Dim-5, and Eu-HMTase mediates methylation of histone H3 at lysine 9 (H3-K9) in mammalian cells. G9a and polycomb group enzymes, EZH1 and EZH2 catalyze methylation of histone H3 at lysine 27 (H3-K27) in mammalian cells (Bannister and Kouzarides 2011). The HDMs include LSD1, LSD2, JARID1A-1D mediates H3K4 demethylation; UTX and JMJD3 demethylate H3K27 marks; LSD1, JHMD2 and JMJD2A-D demethylate H3K9 methylation marks and JMJD1A-C, JHDM1A/B are involved in H3K36 demethylation (Ene et al. 2012).

Numerous studies have established that acetylation and methylation of histones play critical roles in the maintenance of adult stem cells self-renewal and differentiation (Avgustinova and Benitah 2016). For instance conditional ablation of CBP and HAT cofactor TRRAP in HSCs leads to decrement of HSCs population, suggesting that proper histone acetylation is necessary for HSCs self-renewal (Kung et al. 2000; Rebel et al. 2002; Chan et al. 2011; Loizou et al. 2009). Similarly important roles of HATs have been documented in homeostatic maintenance and functions of neural stem and progenitor cells. More precisely CBP and TRRAP are necessary for differentiation of NPCs (Jing Wang et al. 2010; Tapias et al. 2014) and *Moz* and Moz-related factor (MORF) is required for self-renewal of NSCs (Perez-Campo et al. 2014; Sheikh et al. 2012). In addition to HATs, histone deacetylases (HDACs) are also crucial for the maintenance and differentiation of stem cells. Ablation of class I HDACs in the hematopoietic system results in decreased bone marrow cellularity and loss of stem and progenitor cells (Wilting et al. 2010; Heideman et al. 2014). Simultaneous ablation of HDAC1 and HDAC2 in intestinal stem cells results in loss of differentiated cells with altered polarization and increased cell death (Turgeon et al. 2013; Zimberlin et al. 2015). Chemical inhibition of HDACs also causes alterations in differentiation of NPCs with elevation of apoptosis (Hsieh et al. 2004). Simultaneous knockdown of HDAC3, HDAC5, and HDAC7 (class I and II HDACs) results in up-regulation of cyclin-dependent kinase inhibitor, *Cdkn1a* (p21) with concomitant inhibition of NSCs proliferation (G. Sun et al. 2007). Drug-induced inhibition of HDAC activity in MSCs also causes activation of cell cycle regulator p21 and eventually cell cycle arrest (S Lee et al. 2009). Loss of SIRT1 and SIRT2 causes increased self-renewal and proliferation of NSCs (Rafalski et al. 2013). SIRT1 also contribute to directing epidermal stem cell differentiation by promoting keratinocyte production (Ming et al. 2014). In HSCs and satellite cells, SIRT1 ablation leads to premature differentiation implicating that SIRT1 is critical for self-renewal of these stem cells (Ryall et al. 2015; Rimmele et al. 2014; Matsui et al. 2012). Moreover SIRT1 is also required for maintenance of satellite cells in quiescent state (Ryall et al. 2015).

The Trithorax group (TrxG) of methyltransferases, MLL1, MLL5, ASH1L and MEN1 contribute to hematopoiesis by modulating H3K4 methylation. More specifically MLL1 promotes HSC self-renewal and quiescence as genetic ablation of MLL1 in HSCs results in rapid bone marrow failure due to pre-mature cell cycle entry and HSC exhaustion (Jude et al. 2007; McMahon et al. 2007). MLL1-mediated H3K4 methylation is also crucial for NSCs differentiation and lineage specification (Lim et al. 2009). Combined depletion of MLL1 and MLL5 in HSCs primarily impairs stem cell integrity and self-renewal but not lineage specification (McMahon et al. 2007; Madan et al. 2009) suggesting that MLL complexes play different roles in HSCs and NSCs.

The polycomb repressive complex 1 (PRC1) and 2 (PRC2) have also been reported to play important role in HSCs self-renewal and differentiation. BMI1, a component of PRC1, which mediates monoubiquitylation of histone 2A Lys119 (H2AK119) is highly expressed in HSCs. Exogenous expression of BMI1 in adult HSCs enhances their self-renewal potential, while loss of BMI results in cell cycle arrest, premature differentiation, apoptosis and defective self-renewal (Ding et al.

2012). Similar phenotypes have been reported for genetic ablation of other members of PRC1 complex such as MEL18, Phc1, Phc2, RING1A/B and Cbx2 (Sauvageau and Sauvageau 2010; Majewski et al. 2010). Mechanistically, PRC1 maintains long-term self-renewal of HSCs through the repression of the cell cycle inhibitors $p16^{INK4a}$ and $p19^{ARF}$ (Lessard and Sauvageau 2003; Oguro et al. 2010; Iwama et al. 2004). Genetic ablation of BMI1 leads to reduction in proliferative capacity of satellite cells and mammary stem cells (Robson et al. 2011; Pietersen et al. 2008). PRC2 complex mediates H3K27me3, which is critical for self-renewal and differentiation of HSCs, satellite cells and epidermis stem cells (Avgustinova and Benitah 2016). Depletion of PRC2 components including SUZ12, EZH2 or EED in HSCs results in increased self-renewal of hematopoietic stem cells (Majewski et al. 2008; Majewski et al. 2010). EZH1 is indispensable for adult hematopoiesis because it promotes HSC self-renewal and represses cellular senescence in a p16INK4A- and p19ARF- dependent manner (Hidalgo et al. 2012). EZH2 is also required for HSC differentiation towards the lymphoid lineage during adult hematopoiesis (Mochizuki-Kashio et al. 2011; Su et al. 2003). Furthermore important roles of PcG proteins in regulation of skeletal myogenesis have also been documented. EZH2 is exclusively expressed in satellite cells and represses expression of muscle differentiation-specific genes through H3K27me3 mark (Caretti et al. 2004). During maturation of muscle cells, EZH1 replaces EZH2 and promotes myogenesis in satellite cells, suggesting that PRC2 components EZH2 or EZH1 might play distinct roles in undifferentiated versus differentiated myocytes (Caretti et al. 2004; Palacios et al. 2010). Similar observations have been made in the epidermal stem cells (Ezhkova et al. 2011). Histone methyltransferase G9a together with its partner GLP is essential for establishment and maintains the repressive mark H3K9me2. In adult human HSCs, the activity of G9a and GLP is necessary for lineage commitment and differentiation (X. Chen et al. 2012). Similarly, disruption of G9a and GLP in postnatal neurons has been shown to cause impairment of cognitive functions of the brain and its ability to perceive external stimuli (Schaefer et al. 2009). Histone H4K20 methyltransferase Suv4–20h1/h2 regulates the maintenance of the lymphoid progenitor cell pool (Schotta et al. 2008).

The important role of histone demethylase LSD1 (KDM1A), which demethylates H3K4 me1/me2 and H3K9 me1/me2 in the regulation of stem cell state and differentiation has also been documented. The depletion of LSD1 in HSCs reduces the levels of terminally differentiated granulocytes and erythrocytes, whereas the levels of their precursors are increased, which establishes that LSD1 is required for differentiation of HSCs (Y. Guo et al. 2016). Histone demethylase KDM2A (FBXL11) and KDM2B (FBXL10), which demethylates H3K36me2/me3 are essential for mesenchymal stem cell differentiation (Deng et al. 2015). KDM2A interacts with BCOR and inhibits odontogenic differentiation of human stem cells from apical papilla, a type of dental MSCs (Z. Fan et al. 2009). KDM2B has been reported to inhibit adipogenesis of MSCs by recruiting the polycomb repressive complex 1 (PRC1) to repress key genes (e.g., Cdk1, Uhrf1, Pparg1, and Pparg2) required for the conversion of pluripotent cells into the adipogenic lineage (Inagaki et al. 2015). Similarly, KDM4B (JMJD2B) that removes the H3K9me3 marks has been reported to induce osteoblast differentiation of MSCs by regulating the expression of DLX5 (Du et al. 2013; Dong et al. 2013). H3K27 demethylases UTX (KDM6A) is essential for somatic cell reprogramming (Morales Torres, Laugesen, and Helin 2013; C. Wang et al. 2012), whereas JMJD3 (KDM6B) is important for neuronal and epidermal differentiation (W. Zhao et al. 2013). In addition, KDM6A and KDM6B play key role in MSCs lineage specification. While KDM6A promote osteoblast differentiation by regulating the expression of key genes (*RUNX2, Osteopontin, and Osteocalcin*) (Hemming et al. 2014), KDM6B promotes osteogenic differentiation by regulating the expression of BMP (bone morphogenetic protein) and HOX genes (Ye et al. 2012; Xu et al. 2013). Finally, both these proteins inhibit adipogenic differentiation in MSCs as depletion of KDM6A and KDM6B enhances adipogenesis and inhibits osteogenic differentiation in human bone marrow MSCs (Ye et al. 2012).

2.3. Role of Histone Modifications in Stem Cell Aging

Alterations of histone modifications pattern are invariably associated with stem cell aging, which is extensively studied in the context of HSCs (D. Sun et al. 2014). Epigenetic profiling of young and old HSCs reveals that the level of activation mark H3K4me3 is increased across self-renewal genes that result in increased HSCs number and defective differentiation (D. Sun et al. 2014). Interestingly, this gain in H3K4me3 level corroborated with downregulation of H3K4me3 demethylase KDM5b expression (Cellot et al. 2013). Apart from KDM5b, expression levels of several other chromatin modifiers including components of PRC complexes, histone deacetylases, and histone demethylases have also been shown to be altered in aging stem cells (Beerman and Rossi 2015; Y. Wang, Yuan, and Xie 2018; Cakouros and Gronthos 2019). Overexpression of EZH2, a component of PRC2 complex improves long-term repopulating potential HSCs during aging (Chou, Yu, and Hung 2011). Moreover, the levels of both H3K27me3 and H3K4me3 have been shown to increase with age in mouse HSCs (Chambers et al. 2007). Similarly changes in H3K9 methylation during aging can induce HSC differentiation in mouse (Challen et al. 2014; Mayle et al. 2015; Ugarte et al. 2015). Genetic ablation of SIRT6 in mouse HSCs affects HSC proliferation during aging (H. Wang et al. 2016). Genome-wide studies have also revealed that the expressions of several lysine-specific demethylases like KDM3a, KDM3b and UTX are down-regulated during aging (Herzog et al. 2012) (Kidder, Hu, and Zhao 2014; Stalker and Wynder 2012; Thieme et al. 2013). The levels of activating modifications H4K16Ac have been reported to decrease with age in HSCs (Florian et al. 2012).

2.3.1. Role of Histone Modifications in Mesenchymal Stem Cells (MSCs) Aging

Aging MSCs display increased differentiation propensity towards adipogenic lineage in comparison to osteogenic lineage and alterations in several histone modifications have been suggested as possible mechanisms for biased differentiation potential of MSCs (Cakouros and Gronthos 2019). More precisely expression level of HDACs and PcG proteins are down-regulated, while cellular level of H3K27 histone demethylase JMJD3 is up-regulated in aging MSCs (Jung et al. 2010). Mechanistically, alterations in H3 acetylation have been linked to reduced self-renewal and increase osteogenic differentiation of MSCs (Z. Li et al. 2011). The contribution of MSCs in aging process has been studied in patients with Werner syndrome (WS), which exhibits premature cellular aging phenotypes with defects in MSCs (Kudlow, Kennedy, and Monnat 2007). WS is caused by deficiency in WRN protein. $WRN^{-/-}$ ESC (ESC from patients with Werner Syndrome), when differentiated into MSCs, expressed all the MSC markers and properly differentiated into osteoblasts, chondrocytes and adipocytes, however, when these MSCs were serially passaged they showed loss of replicative potential, increased number of senescence and up-regulation of cell cycle inhibitors, p16Ink4A and p21 Waf1 (Cakouros and Gronthos 2019). Genome-wide examination of H3K27me3, H3K9me3, H3K4me3 and 5-methyl cytosine in MSCs differentiated from $WRN^{-/-}$ ESC, revealed no significant changes except for a significant loss of H3K9me3 and heterochromatin organization (Goto et al. 2013). Mechanistically, WRN protein form a multipotent complex that includes H3K9 methyltransferase SUV39H1, HP1, and the nuclear lamina-heterochromatin anchoring protein LAP2 and depletion of WRN protein destabilizes this complex leading to loss of H3K9me3 and heterochromatinization. Knockdown of individual components of the complex also resulted in a significant reduction in H3K9me3 and induction of cellular senescence, while overexpression of these genes in WRN deficient cells caused increased H3K9me3 and maintained cell viability. In agreement to these findings, decreased levels of WRN, SUV39H1, HP1, LAP2b and H3K9me3 marks have also been reported in primary MSCs from older individuals, suggesting that genome instability and heterochromatin disorganization associated with WRN deficiency may be a potential driver of normal MSC aging (W. Zhang et al. 2015). Histone deacetylation also plays an important role in MSCs aging. MSCs deficient in the histone deacetylase SIRT6 displayed accelerated cellular senescence, deregulated redox metabolism and increased sensitivity to oxidative stress. Mechanistically, SIRT6 deficiency increases global levels of H3K56Ac in human MSCs, which impairs the recruitment of the RNAP II complex to promoters of antioxidant NRF2 pathway target genes, thus leading to senescence-associated cellular redox unbalance (Pan et al. 2016).

2.3.2. Role of Histone Modifications in Muscle Stem Cells (MuSCs) and Other Stem Cells Aging

The regeneration potential of muscle stem cells (satellite cells) also declines with aging, which is partly mediated through alterations in histone modifications (Hwang and Brack 2018). For example, the levels of histone methylation mark H3K4me3 have been shown to decrease with age, whereas levels of the repressive histone methylation mark H3K27me3 has been reported to increase with age (L. Liu et al. 2013). This increment in the H3K27me3 level has been linked to downregulation of several genes involved in the regulation of satellite cell function. These observations are consistent with the fact that H3K27me3 demethylase UTX plays important role in maintenance of H3K27me3 level during skeletal muscle regeneration (Faralli et al. 2016). Apart from these epigenetic signatures, methylation of histone 4 at lysine 20 (H4K20 methylation) has also been reported to play important role in maintaining satellite cell quiescence in mice (Boonsanay et al. 2016). Similarly role of broad H3K4me3 domains has been reported to promote self-renewal and differentiation of neuronal stem cells (Benayoun et al. 2014).

2.4. Epigenetic Crosstalk between DNA Methylation and Histone Modifications in Aging Stem Cells

Numerous studies suggest that the crosstalk between epigenetic mechanisms also contribute to the stem cells aging. An antagonistic relationship has been demonstrated between DNA methylation and histone lysine methylation on the promoter region of certain gene loci. The presence H3K4 methylation on certain gene loci restricts DNA methylation by inhibiting recruitment of DNMT3A and DNMT3B (Rose and Klose 2014). In aging stem cells, the expression levels of H3K4 demethylases KDM1a and KDM1b are down-regulated, which results in increased level of H3K4 methylation and inhibition of DNMT3A and DNMT3B recruitment on these loci. For example in HSCs, DNA methylation and H3K4 demethylation are required for repression of certain genes associated with HSCs self-renewal, however loss of KDM1A/LSD1 in these cells leads to increase in H3K4me1/2 methylation on these genes, thus preventing the DNA methylation (Kerenyi et al. 2013). Similarly, an antagonistic relationship has been reported between DNA methylation and H3K27 methylation. In ESCs, H3K27me3 is readily found at promoters with CpG island that are hypo-methylated, however during differentiation many of these regions, which acquire H3K27me3 are replaced by DNA methylation, suggesting DNA methylation as permanent mark of lineage repression in ESCs. Interestingly, the same mechanism may be involved in restricting the differentiation potential of old stem cells because the regions marked by H3K27me in ESCs are preferentially hypermethylated in aged HSCs and MSCs (Beerman et al. 2013; D. Sun et al. 2014; Fernandez et al. 2015). Recently an association between PRC2 complex, DNMT3L (Neri, Krepelova, et al. 2013) and TET1 (Neri, Incarnato, et al. 2013) has been reported to inhibit DNA methylation in stem cells. For example PRC2 core factors are significantly downregulated in aged HSCs, resulting in the loss of PRC2 mediated repression in these cells because of destabilization of PRC2 complex, DNMT3L and TET1.

While the antagonistic relationship of H3K27 and H3K4 methylation with DNA methylation has been reported, a synergistic association of H3K36me3 with de novo DNA methyltransferases have been demonstrated in aging stem cells (Dhayalan et al. 2010; Morselli et al. 2015). In aging HSCs, the genomic regions showing decreased levels of H3K36me3 are also hypomethylated (D. Sun et al. 2014), suggesting that H3K36me3 is required for recruitment of DNA methyltransferases. Collectively, these data suggest that the crosstalk between the DNA methylation and histone modifications play a complex role in maintaining and safeguarding stem cell potential during aging.

2.5. Role of Small Non-coding RNAs in Stem Cell Fate Decision and Aging

Micro RNAs (miRNAs) are small noncoding evolutionarily conserved RNAs that regulate gene expression at the posttranscriptional level (Gangaraju and Lin 2009; Smith-Vikos and Slack 2012). miRNAs serve diverse roles in almost all biological and metabolic processes, including early development, cell proliferation, cell cycle regulation, apoptosis, fat metabolism, signal transduction, aging, and diseases (Davis et al. 2017; Fei et al. 2013; L. Guo, Zhao, and Wu 2011; Hodzic, Naaldijk, and Stolzing 2013) (Yi and Fuchs 2011; Choi, Lee, and Kang 2017; Dietrich et al. 2018). Mechanistically miRNAs function by binding to specific sequences in the 3′ untranslated region (UTR) of their target genes and cause degradation of transcripts by the RNA-induced silencing complex (RISC) (Lagos-Quintana et al. 2001). Functionally, miRNAs work in a complex network in which each miRNA controls hundreds of distinct target genes, where the expression of a single coding gene can be regulated by multiple miRNAs or a single miRNA can regulate expression of multiple genes.

In recent years, it has been established that miRNAs are important regulators of self-renewal and differentiation properties of variety of stem cell types including mammary gland progenitor cells, skin stem cell, neuronal stem cell, muscle stem cells, hematopoietic stem cells, cardiomyocyte progenitor stem cells etc. (Forstemann et al. 2005; Shcherbata et al. 2006; L. Zhang et al. 2011; Z. Yu et al. 2012; Melton, Judson, and Blelloch 2010). Deregulation of miRNAs function in stem cells is associated with developmental defects, cancer, and aging. Critical roles of miRNAs in regulation of aging stem cell functions have been described in Table 3 (Choi, Lee, and Kang 2017; Dietrich et al. 2018).

Table 3. miRNA involved is stem cell aging and senescence (Modified from Dietrich et al. 2018)

Stem cell type	miRNAs	Roles in	Species	References
BM-MSC	let-7f, miR-29c, miR-369-5p, miR-371,miR-499 miR-29c-3p, miR-140, miR-146a/b, miR-195	Senescence	*H. sapiens*	(Wagner et al. 2008; Okada et al. 2016)
	miR-17, miR-19a, miR-19b, miR-20a, miR-519d, miR-199b-5p	Aging	*H. sapiens*	(Hackl et al. 2010)
	miR-543, miR-590-3p	Aging	*M. musculus / H. sapiens*	(Seunghee Lee et al. 2014)
	miR-335	Senescence/aging	*H. sapiens*	(Tome et al. 2014)
	miR-183-5p	Senescence	*M. musculus*	(Davis et al. 2017)
	let-7f, miR-23a, miR-125b, miR-199-3p, miR-222, miR-558, miR-766	Aging	*Rhesus monkey (Macacamulatta)*	(J. M. Yu et al. 2011)
UC-MSC	let-7a1, let-7d, let-7f1, miR-23a, miR-26a,miR-30a, miR-200c, miR-214	Senescence	*H. sapiens*	(Seunghee Lee et al. 2011; So et al. 2011)
	miR-141-3p	Aging	*H. sapiens*	(K.-R. Yu et al. 2013)
BM-HSC	miR-146a miR-125b miR-132, miR-212	Aging	*M. musculus*	(J. L. Zhao et al. 2013; Mehta et al. 2015; Safak et al. 2014)
ASC and BM-MSC	miR-122, miR-510, miR-452, miR-335,miR-935, miR-142-3p, miR-483-3p,miR-203, miR-153, miR-1277, miR-141	Aging	*H. sapiens*	(Pandey et al. 2011)
ASC	miR-27b, miR-106a, miR-199a, let-7	Aging	*H. sapiens*	(Alt et al. 2012)

Table 3. (Continued)

Stem cell type	miRNAs	Roles in	Species	References
ASC	miR-143, miR-204	Aging	*R. norvegicus*	(Fei et al. 2013)
ADSC	miR-17hg, miR-100hg	Senescence	*H. sapiens*	(Lopez and Granados-Lopez 2017)
SC (satellite)	let-7b, let-7e	Aging	*H. sapiens*	(Drummond et al. 2011)
Satellite and myoblast cells	miR-143-3p	Aging	*M. musculus/ H. sapiens*	(Soriano-Arroquia et al. 2016)
Muscle stem cell (MuSC)	miR-1, miR-206, miR-24	Aging	Porcine	(Redshaw, Sweetman, and Loughna 2014)
Tendon stem/ progenitor cell	miR-135a, miR-140-5p	Senescence	*H. sapiens*	(L. Chen, Wang, et al. 2015; L. Chen, Liu, et al. 2015)
NSC	let-7b	Aging	*M. musculus/*	(Nishino et al. 2008)
Cardiac progenitor cells	miR-675	Senescence	*M. musculus*	(Cai et al. 2016)
Human DPSC	miR-152	Senescence	*H. sapiens*	(Gu et al. 2016)

2.5.1. Role of Micro RNAs in Hematopoietic Stem Cell (HSCs) Aging

Micro RNAs, miR-146a, miR-125b, miRNAs 212/132 regulate HSC numbers during aging and contribute to age-related disorders (J. L. Zhao et al. 2013; Mehta et al. 2015; Safak et al. 2014). miR-146a function as a key regulator of HSC aging as its deficiency in young mice has been shown to decline the quality of long-term HSCs. Similarly miR-125b functions as a critical regulator of HSC aging and use of anti-aging interventions can employ positive effects on HSC potential by regulating miR-125b expression (Safak et al. 2014). miR 212/132 cluster, which regulate HSCs self-renewal and survival during aging has been also shown to be upregulated in HSCs during aging (Pandey et al. 2011).

2.5.2. Role of Micro RNAs in Mesenchymal Stem Cell (MSCs) Aging

Similar to HSCs, several miRNAs have been reported to regulate age-associated alterations in MSCs (Seunghee Lee et al. 2014; Shang et al. 2016; Alt et al. 2012; Lopez and Granados-Lopez 2017). miRNAs such as miR-371, miR-369-5p, miR-29c, miR-499, and let-7f are upregulated in MSCs during aging, which is associated with their proliferative potential (Wagner et al. 2008). AIMP3 (aminoacyl-tRNA synthetase-interacting multifunctional protein-3)/p18 regulates cellular aging in MSCs through miR-543 and miR-590-3p (Seunghee Lee et al. 2014). miR-335 is upregulated in aging MSCs that results in cell senescence alterations (Tome et al. 2014). miR-29c-3p has been shown to promote the senescence of MSCs by targeting CNOT6 through p53-p21 and p16-pRB pathways (Shang et al. 2016). The increase of miR-199b-5p expression in aging MSCs resulted in age-related deterioration of MSCs function through regulation of SIRT1, TGFα, and PODXL (Peffers et al. 2016). The increase in level of miR-183-5p in MSC during aging and oxidative stress has been demonstrated to reduce cell proliferation and osteogenic differentiation (Davis et al. 2017).

2.5.3. Role of Micro RNAs in Muscle Stem Cells (MuSCs) and other Stem Cell Aging

Micro RNAs are potential regulators of skeletal muscle mass and function as alternations in their expression during aging have been linked to loss of skeletal muscle mass. Several miRNAs like Let-7b, Let-7e, miR-1, miR-206, miR- 143-3p and miR- 431 have been shown to be altered in aging skeletal muscle stem cells in contrast to young muscle stem cells. Micro RNAs Let-7b and Let-7e are shown to upregulate in older individuals compared to younger, and this increased expression of Let-7 has been linked to decrease in the self-renewal potential of aging muscle stem cells (Drummond et al. 2011). Similarly, miR-1 and miR-206 have been shown to be down-regulated in young muscle stem cells in comparison to old muscle stem cells whereas miR-24 has been shown to be upregulated in aging muscle stem cells (Redshaw, Sweetman, and Loughna 2014). The deregulation of miR-143-3p and its target gene Igfbp5 has been demonstrated to affect the satellite cell function during aging (Soriano-Arroquia et al. 2016).

The proliferation and differentiation potential of tendon stem/progenitor cells (TSPCs) is also regulated by miRNAs (Couppe et al. 2009; Tan, Lui, and Rui 2012). miR-135a that regulates senescence of TSPCs by targeting Rho-associated coiled-coil protein kinase 1 (ROCK1) is down-regulated in aged TSPCs. The overexpression of miR-135a in young TSPCs inhibits senescence and restores their proliferation and differentiation, while loss of miR-135a in aged TSPCs resulted in induction of senescence, suggesting miR-135a regulates TSPCs senescence by repressing ROCK1 (L. Chen, Wang, et al. 2015). Similarly, miR-140-5p has been shown to affect TSPCs aging by regulating the expression of peptidyl-prolyl cis/trans isomerase (Pin1) gene (W. Zhang et al. 2015; L. Chen, Liu, et al. 2015). Similar to TSPCs, several miRNAs are involved in the aging of dental pulp stem cells (DPSCs) (Hara et al. 2013; Vasanthan et al. 2015). In aging human DPSCs, the upregulation of miR-152 has been shown to induce senescence in these cells by downregulating the expression of histone deacetylase SIRT7 (Gu et al. 2016). Micro RNAs have also been shown to play important role in aging of the neural stem cell (NSCs) and cardiac progenitor cells (CPCs). In neuronal stem cells the loss of self-renewal potential is associated with age-dependent upregulation of let-7b (Nishino et al., 2008), whereas in cardiac progenitor cells the H19/miR-675/USP10 pathway is altered (Boon et al. 2013; Small and Olson 2011).

3. Aging Stem Cell Epigenome and Diseases

Functional deregulations of stem cells are frequently documented in age-related human diseases and genetic disorders. For example, a premature depletion of mesenchymal stem cells is observed in Hutchinson Gilford Progeria Syndrome (G.-H. Liu, Barkho, et al. 2011) (G.-H. Liu, Suzuki, et al. 2011), Werner syndrome (W. Zhang et al. 2015) and Fanconi anaemia (G.-H. Liu et al. 2014). Neuronal stem cell differentiation is altered in Parkinson's disease (G.-H. Liu et al. 2012) and Xenoderma pigmentation (Fu et al. 2016). Functional deregulation of HSCs has also been observed in Fanconi Anemia (G.-H. Liu et al. 2014). These observations establish that stem cell functions are compromised during aging. Although human aging is invariably associated with disease burden in all tissue types, however the epigenetic basis of age-related diseases are best characterized in hematopoietic system including myelodysplastic syndrome (MDS), leukemias (AML, CML, CLL, CMML), myeloproliferative disorder (myeloma), lymphoma (Hodgkin's and Non-Hodgkin's lymphoma). In particular, myelodysplastic syndrome is associated with various aging-associated epigenetic deregulations like aberrant DNA methylation induced clonal expansion of HSCs with abnormal differentiation potential (Will et al. 2012). In fact DNA methyltransferase inhibitors; 5-Azacytidine and 5-Aza-2'-deoxycytidine (Decitabine) are frequently used in clinical practice for treatment of MDS.

The clonal evolution of epigenetically dysregulated stem cells appears as a common mechanism underlying pre-disease states (Figure 3), which is driven by critical epigenetic regulators including DNMT3A, TET2, ASXL1 and IDH1/2 (Corces-Zimmerman et al. 2014; Shlush et al. 2014; Jan and Majeti 2013). For example loss of Dnmt3A confers a competitive self-renewal advantage within HSC pool and DNMT3A is frequently mutated in myeloid malignancies including MDS, CML, and myeloproliferative neoplasms (MPNs) (L. Yang, Rau, and Goodell 2015). In addition, HSCs harboring TET2 mutants display selective advantage to clonal expansion and TET2 mutants are enriched in MPNs, AML, MDS, B and T cell lymphomas (Ko et al. 2015; Ko et al. 2011) (Moran-Crusio et al. 2011; Shide et al. 2012; Xie et al. 2014). Collectively, these evidence highlight that epigenetic deregulation plays an important role in establishing pre-disease states.

A significant proportion of hypermethylated loci in aging HSCs and MSCs were found overlapping with loci associated with Polycomb group of Proteins (PcG), which mediates H3K27 methylation (Bork et al. 2010; Fernandez et al. 2015; Maegawa et al. 2010; Beerman et al. 2013; D. Sun et al. 2014). Interestingly, somatic mutations in PcG family member

ASXL1 are frequently observed in aging stem cells which results in loss of PRC2 mediated H3K27me3 whereas complete loss of ASXL1 in mice leads to the global loss of H3K27me3 and H3K4me3 with onset of myelodysplastic syndrome (Jiapeng Wang et al. 2014). Based on these facts, it is plausible to speculate that ASXL1 mutations cause loss of antagonistic methylation marks (H3K27me3 and H3K4me3) that allow for accumulation of aberrant DNA methylation at these loci and contribute to the MDS phenotypes. Furthermore Ezh2 is also frequently mutated in cancer and MDS further implicating a mechanism by which diminished PRC2 regulation can lead to aberrant DNA methylation at histone regulated regions. In addition to mutations of epigenetic regulators, direct mutation of epigenetic marks also occurs during aging. The most frequently identified mutation in human stem and progenitors are cytosine to thymine (C-T) transition that occurs upon deamination of methylcytosine (Welch et al. 2012). The C-T transition is most commonly occurs during aging but also highly prevalent in aged, non-diseased blood (Kandoth et al. 2013; Jaiswal et al. 2014; Xie et al. 2014). The direct conversion of methylcytosine to thymine permanently alters potential DNA methylation at that site. The age-associated loss of methylcytosine through deamination together with epigenetic regulators likely collaborates to underwrite the global DNA hypomethylation associated with cancers (Watanabe and Maekawa 2010). Taken together, mutations of the epigenetic regulators/target sites are key drivers of hematological malignancies from pre-disease states, thus raising the possibility that targeted epigenetic therapies may be effective in treating such diseases (Neff and Armstrong 2013).

REFERENCES

Alt, Eckhard U., Senst, Christiane, Murthy, Subramanyam N, Slakey, Douglas P., Dupin, Charles L., Chaffin, Abigail E., Kadowitz, Philip J., and Izadpanah, Reza. 2012. "Aging Alters Tissue Resident

Mesenchymal Stem Cell Properties." *Stem Cell Research* 8 (2): 215–25. https://doi.org/10.1016/j.scr.2011.11.002.

Armanios, Mary. 2013. "Telomeres and Age-Related Disease: How Telomere Biology Informs Clinical Paradigms." *The Journal of Clinical Investigation* 123 (3): 996–1002. https://doi.org/10.1172/JCI66370.

Avgustinova, Alexandra, and Benitah, Salvador Aznar. 2016. "Epigenetic Control of Adult Stem Cell Function." *Nature Reviews. Molecular Cell Biology* 17 (10): 643–58. https://doi.org/10.1038/nrm.2016.76.

Bannister, Andrew J., and Kouzarides, Tony. 2011. "Regulation of Chromatin by Histone Modifications." *Cell Research* 21 (3): 381–95. https://doi.org/10.1038/cr.2011.22.

Beerman, Isabel, Bock, Christoph, Garrison, Brian S., Smith, Zachary D, Hongcang Gu, Alexander Meissner, and Derrick J Rossi. 2013. "Proliferation-Dependent Alterations of the DNA Methylation Landscape Underlie Hematopoietic Stem Cell Aging." *Cell Stem Cell* 12 (4): 413–25. https://doi.org/10.1016/j.stem.2013.01.017.

Beerman, Isabel, and Derrick J Rossi. 2014. "Epigenetic Regulation of Hematopoietic Stem Cell Aging." *Experimental Cell Research* 329 (2): 192–99. https://doi.org/10.1016/j.yexcr.2014.09.013.

———. 2015. "Epigenetic Control of Stem Cell Potential during Homeostasis, Aging, and Disease." *Cell Stem Cell* 16 (6): 613–25. https://doi.org/10.1016/j.stem.2015.05.009.

Behrens, Axel, Jan M van Deursen, K Lenhard Rudolph, and Bjorn Schumacher. 2014. "Impact of Genomic Damage and Ageing on Stem Cell Function." *Nature Cell Biology* 16 (3): 201–7. https://doi.org/10.1038/ncb2928.

Benayoun, Berenice A, Elizabeth A Pollina, Duygu Ucar, Salah Mahmoudi, Kalpana Karra, Edith D Wong, Keerthana Devarajan, et al. 2014. "H3K4me3 Breadth Is Linked to Cell Identity and Transcriptional Consistency." *Cell* 158 (3): 673–88. https://doi.org/ 10.1016/j.cell.2014.06.027.

Bird, Adrian. 2007. "Perceptions of Epigenetics." *Nature* 447 (7143): 396–98. https://doi.org/10.1038/nature05913.

Bock, Christoph, Isabel Beerman, Wen-Hui Lien, Zachary D Smith, Hongcang Gu, Patrick Boyle, Andreas Gnirke, Elaine Fuchs, Derrick J Rossi, and Alexander Meissner. 2012. "DNA Methylation Dynamics during in Vivo Differentiation of Blood and Skin Stem Cells." *Molecular Cell* 47 (4): 633–47. https://doi.org/10.1016/j.molcel.2012.06.019.

Boon, Reinier A, Kazuma Iekushi, Stefanie Lechner, Timon Seeger, Ariane Fischer, Susanne Heydt, David Kaluza, et al. 2013. "MicroRNA-34a Regulates Cardiac Ageing and Function." *Nature* 495 (7439): 107–10. https://doi.org/10.1038/nature11919.

Boonsanay, Verawan, Ting Zhang, Angelina Georgieva, Sawa Kostin, Hui Qi, Xuejun Yuan, Yonggang Zhou, and Thomas Braun. 2016. "Regulation of Skeletal Muscle Stem Cell Quiescence by Suv4-20h1-Dependent Facultative Heterochromatin Formation." *Cell Stem Cell* 18 (2): 229–42. https://doi.org/10.1016/j.stem.2015.11.002.

Bork, Simone, Stefan Pfister, Hendrik Witt, Patrick Horn, Bernhard Korn, Anthony D Ho, and Wolfgang Wagner. 2010. "DNA Methylation Pattern Changes upon Long-Term Culture and Aging of Human Mesenchymal Stromal Cells." *Aging Cell* 9 (1): 54–63. https://doi.org/10.1111/j.1474-9726.2009.00535.x.

Brack, Andrew S, Michael J Conboy, Sudeep Roy, Mark Lee, Calvin J Kuo, Charles Keller, and Thomas A Rando. 2007. "Increased Wnt Signaling during Aging Alters Muscle Stem Cell Fate and Increases Fibrosis." *Science (New York, N.Y.)* 317 (5839): 807–10. https://doi.org/10.1126/science.1144090.

Brand, Marjorie, Kiran Nakka, Jiayu Zhu, and F Jeffrey Dilworth. 2019. "Polycomb/Trithorax Antagonism: Cellular Memory in Stem Cell Fate and Function." *Cell Stem Cell* 24 (4): 518–33. https://doi.org/10.1016/j.stem.2019.03.005.

Bratic, Ana, and Nils-Goran Larsson. 2013. "The Role of Mitochondria in Aging." *The Journal of Clinical Investigation* 123 (3): 951–57. https://doi.org/10.1172/JCI64125.

Broske, Ann-Marie, Lena Vockentanz, Shabnam Kharazi, Matthew R Huska, Elena Mancini, Marina Scheller, Christiane Kuhl, et al. 2009.

"DNA Methylation Protects Hematopoietic Stem Cell Multipotency from Myeloerythroid Restriction." *Nature Genetics* 41 (11): 1207–15. https://doi.org/10.1038/ng.463.

Cai, Benzhi, Wenya Ma, Chongwei Bi, Fan Yang, Lai Zhang, Zhenbo Han, Qi Huang, et al. 2016. "Long Noncoding RNA H19 Mediates Melatonin Inhibition of Premature Senescence of C-Kit(+) Cardiac Progenitor Cells by Promoting MiR-675." *Journal of Pineal Research* 61 (1): 82–95. https://doi.org/10.1111/jpi.12331.

Cakouros, Dimitrios, and Stan Gronthos. 2019. "Epigenetic Regulation of Bone Marrow Stem Cell Aging: Revealing Epigenetic Signatures Associated with Hematopoietic and Mesenchymal Stem Cell Aging." *Aging and Disease* 10 (1): 174–89. https://doi.org/10.14336/AD.2017.1213.

Caretti, Giuseppina, Monica Di Padova, Bruce Micales, Gary E Lyons, and Vittorio Sartorelli. 2004. "The Polycomb Ezh2 Methyltransferase Regulates Muscle Gene Expression and Skeletal Muscle Differentiation." *Genes & Development* 18 (21): 2627–38. https://doi.org/10.1101/gad.1241904.

Carlson, Morgan E, and Irina M Conboy. 2007. "Regulating the Notch Pathway in Embryonic, Adult and Old Stem Cells." *Current Opinion in Pharmacology* 7 (3): 303–9. https://doi.org/10.1016/j.coph.2007.02.004.

Cellot, Sonia, Kristin J Hope, Jalila Chagraoui, Martin Sauvageau, Eric Deneault, Tara MacRae, Nadine Mayotte, et al. 2013. "RNAi Screen Identifies Jarid1b as a Major Regulator of Mouse HSC Activity." *Blood* 122 (9): 1545–55. https://doi.org/10.1182/blood-2013-04-496281.

Challen, Grant A, Deqiang Sun, Mira Jeong, Min Luo, Jaroslav Jelinek, Jonathan S Berg, Christoph Bock, et al. 2011. "Dnmt3a Is Essential for Hematopoietic Stem Cell Differentiation." *Nature Genetics* 44 (1): 23–31. https://doi.org/10.1038/ng.1009.

Challen, Grant A, Deqiang Sun, Allison Mayle, Mira Jeong, Min Luo, Benjamin Rodriguez, Cates Mallaney, et al. 2014. "Dnmt3a and Dnmt3b Have Overlapping and Distinct Functions in Hematopoietic

Stem Cells." *Cell Stem Cell* 15 (3): 350–64. https://doi.org/10.1016/j.stem.2014.06.018.

Chambers, Stuart M, Chad A Shaw, Catherine Gatza, C Joseph Fisk, Lawrence A Donehower, and Margaret A Goodell. 2007. "Aging Hematopoietic Stem Cells Decline in Function and Exhibit Epigenetic Dysregulation." *PLoS Biology* 5 (8): e201. https://doi.org/10.1371/journal.pbio.0050201.

Chan, Wai-In, Rebecca L Hannah, Mark A Dawson, Clare Pridans, Donna Foster, Anagha Joshi, Berthold Gottgens, Jan M Van Deursen, and Brian J P Huntly. 2011. "The Transcriptional Coactivator Cbp Regulates Self-Renewal and Differentiation in Adult Hematopoietic Stem Cells." *Molecular and Cellular Biology* 31 (24): 5046–60. https://doi.org/10.1128/MCB.05830-11.

Chen, Lei, Junpeng Liu, Xu Tao, Guodong Wang, Qing Wang, and Ximing Liu. 2015. "The Role of Pin1 Protein in Aging of Human Tendon Stem/Progenitor Cells." *Biochemical and Biophysical Research Communications* 464 (2): 487–92. https://doi.org/10.1016/j.bbrc.2015.06.163.

Chen, Lei, Guo-Dong Wang, Jun-Peng Liu, Hua-Song Wang, Xi-Ming Liu, Qing Wang, and Xian-Hua Cai. 2015. "MiR-135a Modulates Tendon Stem/Progenitor Cell Senescence via Suppressing ROCK1." *Bone* 71 (February): 210–16. https://doi.org/10.1016/j.bone.2014. 11.001.

Chen, Xiaoji, Kyobi Skutt-Kakaria, Jerry Davison, Yang-Li Ou, Edward Choi, Punam Malik, Keith Loeb, et al. 2012. "G9a/GLP-Dependent Histone H3K9me2 Patterning during Human Hematopoietic Stem Cell Lineage Commitment." *Genes & Development* 26 (22): 2499–2511. https://doi.org/10.1101/gad.200329.112.

Cho, Rebecca H, Hans B Sieburg, and Christa E Muller-Sieburg. 2008. "A New Mechanism for the Aging of Hematopoietic Stem Cells: Aging Changes the Clonal Composition of the Stem Cell Compartment but Not Individual Stem Cells." *Blood* 111 (12): 5553–61. https://doi.org/10.1182/blood-2007-11-123547.

Choi, Soon Won, Jin Young Lee, and Kyung-Sun Kang. 2017. "MiRNAs in Stem Cell Aging and Age-Related Disease." *Mechanisms of Ageing and Development* 168 (December): 20–29. https://doi.org/10.1016/j.mad.2017.08.013.

Chou, Ruey-Hwang, Yung-Luen Yu, and Mien-Chie Hung. 2011. "The Roles of EZH2 in Cell Lineage Commitment." *American Journal of Translational Research* 3 (3): 243–50.

Cimmino, Luisa, Meelad M Dawlaty, Delphine Ndiaye-Lobry, Yoon Sing Yap, Sofia Bakogianni, Yiting Yu, Sanchari Bhattacharyya, et al. 2015. "TET1 Is a Tumor Suppressor of Hematopoietic Malignancy." *Nature Immunology* 16 (6): 653–62. https://doi.org/10.1038/ni.3148.

Cole, John J, Neil A Robertson, Mohammed Iqbal Rather, John P Thomson, Tony McBryan, Duncan Sproul, Tina Wang, et al. 2017. "Diverse Interventions That Extend Mouse Lifespan Suppress Shared Age-Associated Epigenetic Changes at Critical Gene Regulatory Regions." *Genome Biology* 18 (1): 58. https://doi.org/10.1186/s13059-017-1185-3.

Conboy, Irina M, Michael J Conboy, Gayle M Smythe, and Thomas A Rando. 2003. "Notch-Mediated Restoration of Regenerative Potential to Aged Muscle." *Science (New York, N.Y.)* 302 (5650): 1575–77. https://doi.org/10.1126/science.1087573.

Corces-Zimmerman, M Ryan, Wan-Jen Hong, Irving L Weissman, Bruno C Medeiros, and Ravindra Majeti. 2014. "Preleukemic Mutations in Human Acute Myeloid Leukemia Affect Epigenetic Regulators and Persist in Remission." *Proceedings of the National Academy of Sciences of the United States of America* 111 (7): 2548–53. https://doi.org/10.1073/pnas.1324297111.

Couppe, C., Hansen, P., Kongsgaard, M., Kovanen, V., Suetta, C., Aagaard, P., Kjaer, M., and Magnusson, S. P. 2009. "Mechanical Properties and Collagen Cross-Linking of the Patellar Tendon in Old and Young Men." *Journal of Applied Physiology (Bethesda, Md. : 1985)* 107 (3): 880–86. https://doi.org/10.1152/japplphysiol.00291.2009.

Davis, Colleen, Dukes, Amy, Drewry, Michelle, Helwa, Inas, Johnson, Maribeth H., Isales, Carlos M., Hill, William D., et al. 2017. "MicroRNA-183-5p Increases with Age in Bone-Derived Extracellular Vesicles, Suppresses Bone Marrow Stromal (Stem) Cell Proliferation, and Induces Stem Cell Senescence." *Tissue Engineering. Part A* 23 (21–22): 1231–40. https://doi.org/10.1089/ten.TEA.2016.0525.

Deaton, Aimee M., and Bird, Adrian. 2011. "CpG Islands and the Regulation of Transcription." *Genes & Development* 25 (10): 1010–22. https://doi.org/10.1101/gad.2037511.

Deng, Peng, Qian-Ming Chen, Christine Hong, and Cun-Yu Wang. 2015. "Histone Methyltransferases and Demethylases: Regulators in Balancing Osteogenic and Adipogenic Differentiation of Mesenchymal Stem Cells." *International Journal of Oral Science* 7 (4): 197–204. https://doi.org/10.1038/ijos.2015.41.

Dhayalan, Arunkumar, Arumugam Rajavelu, Philipp Rathert, Raluca Tamas, Renata Z Jurkowska, Sergey Ragozin, and Albert Jeltsch. 2010. "The Dnmt3a PWWP Domain Reads Histone 3 Lysine 36 Trimethylation and Guides DNA Methylation." *The Journal of Biological Chemistry* 285 (34): 26114–20. https://doi.org/10.1074/jbc.M109.089433.

Dietrich, Catharine, Singh, Manish, Kumar, Nishant, and Singh, Shree Ram. 2018. "The Emerging Roles of MicroRNAs in Stem Cell Aging." *Advances in Experimental Medicine and Biology* 1056: 11–26. https://doi.org/10.1007/978-3-319-74470-4_2.

Ding, Xiaolei, Lin, Qiong, Ensenat-Waser, Roberto, Rose-John, Stefan, and Zenke, Martin. 2012. "Polycomb Group Protein Bmi1 Promotes Hematopoietic Cell Development from Embryonic Stem Cells." *Stem Cells and Development* 21 (1): 121–32. https://doi.org/10.1089/scd.2010.0539.

Dong, Rui, Yao, Rui, Du, Juan, Wang, Songlin, and Fan, Zhipeng. 2013. "Depletion of Histone Demethylase KDM2A Enhanced the Adipogenic and Chondrogenic Differentiation Potentials of Stem Cells from Apical Papilla." *Experimental Cell Research* 319 (18): 2874–82. https://doi.org/10.1016/j.yexcr.2013.07.008.

Drummond, Micah J, John J McCarthy, Mala Sinha, Heidi M Spratt, Elena Volpi, Karyn A Esser, and Blake B Rasmussen. 2011. "Aging and MicroRNA Expression in Human Skeletal Muscle: A Microarray and Bioinformatics Analysis." *Physiological Genomics* 43 (10): 595–603. https://doi.org/10.1152/physiolgenomics.00148.2010.

Du, Juan, Ma,Yushi, Ma, Ping, Wang, Songlin, and Fan, Zhipeng. 2013. "Demethylation of Epiregulin Gene by Histone Demethylase FBXL11 and BCL6 Corepressor Inhibits Osteo/Dentinogenic Differentiation." *Stem Cells (Dayton, Ohio)* 31 (1): 126–36. https://doi.org/10.1002/stem.1255.

Dykstra, Brad, Olthof, Sandra, Schreuder, Jaring, Ritsema, Martha, and Haan, Gerald de. 2011. "Clonal Analysis Reveals Multiple Functional Defects of Aged Murine Hematopoietic Stem Cells." *The Journal of Experimental Medicine* 208 (13): 2691–2703. https://doi.org/10.1084/jem.20111490.

Elliott, GiNell, Hong, Chibo, Xing, Xiaoyun, Zhou, Xin, Li, Daofeng, Coarfa, Cristian, Bell, Robert J. A., et al. 2015. "Intermediate DNA Methylation Is a Conserved Signature of Genome Regulation." *Nature Communications* 6 (February): 6363. https://doi.org/10.1038/ncomms7363.

Ene, Chibawanye I., Edwards, Lincoln, Riddick, Gregory, Baysan, Mehmet, Woolard, Kevin, Kotliarova, Svetlana, Chen, Lai, et al. 2012. "Histone Demethylase Jumonji D3 (JMJD3) as a Tumor Suppressor by Regulating P53 Protein Nuclear Stabilization." *PloS One* 7 (12): e51407. https://doi.org/10.1371/journal.pone.0051407.

Ermolaeva, Maria, Neri, Francesco, Ori, Alessandro, and Rudolph, K Lenhard. 2018. "Cellular and Epigenetic Drivers of Stem Cell Ageing." *Nature Reviews. Molecular Cell Biology* 19 (9): 594–610. https://doi.org/10.1038/s41580-018-0020-3.

Ezhkova, Elena, Lien,Wen-Hui, Stokes, Nicole, Pasolli, H. Amalia, Silva, Jose M., and Fuchs, Elaine. 2011. "EZH1 and EZH2 Cogovern Histone H3K27 Trimethylation and Are Essential for Hair Follicle Homeostasis and Wound Repair." *Genes & Development* 25 (5): 485–98. https://doi.org/10.1101/gad.2019811.

Fan, G, Beard, C., Chen, R Z., Csankovszki, G., Sun, Y., Siniaia, M., Biniszkiewicz D., et al. 2001. "DNA Hypomethylation Perturbs the Function and Survival of CNS Neurons in Postnatal Animals." *The Journal of Neuroscience: The Official Journal of the Society for Neuroscience* 21 (3): 788–97.

Fan, Guoping, Martinowich, Keri, Chin, Mark H., He, Fei., Fouse Shaun D., Hutnick, Leah, Hattori, Daisuke, et al. 2005. "DNA Methylation Controls the Timing of Astrogliogenesis through Regulation of JAK-STAT Signaling." *Development (Cambridge, England)* 132 (15): 3345–56. https://doi.org/10.1242/dev.01912.

Fan, Zhipeng, Yamaza, Takayoshi, Lee, Janice S., Yu, Jinhua, Songlin Wang, Guoping Fan, Songtao Shi, and Cun-Yu Wang. 2009. "BCOR Regulates Mesenchymal Stem Cell Function by Epigenetic Mechanisms." *Nature Cell Biology* 11 (8): 1002–9. https://doi. org/10. 1038/ncb1913.

Faralli, Herve, Wang, Chaochen, Nakka, Kiran, Benyoucef, Aissa, Sebastian, Soji, Zhuang, Lenan, Chu, Alphonse, et al. 2016. "UTX Demethylase Activity Is Required for Satellite Cell-Mediated Muscle Regeneration." *The Journal of Clinical Investigation* 126 (4): 1555–65. https://doi.org/10.1172/JCI83239.

Fei, Jia, Tamski, Holly Cook, Carla, and Santanam, Nalini. 2013. "MicroRNA Regulation of Adipose Derived Stem Cells in Aging Rats." *PloS One* 8 (3): e59238. https://doi.org/10.1371/journal.pone. 0059238.

Fernandez, Agustin F., Bayon, Gustavo F., Urdinguio, Rocio G., Torano, Estela G., Garcia, Maria G., Carella, Antonella, Petrus-Reurer, Sandra, et al. 2015. "H3K4me1 Marks DNA Regions Hypomethylated during Aging in Human Stem and Differentiated Cells." *Genome Research* 25 (1): 27–40. https://doi.org/10.1101/gr.169011.113.

Field, Adam E., Robertson, Neil A., Wang, Tina, Havas, Aaron., Ideker Trey, and Adams Peter D., 2018. "DNA Methylation Clocks in Aging: Categories, Causes, and Consequences." *Molecular Cell* 71 (6): 882–95. https://doi.org/10.1016/j.molcel.2018.08.008.

Flach, Johanna, Bakker, Sietske T., Mohrin, Mary, Conroy, Pauline C., Pietras, Eric M., Reynaud, Damien, Alvarez, Silvia, et al. 2014. "Replication Stress Is a Potent Driver of Functional Decline in Ageing Haematopoietic Stem Cells." *Nature* 512 (7513): 198–202. https://doi.org/10.1038/nature13619.

Florian, Maria Carolina, Karin Dorr, Anja Niebel, Deidre Daria, Hubert Schrezenmeier, Markus Rojewski, Marie-Dominique Filippi, et al. 2012. "Cdc42 Activity Regulates Hematopoietic Stem Cell Aging and Rejuvenation." *Cell Stem Cell* 10 (5): 520–30. https://doi.org/10.10 16/j.stem.2012.04.007.

Forstemann, Klaus, Yukihide Tomari, Tingting Du, Vasily V Vagin, Ahmet M Denli, Diana P Bratu, Carla Klattenhoff, William E Theurkauf, and Phillip D Zamore. 2005. "Normal MicroRNA Maturation and Germ-Line Stem Cell Maintenance Requires Loquacious, a Double-Stranded RNA-Binding Domain Protein." *PLoS Biology* 3 (7): e236. https://doi.org/10.1371/journal.pbio.0030236.

Fraga, Mario F, Esteban Ballestar, Maria F Paz, Santiago Ropero, Fernando Setien, Maria L Ballestar, Damia Heine-Suner, et al. 2005. "Epigenetic Differences Arise during the Lifetime of Monozygotic Twins." *Proceedings of the National Academy of Sciences of the United States of America* 102 (30): 10604–9. https://doi.org/10.107 3/pnas.0500398102.

Fu, Lina, Xiuling Xu, Ruotong Ren, Jun Wu, Weiqi Zhang, Jiping Yang, Xiaoqing Ren, et al. 2016. "Modeling Xeroderma Pigmentosum Associated Neurological Pathologies with Patients-Derived IPSCs." *Protein & Cell* 7 (3): 210–21. https://doi.org/10.1007/s13238-016-024 4-y.

Gangaraju, Vamsi K, and Haifan Lin. 2009. "MicroRNAs: Key Regulators of Stem Cells." *Nature Reviews. Molecular Cell Biology* 10 (2): 116–25. https://doi.org/10.1038/nrm2621.

Genovese, Giulio, Anna K Kahler, Robert E Handsaker, Johan Lindberg, Samuel A Rose, Samuel F Bakhoum, Kimberly Chambert, et al. 2014. "Clonal Hematopoiesis and Blood-Cancer Risk Inferred from Blood

DNA Sequence." *The New England Journal of Medicine* 371 (26): 2477–87. https://doi.org/10.1056/NEJMoa1409405.

Goldberg, Aaron D, C David Allis, and Emily Bernstein. 2007. "Epigenetics: A Landscape Takes Shape." *Cell* 128 (4): 635–38. https://doi.org/10.1016/j.cell.2007.02.006.

Goodell, Margaret A, and Thomas A Rando. 2015. "Stem Cells and Healthy Aging." *Science (New York, N.Y.)* 350 (6265): 1199–1204. https://doi.org/10.1126/science.aab3388.

Gopinath, Suchitra D, and Thomas A Rando. 2008. "Stem Cell Review Series: Aging of the Skeletal Muscle Stem Cell Niche." *Aging Cell* 7 (4): 590–98. https://doi.org/10.1111/j.1474-9726.2008.00399.x.

Goriely, Anne, and Andrew O M Wilkie. 2012. "Paternal Age Effect Mutations and Selfish Spermatogonial Selection: Causes and Consequences for Human Disease." *American Journal of Human Genetics* 90 (2): 175–200. https://doi.org/10.1016/j.ajhg.2011.12.017.

Goto, M, Y Ishikawa, M Sugimoto, and Y Furuichi. 2013. "Werner Syndrome: A Changing Pattern of Clinical Manifestations in Japan (1917~2008)." *Bioscience Trends* 7 (1): 13–22.

Gu, Shensheng, Shujun Ran, Bin Liu, and Jingping Liang. 2016. "MiR-152 Induces Human Dental Pulp Stem Cell Senescence by Inhibiting SIRT7 Expression." *FEBS Letters*. England. https://doi.org/10.1002/1873-3468.12138.

Guo, Ling, Robert C H Zhao, and Yaojiong Wu. 2011. "The Role of MicroRNAs in Self-Renewal and Differentiation of Mesenchymal Stem Cells." *Experimental Hematology* 39 (6): 608–16. https://doi.org/10.1016/j.exphem.2011.01.011.

Guo, Yidi, Xueqi Fu, Bo Huo, Yongsen Wang, Jing Sun, Lingyuan Meng, Tian Hao, Zhizhuang Joe Zhao, and Xin Hu. 2016. "GATA2 Regulates GATA1 Expression through LSD1-Mediated Histone Modification." *American Journal of Translational Research* 8 (5): 2265–74.

Hackl, Matthias, Stefan Brunner, Klaus Fortschegger, Carina Schreiner, Lucia Micutkova, Christoph Muck, Gerhard T Laschober, et al. 2010. "MiR-17, MiR-19b, MiR-20a, and MiR-106a Are down-Regulated in

Human Aging." *Aging Cell* 9 (2): 291–96. https://doi.org/10.1111/j.1474-9726.2010.00549.x.

Hahn, Oliver, Sebastian Gronke, Thomas M Stubbs, Gabriella Ficz, Oliver Hendrich, Felix Krueger, Simon Andrews, et al. 2017. "Dietary Restriction Protects from Age-Associated DNA Methylation and Induces Epigenetic Reprogramming of Lipid Metabolism." *Genome Biology* 18 (1): 56. https://doi.org/10.1186/s13059-017-1187-1.

Hara, Emilio Satoshi, Mitsuaki Ono, Takanori Eguchi, Satoshi Kubota, Hai Thanh Pham, Wataru Sonoyama, Shoji Tajima, Masaharu Takigawa, Stuart K Calderwood, and Takuo Kuboki. 2013. "MiRNA-720 Controls Stem Cell Phenotype, Proliferation and Differentiation of Human Dental Pulp Cells." *PloS One* 8 (12): e83545. https://doi.org/10.1371/journal.pone.0083545.

Heideman, Marinus R, Cesare Lancini, Natalie Proost, Eva Yanover, Heinz Jacobs, and Jan-Hermen Dannenberg. 2014. "Sin3a-Associated Hdac1 and Hdac2 Are Essential for Hematopoietic Stem Cell Homeostasis and Contribute Differentially to Hematopoiesis." *Haematologica* 99 (8): 1292–1303. https://doi.org/10.3324/haematol.2013.092643.

Hemming, Sarah, Dimitrios Cakouros, Sandra Isenmann, Lachlan Cooper, Danijela Menicanin, Andrew Zannettino, and Stan Gronthos. 2014. "EZH2 and KDM6A Act as an Epigenetic Switch to Regulate Mesenchymal Stem Cell Lineage Specification." *Stem Cells (Dayton, Ohio)* 32 (3): 802–15. https://doi.org/10.1002/stem.1573.

Herzog, Marielle, Eleonore Josseaux, Sarah Dedeurwaerder, Emilie Calonne, Michael Volkmar, and Francois Fuks. 2012. "The Histone Demethylase Kdm3a Is Essential to Progression through Differentiation." *Nucleic Acids Research* 40 (15): 7219–32. https://doi.org/10.1093/nar/gks399.

Hidalgo, Isabel, Antonio Herrera-Merchan, Jose Manuel Ligos, Laura Carramolino, Javier Nunez, Fernando Martinez, Orlando Dominguez, Miguel Torres, and Susana Gonzalez. 2012. "Ezh1 Is Required for Hematopoietic Stem Cell Maintenance and Prevents Senescence-like Cell Cycle Arrest." *Cell Stem Cell* 11 (5): 649–62. https://doi.org/10.1016/j.stem.2012.08.001.

Hodges, Emily, Antoine Molaro, Camila O Dos Santos, Pramod Thekkat, Qiang Song, Philip J Uren, Jin Park, et al. 2011. "Directional DNA Methylation Changes and Complex Intermediate States Accompany Lineage Specificity in the Adult Hematopoietic Compartment." *Molecular Cell* 44 (1): 17–28. https://doi.org/10.1016/j.molcel.2011.08.026.

Hodzic, M, Y Naaldijk, and A Stolzing. 2013. "Regulating Aging in Adult Stem Cells with MicroRNA." *Zeitschrift Fur Gerontologie Und Geriatrie* 46 (7): 629–34. https://doi.org/10.1007/s00391-013-0531-7.

Hon, Gary C, Chun-Xiao Song, Tingting Du, Fulai Jin, Siddarth Selvaraj, Ah Young Lee, Chia-An Yen, et al. 2014. "5mC Oxidation by Tet2 Modulates Enhancer Activity and Timing of Transcriptome Reprogramming during Differentiation." *Molecular Cell* 56 (2): 286–97. https://doi.org/10.1016/j.molcel.2014.08.026.

Hsieh, Jenny, Kinichi Nakashima, Tomoko Kuwabara, Eunice Mejia, and Fred H Gage. 2004. "Histone Deacetylase Inhibition-Mediated Neuronal Differentiation of Multipotent Adult Neural Progenitor Cells." *Proceedings of the National Academy of Sciences of the United States of America* 101 (47): 16659–64. https://doi.org/10.1073/pnas.0407643101.

Huynh, Nam Cong-Nhat, Vincent Everts, and Ruchanee Salingcarnboriboon Ampornaramveth. 2017. "Histone Deacetylases and Their Roles in Mineralized Tissue Regeneration." *Bone Reports* 7 (December): 33–40. https://doi.org/10.1016/j.bonr.2017.08.001.

Hwang, Ara B, and Andrew S Brack. 2018. "Muscle Stem Cells and Aging." *Current Topics in Developmental Biology* 126: 299–322. https://doi.org/10.1016/bs.ctdb.2017.08.008.

Inagaki, Takeshi, Satoshi Iwasaki, Yoshihiro Matsumura, Takeshi Kawamura, Toshiya Tanaka, Yohei Abe, Ayumu Yamasaki, et al. 2015. "The FBXL10/KDM2B Scaffolding Protein Associates with Novel Polycomb Repressive Complex-1 to Regulate Adipogenesis." *The Journal of Biological Chemistry* 290 (7): 4163–77. https://doi.org/10.1074/jbc.M114.626929.

Iwama, Atsushi, Hideyuki Oguro, Masamitsu Negishi, Yuko Kato, Youhei Morita, Hiroko Tsukui, Hideo Ema, et al. 2004. "Enhanced Self-Renewal of Hematopoietic Stem Cells Mediated by the Polycomb Gene Product Bmi-1." *Immunity* 21 (6): 843–51. https://doi.org/10.1016/j.immuni.2004.11.004.

Jaiswal, Siddhartha, Pierre Fontanillas, Jason Flannick, Alisa Manning, Peter V Grauman, Brenton G Mar, R Coleman Lindsley, et al. 2014. "Age-Related Clonal Hematopoiesis Associated with Adverse Outcomes." *The New England Journal of Medicine* 371 (26): 2488–98. https://doi.org/10.1056/NEJMoa1408617.

Jan, M., and Majeti, R. 2013. "Clonal Evolution of Acute Leukemia Genomes." *Oncogene* 32 (2): 135–40. https://doi.org/10.1038/onc.2012.48.

Ji, Hong, Lauren I R Ehrlich, Jun Seita, Peter Murakami, Akiko Doi, Paul Lindau, Hwajin Lee, et al. 2010. "Comprehensive Methylome Map of Lineage Commitment from Haematopoietic Progenitors." *Nature* 467 (7313): 338–42. https://doi.org/10.1038/nature09367.

Jude, Craig D., Climer, Leslie, Xu, Diyong, Artinger, Erika, Fisher, Jill K., and Ernst, Patricia. 2007. "Unique and Independent Roles for MLL in Adult Hematopoietic Stem Cells and Progenitors." *Cell Stem Cell* 1 (3): 324–37. https://doi.org/10.1016/j.stem.2007.05.019.

Jung, Ji-Won, Seunghee Lee, Min-Soo Seo, Sang-Bum Park, Andreas Kurtz, Soo-Kyung Kang, and Kyung-Sun Kang. 2010. "Histone Deacetylase Controls Adult Stem Cell Aging by Balancing the Expression of Polycomb Genes and Jumonji Domain Containing 3." *Cellular and Molecular Life Sciences: CMLS* 67 (7): 1165–76. https://doi.org/10.1007/s00018-009-0242-9.

Kaaij, Lucas T J, Wetering, Marc van de, Fang Fang, Decato, Benjamin, Molaro, Antoine, Werken, Harmen J G van de, Es, Johan H van et al. 2013. "DNA Methylation Dynamics during Intestinal Stem Cell Differentiation Reveals Enhancers Driving Gene Expression in the Villus." *Genome Biology* 14 (5): R50. https://doi.org/10.1186/gb-2013-14-5-r50.

Kandoth, Cyriac, McLellan, Michael D., Vandin, Fabio, Ye, Kai, Niu, Beifang, Lu, Charles, Xie, Mingchao, et al. 2013. "Mutational Landscape and Significance across 12 Major Cancer Types." *Nature* 502 (7471): 333–39. https://doi.org/10.1038/nature12634.

Kerenyi, Marc A., Shao, Zhen, Hsu, Yu-Jung, Guo, Guoji, Luc, Sidinh, O'Brien, Kassandra, Fujiwara, Yuko, Peng, Cong, Nguyen, Minh and Orkin, Stuart H. 2013. "Histone Demethylase Lsd1 Represses Hematopoietic Stem and Progenitor Cell Signatures during Blood Cell Maturation." *ELife* 2 (June): e00633. https://doi.org/10.7554/eLife.00633.

Keyes, Brice E, and Elaine Fuchs. 2018. "Stem Cells: Aging and Transcriptional Fingerprints." *The Journal of Cell Biology* 217 (1): 79–92. https://doi.org/10.1083/jcb.201708099.

Kidder, Benjamin L, Hu, Gangqing and Zhao, Keji. 2014. "KDM5B Focuses H3K4 Methylation near Promoters and Enhancers during Embryonic Stem Cell Self-Renewal and Differentiation." *Genome Biology* 15 (2): R32. https://doi.org/10.1186/gb-2014-15-2-r32.

Ko, Myunggon, An, Jungeun, Pastor, William A., Koralov, Sergei B, Rajewsky, Klaus and Rao, Anjana. 2015. "TET Proteins and 5-Methylcytosine Oxidation in Hematological Cancers." *Immunological Reviews* 263 (1): 6–21. https://doi.org/10.1111/imr.12239.

Ko, Myunggon, Bandukwala, Hozefa S., An, Jungeun, Lamperti, Edward D., Thompson, Elizabeth C., Hastie, Ryan, Tsangaratou, Angeliki, Rajewsky, Klaus, Koralov, Sergei B., and Rao, Anjana. 2011. "Ten-Eleven-Translocation 2 (TET2) Negatively Regulates Homeostasis and Differentiation of Hematopoietic Stem Cells in Mice." *Proceedings of the National Academy of Sciences of the United States of America* 108 (35): 14566–71. https://doi.org/10.1073/pnas.1112317108.

Kudlow, Brian A., Kennedy, Brian K., and Raymond J Jr, Monnat. 2007. "Werner and Hutchinson-Gilford Progeria Syndromes: Mechanistic Basis of Human Progeroid Diseases." *Nature Reviews. Molecular Cell Biology* 8 (5): 394–404. https://doi.org/10.1038/nrm2161.

Kung, A L, Rebel, V I., Bronson, R T., Ch'ng, L E., Sieff, C A., Livingston, D M., and Yao, T P. 2000. "Gene Dose-Dependent Control of Hematopoiesis and Hematologic Tumor Suppression by CBP." *Genes & Development* 14 (3): 272–77.

Lagos-Quintana, M, Rauhut, R., Lendeckel, W, and Tuschl, T. 2001. "Identification of Novel Genes Coding for Small Expressed RNAs." *Science (New York, N.Y.)* 294 (5543): 853–58. https://doi.org/10.1126/science.1064921.

Lee, S., Park, J-R., Seo, M-S., Roh, K-H., Park, S-B., Hwang, J-W., Sun B. , et al. 2009. "Histone Deacetylase Inhibitors Decrease Proliferation Potential and Multilineage Differentiation Capability of Human Mesenchymal Stem Cells." *Cell Proliferation* 42 (6): 711–20. https://doi.org/10.1111/j.1365-2184.2009.00633.x.

Lee, Seunghee, Jung, Ji-Won., Park, Sang-Bum., Roh, Kyounghwan., Lee, Su Yeon, Han Kim, Ju, Kang, Soo-Kyung and Kang, Kyung-Sun. 2011. "Histone Deacetylase Regulates High Mobility Group A2-Targeting MicroRNAs in Human Cord Blood-Derived Multipotent Stem Cell Aging." *Cellular and Molecular Life Sciences : CMLS* 68 (2): 325–36. https://doi.org/10.1007/s00018-010-0457-9.

Lee, Seunghee, Kyung-Rok Yu, Young-Sil Ryu, Young Sun Oh, In-Sun Hong, Hyung-Sik Kim, Jin Young Lee, Sunghoon Kim, Kwang-Won Seo, and Kyung-Sun Kang. 2014. "MiR-543 and MiR-590-3p Regulate Human Mesenchymal Stem Cell Aging via Direct Targeting of AIMP3/P18." *Age (Dordrecht, Netherlands)* 36 (6): 9724. https://doi.org/10.1007/s11357-014-9724-2.

Lessard, Julie, and Sauvageau, Guy. 2003. "Bmi-1 Determines the Proliferative Capacity of Normal and Leukaemic Stem Cells." *Nature* 423 (6937): 255–60. https://doi.org/10.1038/nature01572.

Li, Ji, Ting-Xin Jiang, Hughes, Michael W., Wu, Ping, Yu, Juehua, Widelitz, Randall B., Fan, Guoping and Chuong, Cheng-Ming. 2012. "Progressive Alopecia Reveals Decreasing Stem Cell Activation Probability during Aging of Mice with Epidermal Deletion of DNA Methyltransferase 1." *The Journal of Investigative Dermatology* 132 (12): 2681–90. https://doi.org/10.1038/jid.2012.206.

Li, Ting, Yang, Dehua, Li, Jia, Tang, Yu, Yang, Juan and Le, Weidong. 2015. "Critical Role of Tet3 in Neural Progenitor Cell Maintenance and Terminal Differentiation." *Molecular Neurobiology* 51 (1): 142–54. https://doi.org/10.1007/s12035-014-8734-5.

Li, Zhilong, Liu, Chenxiong, Xie, Zhenhua, Song, Pengyue, Zhao, Robert C H., Guo, Ling, Liu, Zhigang and Wu, Yaojiong. 2011. "Epigenetic Dysregulation in Mesenchymal Stem Cell Aging and Spontaneous Differentiation." *PloS One* 6 (6): e20526. https://doi.org/10.1371/journal.pone.0020526.

Lim, Daniel A., Huang, Yin-Cheng, Swigut,Tomek, Mirick, Anika L., Garcia-Verdugo, Jose Manuel, Wysocka, Joanna, Ernst, Patricia and Alvarez-Buylla, Arturo. 2009. "Chromatin Remodelling Factor Mll1 Is Essential for Neurogenesis from Postnatal Neural Stem Cells." *Nature* 458 (7237): 529–33. https://doi.org/10.1038/nature07726.

Liu, Guang-Hui, Barkho, Basam Z., Ruiz, Sergio., Diep, Dinh., Qu, Jing, Yang, Sheng-Lian, Panopoulos, Athanasia D., et al. 2011. "Recapitulation of Premature Ageing with IPSCs from Hutchinson-Gilford Progeria Syndrome." *Nature* 472 (7342): 221–25. https://doi.org/10.1038/nature09879.

Liu, Guang-Hui, Qu, Jing, Suzuki, Keiichiro, Nivet, Emmanuel, Li, Mo, Montserrat, Nuria, Yi, Fei et al. 2012. "Progressive Degeneration of Human Neural Stem Cells Caused by Pathogenic LRRK2." *Nature* 491 (7425): 603–7. https://doi.org/10.1038/nature11557.

Liu, Guang-Hui, Suzuki, Keiichiro, Li, Mo, Qu, Jing, Montserrat, Nuria, Tarantino, Carolina, Gu,Ying et al. 2014. "Modelling Fanconi Anemia Pathogenesis and Therapeutics Using Integration-Free Patient-Derived IPSCs." *Nature Communications* 5 (July): 4330. https://doi.org/10.1038/ncomms5330.

Liu, Guang-Hui, Suzuki, Keiichiro, Qu, Jing, Sancho-Martinez, Ignacio, Yi, Fei, Li, Mo, Kumar, Sachin et al. 2011. "Targeted Gene Correction of Laminopathy-Associated LMNA Mutations in Patient-Specific IPSCs." *Cell Stem Cell* 8 (6): 688–94. https://doi.org/10.1016/j.stem.2011.04.019.

Liu, Ling, Cheung, Tom H., Charville, Gregory W., Hurgo, Bernadette Marie Ceniza, Leavitt, Tripp, Shih, Johnathan, Brunet, Anne and Rando, Thomas A. 2013. "Chromatin Modifications as Determinants of Muscle Stem Cell Quiescence and Chronological Aging." *Cell Reports* 4 (1): 189–204. https://doi.org/10.1016/j.celrep.2013.05.043.

Liu, Ling, and Rando, Thomas A. 2011. "Manifestations and Mechanisms of Stem Cell Aging." *The Journal of Cell Biology* 193 (2): 257–66. https://doi.org/10.1083/jcb.201010131.

Loizou, Joanna I., Oser, Gabriela, Shukla,Vivek, Sawan, Carla, Murr, Rabih, Wang, Zhao-Qi, Trumpp, Andreas, and Herceg, Zdenko. 2009. "Histone Acetyltransferase Cofactor Trrap Is Essential for Maintaining the Hematopoietic Stem/Progenitor Cell Pool." *Journal of Immunology (Baltimore, Md. : 1950)* 183 (10): 6422–31. https://doi.org/10.4049/jimmunol.0901969.

Lopez, Jesus Adrian, and Granados-Lopez, Angelica Judith. 2017. "Future Directions of Extracellular Vesicle-Associated MiRNAs in Metastasis." *Annals of Translational Medicine*. China. https://doi.org/10.21037/atm.2017.01.26.

Madan, Vikas, Madan, Babita, Brykczynska, Urszula, Zilbermann, Frederic, Hogeveen, Kevin, Dohner, Konstanze, Dohner, Hartmut et al. 2009. "Impaired Function of Primitive Hematopoietic Cells in Mice Lacking the Mixed-Lineage-Leukemia Homolog MLL5." *Blood* 113 (7): 1444–54. https://doi.org/10.1182/blood-2008-02-142638.

Maegawa, Shinji, Hinkal, George, Kim, Hyun Soo, Shen, Lanlan, Zhang, Li, Zhang, Jiexin, Zhang, Nianxiang, Liang, Shoudan, Donehower, Lawrence A., and Issa, Jean-Pierre J. 2010. "Widespread and Tissue Specific Age-Related DNA Methylation Changes in Mice." *Genome Research* 20 (3): 332–40. https://doi.org/10.1101/gr.096826.109.

Maegawa, Shinji, Lu,Yue, Tahara, Tomomitsu, Lee, Justin T., Madzo, Jozef, Liang, Shoudan, Jelinek, Jaroslav, Colman, Ricki J., and Issa, Jean-Pierre J. 2017. "Caloric Restriction Delays Age-Related Methylation Drift." *Nature Communications* 8 (1): 539. https://doi.org/10.1038/s41467-017-00607-3.

Majewski, Ian J, Blewitt, Marnie E., Graaf, Carolyn A de., McManus, Edward J., Bahlo, Melanie, Hilton, Adrienne A., Hyland, Craig D., et al. 2008. "Polycomb Repressive Complex 2 (PRC2) Restricts

Hematopoietic Stem Cell Activity." *PLoS Biology* 6 (4):e93. https://doi.org/10.1371/journal.pbio.0060093.

Majewski, Ian J., Ritchie, Matthew E., Phipson, Belinda, Corbin, Jason, Pakusch, Miha, Ebert, Anja, Busslinger, Meinrad et al. 2010. "Opposing Roles of Polycomb Repressive Complexes in Hematopoietic Stem and Progenitor Cells." *Blood* 116 (5): 731–39. https://doi.org/10.1182/blood-2009-12-260760.

Martincorena, Inigo, Roshan, Amit, Gerstung, Moritz, Ellis, Peter, Van Loo, Peter, McLaren, Stuart, Wedge, David C., et al. 2015. "Tumor Evolution. High Burden and Pervasive Positive Selection of Somatic Mutations in Normal Human Skin." *Science (New York, N.Y.)* 348 (6237): 880–86. https://doi.org/10.1126/science.aaa6806.

Matsui, Keiko, Ezoe, Sachiko, Oritani, Kenji, Shibata, Masaru, Tokunaga, Masahiro, Fujita, Natsuko, Tanimura, Akira et al. 2012. "NAD-Dependent Histone Deacetylase, SIRT1, Plays Essential Roles in the Maintenance of Hematopoietic Stem Cells." *Biochemical and Biophysical Research Communications* 418 (4): 811–17. https://doi.org/10.1016/j.bbrc.2012.01.109.

Mayle, Allison, Yang, Liubin, Rodriguez, Benjamin, Zhou, Ting, Chang, Edmund, Curry, Choladda V., Challen, Grant A., et al. 2015. "Dnmt3a Loss Predisposes Murine Hematopoietic Stem Cells to Malignant Transformation." *Blood* 125 (4): 629–38. https://doi.org/10.1182/blood-2014-08-594648.

McKerrell, Thomas, Park, Naomi, Moreno, Thaidy, Grove, Carolyn S., Ponstingl, Hannes, Stephens, Jonathan, Crawley, Charles, et al. 2015. "Leukemia-Associated Somatic Mutations Drive Distinct Patterns of Age-Related Clonal Hemopoiesis." *Cell Reports* 10 (8): 1239–45. https://doi.org/10.1016/j.celrep.2015.02.005.

McMahon, Kathryn A., Hiew, Samantha Y-L., Hadjur, Suzana, Veiga-Fernandes, Henrique, Menzel, Ursula, Price, Amanda J, Kioussis, Dimitris, Williams, Owen and Brady, Hugh J. M. 2007. "Mll Has a Critical Role in Fetal and Adult Hematopoietic Stem Cell Self-Renewal." *Cell Stem Cell* 1 (3): 338–45. https://doi.org/10.1016/j.stem.2007.07.002.

Mehta, Arnav, Zhao, Jimmy L., Sinha, Nikita, Marinov, Georgi K., Mann, Mati, Kowalczyk, Monika S., Galimidi, Rachel P., et al. 2015. "The MicroRNA-132 and MicroRNA-212 Cluster Regulates Hematopoietic Stem Cell Maintenance and Survival with Age by Buffering FOXO3 Expression." *Immunity* 42 (6): 1021–32. https://doi.org/10.1016/j.immuni.2015.05.017.

Melton, Collin, Judson, Robert L., and Blelloch, Robert. 2010. "Opposing MicroRNA Families Regulate Self-Renewal in Mouse Embryonic Stem Cells." *Nature* 463 (7281): 621–26. https://doi.org/10.1038/nature08725.

Ming, Mei, Qiang, Lei, Zhao, Baozhong and He, Yu-Ying. 2014. "Mammalian SIRT2 Inhibits Keratin 19 Expression and Is a Tumor Suppressor in Skin." *Experimental Dermatology*. Denmark. https://doi.org/10.1111/exd.12323.

Mochizuki-Kashio, Makiko, Mishima, Yuta, Miyagi, Satoru, Negishi, Masamitsu, Saraya, Atsunori, Konuma, Takaaki, Shinga, Jun, Koseki, Haruhiko and Iwama, Atsushi. 2011. "Dependency on the Polycomb Gene Ezh2 Distinguishes Fetal from Adult Hematopoietic Stem Cells." *Blood* 118 (25): 6553–61. https://doi.org/10.1182/blood-2011-03-340554.

Morales Torres, Cristina, Laugesen, Anne and Helin, Kristian. 2013. "Utx Is Required for Proper Induction of Ectoderm and Mesoderm during Differentiation of Embryonic Stem Cells." *PloS One* 8 (4): e60020. https://doi.org/10.1371/journal.pone.0060020.

Moran-Crusio, Kelly, Reavie, Linsey, Shih, Alan, Abdel-Wahab, Omar, Ndiaye-Lobry, Delphine, Lobry, Camille, Figueroa, Maria E., et al. 2011. "Tet2 Loss Leads to Increased Hematopoietic Stem Cell Self-Renewal and Myeloid Transformation." *Cancer Cell* 20 (1): 11–24. https://doi.org/10.1016/j.ccr.2011.06.001.

Morselli, Marco, Pastor, William A., Montanini, Barbara, Nee, Kevin, Ferrari, Roberto, Fu, Kai, Bonora, Giancarlo et al. 2015. "In Vivo Targeting of de Novo DNA Methylation by Histone Modifications in Yeast and Mouse." *ELife* 4 (April): e06205. https://doi.org/10.7554/eLife.06205.

Neff, Tobias, and Armstrong, Scott A. 2013. "Recent Progress toward Epigenetic Therapies: The Example of Mixed Lineage Leukemia." *Blood* 121 (24): 4847–53. https://doi.org/10.1182/blood-2013-02-474833.

Neri, Francesco, Incarnato, Danny, Krepelova, Anna, Rapelli, Stefania, Pagnani, Andrea, Zecchina, Riccardo, Parlato, Caterina and Oliviero, Salvatore. 2013. "Genome-Wide Analysis Identifies a Functional Association of Tet1 and Polycomb Repressive Complex 2 in Mouse Embryonic Stem Cells." *Genome Biology* 14 (8): R91. https://doi.org/10.1186/gb-2013-14-8-r91.

Neri, Francesco, Krepelova, Anna, Incarnato, Danny, Maldotti, Mara, Parlato, Caterina, Galvagni, Federico, Matarese, Filomena, Stunnenberg, Hendrik G., and Oliviero, Salvatore. 2013. "Dnmt3L Antagonizes DNA Methylation at Bivalent Promoters and Favors DNA Methylation at Gene Bodies in ESCs." *Cell* 155 (1): 121–34. https://doi.org/10.1016/j.cell.2013.08.056.

Neri, Francesco, Rapelli, Stefania, Krepelova, Anna, Incarnato, Danny, Parlato, Caterina, Basile, Giulia, Maldotti, Mara, Anselmi, Francesca, and Oliviero, Salvatore. 2017. "Intragenic DNA Methylation Prevents Spurious Transcription Initiation." *Nature* 543 (7643): 72–77. https://doi.org/10.1038/nature21373.

Nishino, Jinsuke, Kim, Injune, Chada, Kiran and Morrison, Sean J. 2008. "Hmga2 Promotes Neural Stem Cell Self-Renewal in Young but Not Old Mice by Reducing P16Ink4a and P19Arf Expression." *Cell* 135 (2): 227–39. https://doi.org/10.1016/j.cell.2008.09.017.

Oguro, Hideyuki, Yuan, Jin., Ichikawa, Hitoshi, Ikawa, Tomokatsu, Yamazaki, Satoshi, Kawamoto, Hiroshi, Nakauchi, Hiromitsu and Iwama, Atsushi. 2010. "Poised Lineage Specification in Multipotential Hematopoietic Stem and Progenitor Cells by the Polycomb Protein Bmi1." *Cell Stem Cell* 6 (3): 279–86. https://doi.org/10.1016/j.stem.2010.01.005.

Oh, Juhyun, Lee,Yang David and Wagers, Amy J. 2014. "Stem Cell Aging: Mechanisms, Regulators and Therapeutic Opportunities." *Nature Medicine* 20 (8): 870–80. https://doi.org/10.1038/nm.3651.

Okada, Motoi, Kim, Ha Won, Matsu-ura, Kaoru, Wang, Yi-Gang, Xu, Meifeng and Ashraf, Muhammad. 2016. "Abrogation of Age-Induced MicroRNA-195 Rejuvenates the Senescent Mesenchymal Stem Cells by Reactivating Telomerase." *Stem Cells (Dayton, Ohio)* 34 (1): 148–59. https://doi.org/10.1002/stem.2211.

Okuchi, Yoshihisa, Imajo, Masamichi, Mizuno, Rei, Kamioka, Yuji, Miyoshi, Hiroyuki, Mark Taketo, Makoto, Nagayama, Satoshi, Sakai, Yoshiharu and Matsuda, Michiyuki. 2016. "Identification of Aging-Associated Gene Expression Signatures That Precede Intestinal Tumorigenesis." *PloS One* 11 (9): e0162300. https://doi.org/10.1371/journal.pone.0162300.

Palacios, Daniela, Mozzetta, Chiara, Consalvi, Silvia, Caretti, Giuseppina, Saccone, Valentina, Proserpio, Valentina, Marquez, Victor E., et al. 2010. "TNF/P38alpha/Polycomb Signaling to Pax7 Locus in Satellite Cells Links Inflammation to the Epigenetic Control of Muscle Regeneration." *Cell Stem Cell* 7 (4): 455–69. https://doi.org/10.1016/j.stem.2010.08.013.

Pan, Huize, Guan, Di., Liu, Xiaomeng, Jingyi Li, Lixia Wang, Jun Wu, Junzhi Zhou, et al. 2016. "SIRT6 Safeguards Human Mesenchymal Stem Cells from Oxidative Stress by Coactivating NRF2." *Cell Research* 26 (2): 190–205. https://doi.org/10.1038/cr.2016.4.

Pandey, Amitabh C, Julie A Semon, Deepak Kaushal, Regina P O'Sullivan, Julie Glowacki, Jeffery M Gimble, and Bruce A Bunnell. 2011. "MicroRNA Profiling Reveals Age-Dependent Differential Expression of Nuclear Factor KappaB and Mitogen-Activated Protein Kinase in Adipose and Bone Marrow-Derived Human Mesenchymal Stem Cells." *Stem Cell Research & Therapy* 2 (6): 49. https://doi.org/10.1186/scrt90.

Peffers, M J, Collins, J., Fang, Y., Goljanek-Whysall, K., Rushton, M., Loughlin J., Proctor, C., and Clegg, P. D. 2016. "Age-Related Changes in Mesenchymal Stem Cells Identified Using a Multi-Omics Approach." *European Cells & Materials* 31 (February): 136–59.

Perez-Campo, Flor, M, Costa, Guilherme, Lie-A-Ling, Michael, Stifani, Stefano, Kouskoff, Valerie and Lacaud, Georges. 2014. "MOZ-

Mediated Repression of P16(INK) (4) (a) Is Critical for the Self-Renewal of Neural and Hematopoietic Stem Cells." *Stem Cells (Dayton, Ohio)* 32 (6): 1591–1601. https://doi.org/10.1002/stem.1606.

Petkovich, Daniel A, Dmitriy I Podolskiy, Alexei V Lobanov, Sang-Goo Lee, Richard A Miller, and Vadim N Gladyshev. 2017. "Using DNA Methylation Profiling to Evaluate Biological Age and Longevity Interventions." *Cell Metabolism* 25 (4): 954-960.e6. https://doi.org/10.1016/j.cmet.2017.03.016.

Pietersen, Alexandra M, Evers, Bastiaan, Prasad, Asheeta A., Tanger, Ellen, Cornelissen-Steijger, Paulien, Jonkers, Jos and Lohuizen, Maarten van. 2008. "Bmi1 Regulates Stem Cells and Proliferation and Differentiation of Committed Cells in Mammary Epithelium." *Current Biology : CB* 18 (14): 1094–99. https://doi.org/10.1016/j.cub.20 08.06.070.

Rafalski, Victoria A, Ho, Peggy P., Brett, Jamie O., Ucar, Duygu, Dugas, Jason C., Pollina, Elizabeth A., Chow, Lionel M L., et al. 2013. "Expansion of Oligodendrocyte Progenitor Cells Following SIRT1 Inactivation in the Adult Brain." *Nature Cell Biology* 15 (6): 614–24. https://doi.org/10.1038/ncb2735.

Rebel, Vivienne I, Kung, Andrew L., Tanner, Elizabeth A., Yang, Hong Bronson, Roderick T., and Livingston, David M. 2002. "Distinct Roles for CREB-Binding Protein and P300 in Hematopoietic Stem Cell Self-Renewal." *Proceedings of the National Academy of Sciences of the United States of America* 99 (23): 14789–94. https://doi.org/10.1073/pnas.232568499.

Reddington, James P, Pennings, Sari and Meehan, Richard R.. 2013. "Non-Canonical Functions of the DNA Methylome in Gene Regulation." *The Biochemical Journal* 451 (1): 13–23. https://doi.org/10.1042/BJ2 0121585.

Redshaw, Zoe, Sweetman, Dylan and Loughna, Paul T. 2014. "The Effects of Age upon the Expression of Three MiRNAs in Muscle Stem Cells Isolated from Two Different Porcine Skeletal Muscles." *Differentiation; Research in Biological Diversity* 88 (4–5): 117–23. https://doi.org/10.1016/j.diff.2014.12.001.

Rimmele, Pauline, Bigarella, Carolina L., Liang, Raymond, Izac, Brigitte, Dieguez-Gonzalez, Rebeca, Barbet, Gaetan, Donovan, Michael et al. 2014. "Aging-like Phenotype and Defective Lineage Specification in SIRT1-Deleted Hematopoietic Stem and Progenitor Cells." *Stem Cell Reports* 3 (1): 44–59. https://doi.org/10.1016/j.stemcr.2014.04.015.

Rinaldi, Lorenzo, and Benitah, Salvador Aznar. 2015. "Epigenetic Regulation of Adult Stem Cell Function." *The FEBS Journal* 282 (9): 1589–1604. https://doi.org/10.1111/febs.12946.

Robson, Lesley G, Foggia, Valentina Di, Radunovic, Aleksandar, Bird, Katy, Zhang, Xinyu and Marino, Silvia. 2011. "Bmi1 Is Expressed in Postnatal Myogenic Satellite Cells, Controls Their Maintenance and Plays an Essential Role in Repeated Muscle Regeneration." *PloS One* 6 (11): e27116. https://doi.org/10.1371/journal.pone.0027116.

Rose, Nathan R, and Klose, Robert J. 2014. "Understanding the Relationship between DNA Methylation and Histone Lysine Methylation." *Biochimica et Biophysica Acta* 1839 (12): 1362–72. https://doi.org/10.1016/j.bbagrm.2014.02.007.

Rossi, Derrick J., Bryder, David, Seita, Jun, Nussenzweig, Andre, Hoeijmakers, Jan and Weissman, Irving L. 2007. "Deficiencies in DNA Damage Repair Limit the Function of Haematopoietic Stem Cells with Age." *Nature* 447 (7145): 725–29. https://doi.org/10.1038/nature05862.

Rossi, Derrick J, Bryder, David, Zahn, Jacob M., Ahlenius, Henrik, Sonu, Rebecca, Wagers, Amy J and Weissman, Irving L. 2005. "Cell Intrinsic Alterations Underlie Hematopoietic Stem Cell Aging." *Proceedings of the National Academy of Sciences of the United States of America* 102 (26): 9194–99. https://doi.org/10.1073/pnas.0503280102.

Rossi, Derrick J, Jamieson, Catriona H M and Weissman, Irving L. 2008. "Stems Cells and the Pathways to Aging and Cancer." *Cell* 132 (4): 681–96. https://doi.org/10.1016/j.cell.2008.01.036.

Ryall, James G, Dell'Orso, Stefania, Derfoul, Assia, Juan, Aster, Zare, Hossein, Feng, Xuesong, Clermont, Daphney et al. 2015. "The NAD(+)-Dependent SIRT1 Deacetylase Translates a Metabolic Switch into Regulatory Epigenetics in Skeletal Muscle Stem Cells." *Cell Stem Cell* 16 (2): 171–83. https://doi.org/10.1016/j.stem.2014.12.004.

Sadakierska-Chudy, Anna, and Malgorzata, Filip. 2015. "A Comprehensive View of the Epigenetic Landscape. Part II: Histone Post-Translational Modification, Nucleosome Level, and Chromatin Regulation by NcRNAs." *Neurotoxicity Research* 27 (2): 172–97. https://doi.org/10.1007/s12640-014-9508-6.

Safak, Yalcin, Carty, Mark, Shin, Joseph Yusup, Miller, Richard A., Leslie, Christina and Park, Christopher Y. 2014. "Microrna Mediated Regulation of Hematopoietic Stem Cell Aging." *Blood* 124 (21): 602.

Sauvageau, Martin, and Sauvageau, Guy. 2010. "Polycomb Group Proteins: Multi-Faceted Regulators of Somatic Stem Cells and Cancer." *Cell Stem Cell* 7 (3): 299–313. https://doi.org/10.1016/j.stem.2010.08.002.

Schaefer, Anne, Sampath, Srihari C., Intrator, Adam, Min, Alice, Gertler, Tracy S., Surmeier, D James, Tarakhovsky, Alexander and Greengard, Paul. 2009. "Control of Cognition and Adaptive Behavior by the GLP/G9a Epigenetic Suppressor Complex." *Neuron* 64 (5): 678–91. https://doi.org/10.1016/j.neuron.2009.11.019.

Schotta, Gunnar, Sengupta, Roopsha, Kubicek, Stefan, Malin, Stephen, Kauer, Monika, Callen, Elsa, Celeste, Arkady et al. 2008. "A Chromatin-Wide Transition to H4K20 Monomethylation Impairs Genome Integrity and Programmed DNA Rearrangements in the Mouse." *Genes & Development* 22 (15): 2048–61. https://doi.org/10.1101/gad.476008.

Schubeler, Dirk. 2015. "Function and Information Content of DNA Methylation." *Nature* 517 (7534): 321–26. https://doi.org/10.1038/nature14192.

Sen, George L, Reuter, Jason A., Webster, Daniel E., Zhu, Lilly and Khavari, Paul A. 2010. "DNMT1 Maintains Progenitor Function in Self-Renewing Somatic Tissue." *Nature* 463 (7280): 563–67. https://doi.org/10.1038/nature08683.

Shang, Jin, Yao,Yuan, Fan, Xin, Shangguan, Lei, Li, Jie, Liu, Huan and Zhou, Yue. 2016. "MiR-29c-3p Promotes Senescence of Human

Mesenchymal Stem Cells by Targeting CNOT6 through P53-P21 and P16-PRB Pathways." *Biochimica et Biophysica Acta* 1863 (4): 520–32. https://doi.org/10.1016/j.bbamcr.2016.01.005.

Shcherbata, H R, Hatfield, S., Ward, E J., Reynolds, S., Fischer, K. A., and Ruohola-Baker, H. 2006. "The MicroRNA Pathway Plays a Regulatory Role in Stem Cell Division." *Cell Cycle (Georgetown, Tex.)* 5 (2): 172–75. https://doi.org/10.4161/cc.5.2.2343.

Sheaffer, Karyn L, Kim, Rinho, Aoki, Reina, Elliott, Ellen N., Schug, Jonathan, Burger, Lukas, Schubeler, Dirk and Kaestner, Klaus H. 2014. "DNA Methylation Is Required for the Control of Stem Cell Differentiation in the Small Intestine." *Genes & Development* 28 (6): 652–64. https://doi.org/10.1101/gad.230318.113.

Sheikh, Bilal N, Dixon, Mathew P., Thomas, Tim, and Voss, Anne K. 2012. "Querkopf Is a Key Marker of Self-Renewal and Multipotency of Adult Neural Stem Cells." *Journal of Cell Science* 125 (Pt 2): 295–309. https://doi.org/10.1242/jcs.077271.

Shide, K, T Kameda, Shimoda, H., Yamaji, T., Abe, H., Kamiunten, A., Sekine, M., et al. 2012. "TET2 Is Essential for Survival and Hematopoietic Stem Cell Homeostasis." *Leukemia* 26 (10): 2216–23. https://doi.org/10.1038/leu.2012.94.

Shlush, Liran I, Zandi, Sasan, Mitchell, Amanda, Chen, Weihsu Claire, Brandwein, Joseph M., Gupta, Vikas, Kennedy, James A., et al. 2014. "Identification of Pre-Leukaemic Haematopoietic Stem Cells in Acute Leukaemia." *Nature* 506 (7488): 328–33. https://doi.org/10.1038/nature13038.

Small, Eric M., and Olson, Eric N. 2011. "Pervasive Roles of MicroRNAs in Cardiovascular Biology." *Nature* 469 (7330): 336–42. https://doi.org/10.1038/nature09783.

Smith-Vikos, Thalyana, and Slack, Frank J. 2012. "MicroRNAs and Their Roles in Aging." *Journal of Cell Science* 125 (Pt 1): 7–17. https://doi.org/10.1242/jcs.099200.

So, Ah-Young, Ji-Won Jung, Lee, Seunghee, Kim, Hyung-Sik and Kang, Kyung-Sun. 2011. "DNA Methyltransferase Controls Stem Cell Aging by Regulating BMI1 and EZH2 through MicroRNAs." *PloS One* 6 (5): e19503. https://doi.org/10.1371/journal.pone.0019503.

Soriano-Arroquia, Ana, McCormick, Rachel, Molloy, Andrew P., McArdle, Anne, and Goljanek-Whysall, Katarzyna. 2016. "Age-Related Changes in MiR-143-3p:Igfbp5 Interactions Affect Muscle Regeneration." *Aging Cell* 15 (2): 361–69. https://doi.org/10.1111/acel.12442.

Stadler, Michael B, Rabih Murr, Lukas Burger, Robert Ivanek, Florian Lienert, Anne Scholer, Erik van Nimwegen, et al. 2011. "DNA-Binding Factors Shape the Mouse Methylome at Distal Regulatory Regions." *Nature* 480 (7378): 490–95. https://doi.org/10.1038/nature10716.

Stalker, Leanne, and Wynder, Christopher. 2012. "Evaluation of Histone-Modifying Enzymes in Stem Cell Populations." *Methods in Molecular Biology (Clifton, N.J.)* 809: 411–26. https://doi.org/10.1007/978-1-61779-376-9_27.

Stubbs, Thomas M, Bonder, Marc Jan, Stark, Anne-Katrien, Krueger, Felix, Meyenn, Ferdinand von, Stegle, Oliver and Reik, Wolf. 2017. "Multi-Tissue DNA Methylation Age Predictor in Mouse." *Genome Biology* 18 (1): 68. https://doi.org/10.1186/s13059-017-1203-5.

Su, I-Hsin, Basavaraj, Ashwin, Krutchinsky, Andrew N., Hobert, Oliver, Ullrich, Axel, Chait, Brian T., and Tarakhovsky, Alexander. 2003. "Ezh2 Controls B Cell Development through Histone H3 Methylation and Igh Rearrangement." *Nature Immunology* 4 (2): 124–31. https://doi.org/10.1038/ni876.

Sudo, K, Ema, H, Morita, Y, and Nakauchi, H. 2000. "Age-Associated Characteristics of Murine Hematopoietic Stem Cells." *The Journal of Experimental Medicine* 192 (9): 1273–80. https://doi.org/10.1084/jem.192.9.1273.

Sun, Deqiang, Luo,Min, Jeong, Mira, Rodriguez, Benjamin, Xia, Zheng, Hannah, Rebecca, Wang, Hui, et al. 2014. "Epigenomic Profiling of Young and Aged HSCs Reveals Concerted Changes during Aging That Reinforce Self-Renewal." *Cell Stem Cell* 14 (5): 673–88. https://doi.org/10.1016/j.stem.2014.03.002.

Sun, Guoqiang, Yu, Ruth T., Evans, Ronald M., and Shi, Yanhong. 2007. "Orphan Nuclear Receptor TLX Recruits Histone Deacetylases to Repress Transcription and Regulate Neural Stem Cell Proliferation." *Proceedings of the National Academy of Sciences of the United States of America* 104 (39): 15282–87. https://doi.org/10.1073/pnas.0704089104.

Tan, Qi, Lui, Pauline Po Yee and Rui, Yun Feng. 2012. "Effect of in Vitro Passaging on the Stem Cell-Related Properties of Tendon-Derived Stem Cells-Implications in Tissue Engineering." *Stem Cells and Development* 21 (5): 790–800. https://doi.org/10.1089/scd.2011.0160.

Tapias, Alicia, Zhou, Zhong-Wei, Shi, Yue, Chong, Zechen, Wang, Pei, Groth, Marco, Platzer, Matthias et al. 2014. "Trrap-Dependent Histone Acetylation Specifically Regulates Cell-Cycle Gene Transcription to Control Neural Progenitor Fate Decisions." *Cell Stem Cell* 14 (5): 632–43. https://doi.org/10.1016/j.stem.2014.04.001.

Taylor-Jones, Jane M, Robert E McGehee, Thomas A Rando, Beata Lecka-Czernik, Lipschitz, David A., and Peterson, Charlotte A. 2002. "Activation of an Adipogenic Program in Adult Myoblasts with Age." *Mechanisms of Ageing and Development* 123 (6): 649–61.

Thieme, Sebastian, Gyarfas, Tobias, Richter, Cornelia, Ozhan, Gunes, Fu, Jun, Alexopoulou, Dimitra, Muders, Michael H., et al. 2013. "The Histone Demethylase UTX Regulates Stem Cell Migration and Hematopoiesis." *Blood* 121 (13): 2462–73. https://doi.org/10.1182/blood-2012-08-452003.

Tome, Maria, Sepulveda, Juan Carlos, Delgado, Mario, Andrades, Jose A., Campisi, Judith, Gonzalez, Manuel A., and Bernad, Antonio. 2014. "MiR-335 Correlates with Senescence/Aging in Human Mesenchymal Stem Cells and Inhibits Their Therapeutic Actions through Inhibition of AP-1 Activity." *Stem Cells (Dayton, Ohio)* 32 (8): 2229–44. https://doi.org/10.1002/stem.1699.

Trisciuoglio, Daniela, Martile, Di, Marta and Bufalo, Donatella Del. 2018. "Emerging Role of Histone Acetyltransferase in Stem Cells and Cancer." *Stem Cells International* 2018: 8908751. https://doi.org/10.1155/2018/8908751.

Trowbridge, Jennifer J., Snow, Jonathan W., Kim, Jonghwan and Orkin, Stuart H. 2009. "DNA Methyltransferase 1 Is Essential for and Uniquely Regulates Hematopoietic Stem and Progenitor Cells." *Cell Stem Cell* 5 (4): 442–49. https://doi.org/10.1016/j.stem.2009.08.016.

Turgeon, Naomie, Blais, Mylene, Gagne, Julie-Moore, Tardif,Veronique, Boudreau, Francois, Perreault, Nathalie and Asselin, Claude. 2013. "HDAC1 and HDAC2 Restrain the Intestinal Inflammatory Response by Regulating Intestinal Epithelial Cell Differentiation." *PloS One* 8 (9): e73785. https://doi.org/10.1371/journal.pone.0073785.

Ugarte, Fernando, Sousae, Rebekah, Cinquin, Bertrand, Martin, Eric W., Krietsch, Jana, Sanchez, Gabriela, Inman, Margaux et al. 2015. "Progressive Chromatin Condensation and H3K9 Methylation Regulate the Differentiation of Embryonic and Hematopoietic Stem Cells." *Stem Cell Reports* 5 (5): 728–40. https://doi.org/10.1016/j.stemcr.2015.09.009.

Vasanthan, Punitha, Govindasamy, Vijayendran, Gnanasegaran, Nareshwaran, Kunasekaran, Wijenthiran, Musa, Sabri and Kasim, Noor Hayaty Abu. 2015. "Differential Expression of Basal Micro-RNAs' Patterns in Human Dental Pulp Stem Cells." *Journal of Cellular and Molecular Medicine* 19 (3): 566–80. https://doi.org/10.1111/jcmm.12381.

Waddington, C H. 2012. "The Epigenotype. 1942." *International Journal of Epidemiology* 41 (1): 10–13. https://doi.org/10.1093/ije/dyr184.

Wagner, Wolfgang, Horn, Patrick, Castoldi, Mirco, Diehlmann, Anke, Bork, Simone, Saffrich, Rainer, Benes, Vladimir et al. 2008. "Replicative Senescence of Mesenchymal Stem Cells: A Continuous and Organized Process." *PloS One* 3 (5): e2213. https://doi.org/10.1371/journal.pone.0002213.

Wang, Chaochen, Lee, Ji-Eun, Cho, Young-Wook, Xiao,Ying, Jin, Qihuang, Liu, Chengyu and Ge, Kai. 2012. "UTX Regulates Mesoderm Differentiation of Embryonic Stem Cells Independent of H3K27 Demethylase Activity." *Proceedings of the National Academy of Sciences of the United States of America* 109 (38): 15324–29. https://doi.org/10.1073/pnas.1204166109.

Wang, Hu, Diao, Daojun, Shi, Zhencan, Zhu, Xudong, Gao, Yawei, Gao, Shaorong, Liu, Xiaoyu et al. 2016. "SIRT6 Controls Hematopoietic Stem Cell Homeostasis through Epigenetic Regulation of Wnt Signaling." *Cell Stem Cell* 18 (4): 495–507. https://doi.org/10.1016/j.stem.2016.03.005.

Wang, Jiapeng, Li, Zhaomin, He,Yongzheng, Pan, Feng, Chen, Shi, Rhodes, Steven, Nguyen, Lihn et al. 2014. "Loss of Asxl1 Leads to Myelodys-plastic Syndrome-like Disease in Mice." *Blood* 123 (4): 541–53. https: //doi.org/10.1182/blood-2013-05-500272.

Wang, Jing, Weaver, Ian C G., Gauthier-Fisher, Andree, Wang, Haoran, He, Ling, Yeomans, John, Wondisford, Frederic, Kaplan, David R and Miller, Freda D. 2010. "CBP Histone Acetyltransferase Activity Regulates Embryonic Neural Differentiation in the Normal and Rubinstein-Taybi Syndrome Brain." *Developmental Cell* 18 (1): 114–25. https://doi.org/10.1016/j.devcel.2009.10.023.

Wang, Yuan, Yuan, Quan and Xie, Liang. 2018. "Histone Modifications in Aging: The Underlying Mechanisms and Implications." *Current Stem Cell Research & Therapy* 13 (2): 125–35. https://doi.org/10.2174/1574888X12666170817141921.

Warr, Matthew R, Binnewies, Mikhail, Flach, Johanna, Reynaud, Damien, Garg, Trit, Malhotra, Ritu, Debnath, Jayanta, and Passegue, Emmanuelle. 2013. "FOXO3A Directs a Protective Autophagy Program in Haematopoietic Stem Cells." *Nature* 494 (7437): 323–27. https://doi.org/10.1038/nature11895.

Watanabe, Yoshihisa, and Maekawa, Masato. 2010. "Methylation of DNA in Cancer." *Advances in Clinical Chemistry* 52: 145–67.

Welch, John S, Ley, Timothy J, Link, Daniel C., Miller, Christopher A, Larson, David E, Koboldt, Daniel C., Wartman, Lukas D, et al. 2012. "The Origin and Evolution of Mutations in Acute Myeloid Leukemia." *Cell* 150 (2): 264–78. https://doi.org/10.1016/j.cell.2012.06.023.

Will, Britta, Li Zhou, Vogler, Thomas O, Ben-Neriah, Susanna, Schinke, Tamari, Carolina Roni, Yu, Yiting et al. 2012. "Stem and Progenitor Cells in Myelodysplastic Syndromes Show Aberrant Stage-Specific

Expansion and Harbor Genetic and Epigenetic Alterations." *Blood* 120 (10): 2076–86. https://doi.org/10.1182/blood-2011-12-399683.

Wilting, Roel H., Yanover, Eva, Heideman, Marinus R., Jacobs, Heinz, Horner, James, Torre, Jaco van der, DePinho, Ronald A., and Dannenberg, Jan-Hermen. 2010. "Overlapping Functions of Hdac1 and Hdac2 in Cell Cycle Regulation and Haematopoiesis." *The EMBO Journal* 29 (15): 2586–97. https://doi.org/10.1038/emboj.2010.136.

Wu, Hao, Coskun, Volkan, Tao, Jifang, Xie, Wei, Ge,Weihong, Yoshikawa, Kazuaki, Li, En, Zhang,Yi and Sun, Yi Eve . 2010. "Dnmt3a-Dependent Nonpromoter DNA Methylation Facilitates Transcription of Neurogenic Genes." *Science (New York, N.Y.)* 329 (5990): 444–48. https://doi.org/10.1126/science.1190485.

Wu, Xiaoji, and Zhang, Yi. 2017. "TET-Mediated Active DNA Demethylation: Mechanism, Function and Beyond." *Nature Reviews. Genetics* 18 (9): 517–34. https://doi.org/10.1038/nrg.2017.33.

Xie, Mingchao, Charles Lu, Wang, Jiayin, McLellan, Michael D., Johnson, Kimberly J., Wendl, Michael C., McMichael, Joshua F., et al. 2014. "Age-Related Mutations Associated with Clonal Hematopoietic Expansion and Malignancies." *Nature Medicine* 20 (12): 1472–78. http s://doi.org/10.1038/nm.3733.

Xu, Juan, Yu, Bo, Hong, Christine and Wang, Cun-Yu. 2013. "KDM6B Epigenetically Regulates Odontogenic Differentiation of Dental Mesenchymal Stem Cells." *International Journal of Oral Science* 5 (4): 200–205. https://doi.org/10.1038/ijos.2013.77.

Yahata, Takashi, Takanashi, Tomomi, Muguruma, Yukari, Ibrahim, Abd Aziz, Matsuzawa, Hideyuki, Uno, Tomoko, Sheng, Yin et al. 2011. "Accumulation of Oxidative DNA Damage Restricts the Self-Renewal Capacity of Human Hematopoietic Stem Cells." *Blood* 118 (11): 2941–50. https://doi.org/10.1182/blood-2011-01-330050.

Yang, Liubin, Rau, Rachel and Goodell, Margaret A. 2015. "DNMT3A in Haematological Malignancies." *Nature Reviews. Cancer* 15 (3): 152–65. https://doi.org/10.1038/nrc3895.

Yang, Xiaojing, Han, Han, Carvalho, Daniel D De, Lay, Fides D., Jones, Peter A and Liang, Gangning. 2014. "Gene Body Methylation Can

Alter Gene Expression and Is a Therapeutic Target in Cancer." *Cancer Cell* 26 (4): 577–90. https://doi.org/10.1016/j.ccr.2014.07.028.

Ye, Ling, Fan, Zhipeng, Bo Yu, Chang, Jia, Hezaimi, Khalid Al, Zhou, Xuedong, Park, No-Hee and Wang, Cun-Yu. 2012. "Histone Demethylases KDM4B and KDM6B Promotes Osteogenic Differentiation of Human MSCs." *Cell Stem Cell* 11 (1): 50–61. https://doi.org/10.1016/j.stem.2012.04.009.

Yi, Rui, and Fuchs, Elaine. 2011. "MicroRNAs and Their Roles in Mammalian Stem Cells." *Journal of Cell Science* 124 (Pt 11): 1775–83. https://doi.org/10.1242/jcs.069104.

Yin, Yimeng, Morgunova, Ekaterina, Jolma, Arttu, Kaasinen, Eevi, Sahu, Biswajyoti, Khund-Sayeed, Syed, Das, Pratyush K., et al. 2017. "Impact of Cytosine Methylation on DNA Binding Specificities of Human Transcription Factors." *Science (New York, N.Y.)* 356 (6337). https://doi.org/10.1126/science.aaj2239.

Yu, Ji Min, Wu, Xiying, Gimble, Jeffrey M., Guan, Xiaoyan, Freitas, Michael A, and Bunnell, Bruce A. 2011. "Age-Related Changes in Mesenchymal Stem Cells Derived from Rhesus Macaque Bone Marrow." *Aging Cell* 10 (1): 66–79. https://doi.org/10.1111/j.1474-9726.2010.00646.x.

Yu, Kyung-Rok, Lee, Seunghee, Jung, Ji-Won, Hong, Kim, In-Sun Hyung-Sik Yoojin Seo, Shin, Tae-Hoon and Kang Kyung-Sun. 2013. "MicroRNA-141-3p Plays a Role in Human Mesenchymal Stem Cell Aging by Directly Targeting ZMPSTE24." *Journal of Cell Science* 126 (Pt 23): 5422–31. https://doi.org/10.1242/jcs.133314.

Yu, Zuoren, Li, Yuan, Fan, Huimin, Liu, Zhongmin, and Pestell, Richard G. 2012. "MiRNAs Regulate Stem Cell Self-Renewal and Differentiation." *Frontiers in Genetics* 3: 191. https://doi.org/10.3389/fgene. 2012.00191.

Zhang, Liang, Stokes, Polak, Nicole Lisa and Fuchs, Elaine. 2011. "Specific MicroRNAs Are Preferentially Expressed by Skin Stem Cells to Balance Self-Renewal and Early Lineage Commitment." *Cell Stem Cell* 8 (3): 294–308. https://doi.org/10.1016/j.stem.2011.01.014.

Zhang, Run-Rui, Cui, Qing-Yan, Murai, Kiyohito, Lim, Yen Ching, Smith, Zachary D., Jin, Shengnan, Ye, Peng, et al. 2013. "Tet1 Regulates Adult Hippocampal Neurogenesis and Cognition." *Cell Stem Cell* 13 (2): 237–45. https://doi.org/10.1016/j.stem.2013.05.006.

Zhang, Weiqi, Li, Jingyi, Suzuki, Keiichiro, Qu, Jing, Wang, Ping, Zhou, Junzhi, Liu, Xiaomeng et al. 2015. "Aging Stem Cells. A Werner Syndrome Stem Cell Model Unveils Heterochromatin Alterations as a Driver of Human Aging." *Science (New York, N.Y.)* 348 (6239): 1160–63. https://doi.org/10.1126/science.aaa1356.

Zhao, Jimmy L., Rao, Dinesh S., O'Connell, Ryan M., Garcia-Flores, Yvette and Baltimore, David. 2013. "MicroRNA-146a Acts as a Guardian of the Quality and Longevity of Hematopoietic Stem Cells in Mice." *ELife* 2 (May): e00537. https://doi.org/10.7554/eLife.00537.

Zhao, Wei, Li, Qingtian, Ayers, Stephen, Gu,Yifeng, Shi, Zhong, Zhu, Qingyuan, Chen, Yidong, Wang, Helen Y and Wang, Rong-Fu. 2013. "Jmjd3 Inhibits Reprogramming by Upregulating Expression of INK4a/Arf and Targeting PHF20 for Ubiquitination." *Cell* 152 (5): 10 37–50. https://doi.org/10.1016/j.cell.2013.02.006.

Zimberlin, Cheryl D., Lancini, Cesare, Sno, Rachel, Rosekrans, Sanne L., McLean, Chelsea M, Vlaming, Hanneke, Brink, Gijs R van den, Bots, Michael, Medema, Jan Paul and Dannenberg, Jan-Hermen. 2015. "HDAC1 and HDAC2 Collectively Regulate Intestinal Stem Cell Homeostasis." *FASEB Journal : Official Publication of the Federation of American Societies for Experimental Biology* 29 (5): 2070–80. https://doi.org/10.1096/fj.14-257931.

In: Current Challenges and Management … ISBN: 978-1-53617-304-8
Editor: Abhai Kumar

Chapter 2

FAILURE OF OPTIMUM ACTIVATION IN AGED T CELLS COMPROMISES THEIR RESPONSE TO ANTIGENS

Amit Kumar Kureel, Bharat Singh and Ambak Kumar Rai**, PhD
Department of Biotechnology,
Motilal Nehru National Institute of Technology Allahabad,
Prayagraj, India

ABSTRACT

The increased susceptibility of the elderly to infection presents a major challenge worldwide. Aged persons frequently manifest a declining parameter of innate and adaptive immune system that protects the young against disease. T cells are important key executors of cell-mediated immunity and their activation is important for the initiation and regulation of immune response. Failure of T cell activation in aged T cells is one of the reasons for compromised immune response in aged persons. In this chapter, we have discussed about failure of T cell

* Corresponding Author's Email: ambakrai@mnnit.ac.in.

activation and function(s) in aged person along with expression of costimulatory molecules, cytokine production and their receptors and outcome of impaired T cell activation in aged T cells. we have also discussed various approaches to overcome the impaired T cell activation in aged T cells.

Keywords: aged T cell, T cell activation, TCR signaling

1. INTRODUCTION

Aging is among the greatest known and inevitable risk factor in human life. On the increasing life expectancy, the number of aged people is steeply rising. According to WHO, the world population aged 60 years and older was 900 million in 2015, but it will be almost 2 billion by the 2050. Currently, 125 million people are aged 80 years or older and this would increase up to 434 million people by 2050 (WHO 2018). Out of total deaths of 1, 51,600 people per day across the globe (Ecological global network 2019), approximately two-third die from age-related causes (De Grey 2007). Aged people are susceptible to several infections; against which they used to mount fairly good immune response at their young age. However, numbers of reasons are attributed to the declining state of immune response among elderly, but impaired T cell response is considered one of the most significant.

Developing thymocytes travel from bone marrow (BM) to thymus for the rest of the developmental process and emerge as naïve T cells, which have not been exposed to any sort of foreign antigens. These naïve T cells are housed in secondary lymphoid organs and are competent to recognize and respond to an antigenic challenge. In response to an antigen challenge, they can first get activated, proliferate, migrate to the site of infection/disease from the nearest lymph node and mount the immune response in order to protect the host. The antigen recognition and presentation are performed by the antigen presenting cells (APCs). However, the robustness of the immune response depends on the quality of T cell response, which is proportional to the extent of their optimum activation. Upon presentation of foreign antigen by Major Histo-compatibility Complex (MHC), T cells initiate a series of signaling events, which end up in optimum activation. Thus, the immune response depends on the activation of T cells, which in turn indispensably depends on the antigen presentation by APCs i.e., macrophages (mφ).

Inside the thymus, the developing thymocytes are exposed to various degrees of checks/gateways and the successfully completing thymocytes are destined to become T cells and then released and function in the periphery. These T cells are presented with self MHC-peptide complex inside the thymus. Briefly, thymocytes recognizing and binding to self MHC-peptide complex are selected in the cortical region of the thymus. The non-recognizing thymocytes, possibly having low affinity to self MHC complex, would be clonally deleted at this stage. The selected thymocytes (of mid and high affinity) are presented to cells expressing another set of self MHC-peptide complex in the medullary region of thymus. Here, thymocytes having high affinity, i.e., strongly binding to this self MHC-peptide complex, are clonally deleted. Thus, T cells having mid affinity are generally passed through this two-steps selection process. Ironically, cells which were trained against self MHC-peptide complex, are expected to recognize and respond to self MHC-foreign peptide complex. It is expected from T cells to choose a middle path to avoid autoimmunity (recognizing self MHC-peptide complex with high affinity) and alloreactivity (recognizing self MHC-peptide complex with poor affinity and thus may recognize foreign MHC-peptide complex) (Koch and Radtke 2011). Thus, T cells activation has a prerequisite of rightful presentation of foreign antigen on self MHC. Besides this, various co-stimulatory and adhesion markers are also involved in the optimum activation of T cells. Failing to this, T cells may not receive signal leading to poor activation. This has been discussed in detail later on.

A general notion is that the T cells are not optimally activated among the aged population. Aging, which may also be referred as cellular senescence at the cell level, results from the gradual accumulation of functional losses due to exposure to several stresses/ stimuli (Wang and Dreesen 2018). At a young age, our cells are exposed to various stresses/stimuli and show adaptation (i.e., adjustment to the altered environment). If the stresses/stimuli are not removed, cells may undergo injury. Injury may be of reversible or irreversible in nature, which depends on the type of stresses/stimuli as well as the type and status of exposed cells. Theoretically, cells undergoing adaptation revert back to its original state, if the stresses/stimuli are removed. However, this may not be true practically, because cells show losses of functions at every round of adaptation and reversal to normal state. However, it gets manifested only upon significant accumulation of such losses in a given function. Thus, cellular senescence i.e., cell aging, is a gradual accumulation of experiences of every exposure to stimuli/stresses which results in loss of functions (Wang and Dreesen 2018).

Ageing is also accompanied by a progressive loss of immune competence demonstrated by loss in both humoral and cell mediated immunity. Age related decline in the immune system is also often termed as immune-senescence (Ponnappan and Ponnappan 2011). It is associated with numerous functional and phenotypic changes in T cells, B cells and monocyte/macrophage. Furthermore, there is an increased susceptibility to bacterial and viral infection and reduced vaccine responses (Gardner 1980). Moreover, occurrences of cancer have been widely reported in aged people (White et al. 2014). Age-related impairments are predominantly demonstrated in T cell, because T cell plays a central role in immune responses and has been in the spotlight of research. Failure of T cell activation continues to be a major concern among the scientific community working in the field of immune-aging/senescence (Coffman and Cohen 1989). Greater the extent of aging, higher the level of impairment will be in T cell activation and their response to recall antigen.

In this chapter, we briefly review the cellular and molecular events that lead to the activation of the T cell. Besides this, we will also lay down our focus on expressions and interactions of costimulatory as well as accessory molecules. These molecules play an important role in determining the outcome of T cell-APC interaction. Thereafter, we will discuss T cell activation in aged T cells and how it is impaired. In the later part of the chapter, we will discuss the outcome of impaired T cell activation in aged T cell and different approaches to overcome the same.

2. ACTIVATION OF T CELLS

The developed T cells released from the thymus are stored in secondary lymphoid organs. These naïve T cells (i.e., competent and unexposed) are very dynamic in their pool and should not be considered homogeneous. During their stay, they may get an opportunity to interact with any antigen. If that does not happen, they complete their life cycle either in one lymphoid organ and/or being circulated among different lymphoid organs through blood and lymph. At last, they die to create space for freshly generated naïve T cells. Otherwise, they encounter the antigenic challenge and get activated and move out of the lymphoid tissues. With the growing age and regression of thymus function, the renewal of naïve T cells pool gets slowed down. The continuous supply of fully prepared naïve T cells (i.e., thymic output) decreases with regression in T cell function. However, contrary to reduced thymic output, naïve T cells pool is found constant in aged conditions and this may vary in terms of age of the individual cell, their response to new antigens, their fragility to robust challenges etc. (Salam et al. 2013). The maintenance of naïve T cells pool in aged individuals is plausibly due to either increased longevity of these cells and/or progeny derived from these long-standing cells in lymphoid tissues (Tsukamoto et al. 2009).

Activation of T cell is a result of their encounter with mature APCs loaded with their cognate antigen (Figure 1). As a result of the downstream signaling cascade, they become activated. However, it's not only TCR-MHC-peptide interaction, but several co-stimulatory and accessory molecules interactions are involved in the T cells-APC conjugate. Firstly, synapse formation between T cells and APC is the prerequisite for efficient signaling leading to positive cell responses such as cell survival, proliferation, cytoskeleton rearrangement, changes in gene expression, and increased metabolic activity (Lever et al. 2014). An inefficient synapse i.e., loosely conjugated T cell- APC pair, may lead to functional unresponsiveness and/or apoptotic pathway to delete such clone (Fooksman et al. 2009). Response (s) of T cells are generally regulated by positive and negative regulators. These are together involved in the maintenance of a balanced T cells response. Gradually over time, these experiences of tackling diverse antigens are stored in the form of their respective TCR V-D-J combinations i.e., memory T cells. Furthermore, the TCR diversity and clonal expansion upon antigenic challenge are the hallmark of the T cell mediated response. The size and diversity of the TCR repertoire determine the successful elimination of pathogens from the system. However, with the increasing age, a decline in TCR diversity has been observed (Nikolich-Žugich 2008).

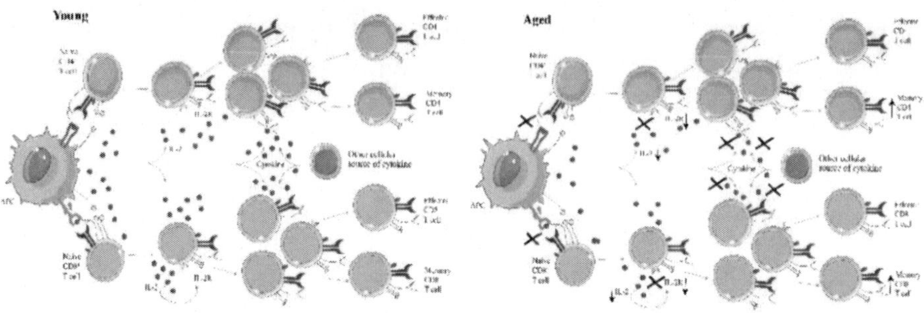

Figure 1. Differences in the development of immune response in young and elderly. In the secondary lymphoid organ of young, APC induced activation of naïve T cells is strengthened by the release of cytokines i.e., IL-2 and presence of costimulatory molecules in the synapse. As a result, there is the clonal expansion of activated effector T-cells and gradually attaining a significant number. However, in aged as compared to young, lack of strong costimulatory signal accompanied by low levels of proliferative cytokines [i.e., IL 2] and their receptors leads to an imbalanced ratio of effector and memory T-cells. This is clearly manifested in the higher frequency of memory T-cells than effector cells.

3. Prerequisite for T Cell Activation

An efficient T cell-APC interaction is the prerequisite of optimum T cell activation. Firstly, APCs i.e., mφ and DC, express the foreign peptide on self MHC along with other costimulatory molecules. It is already established that the downregulation of MHC molecules impairs the antigen presentation and thus the T cell activation. As we all know, $CD4^+$ T cells (T_H cells) are presented with foreign exogenous antigen via MHC class-II molecules. Activation of T_H cells initiates the cascade of events which further activates other effectors subsets. Importantly, it also activates mφ to express a higher level of MHC and co-stimulatory molecules. Decreased expression of MHC class II is well documented in aged cases, suggesting an impaired activation of T cells (Janick-Buckner et al. 1991).

A definite combination of V-D-J in TCR defines specificity for a given type of antigen. TCR is supposed to discriminate/identify the foreign peptide-self MHC (fP-sMHC) complex over self-peptide-self MHC (sP-sMHC) complex. There are two issues pertaining to this recognition. First, as briefed above, T cells are trained against sP-sMHC complex with moderate affinity and are being encountered with fP-sMHC complex upon infection. The recognition process seems to be performed by '*Gods' Hand*' that it selectively as well as efficiently discriminate sP-sMHC over fP-sMHC complex. Secondly, this must be noted that the proportional presence of fP-sMHC complex on the surface of mφ in low at the early stage of infection. At a later stage, its expression gets increased in comparison to the initial level and gradually outnumbers the sP-sMHC complex. At an early stage of infection, it is very challenging for T cells to recognize fP-sMHC on a cell surface which is dominantly populated with sP-sMHC complex. Thus, the outcome of T cells-APC interaction depends on their stable cognate pairing as well as the organization of signaling molecule in the immune synapse.

In the central part of the immune synapse (cSMAC), the TCR /MHC – peptide complex and coreceptors are assembled and this plays a critical role in establishing T cell-APC conjugate (Figure 2). CD4 and CD8 co-receptors stabilize the interaction between TCR and MHC molecule in cSMAC (Dustin, Chakraborty, and Shaw 2010). Interaction between costimulatory receptor (s) on T cell and their ligand (s) on dendritic cells (CD80/86) provide a second signal. Interaction of adhesion molecules (LFA-1/ICAM-1 and CD2/LFA-3) are also critical for the signal generated by TCR-MHC interaction. These accessory interactions are aggregated in the mantle region around the cSMACi.epSMAC (Dustin, Chakraborty, and Shaw 2010). At a young age, the formation of the immune synapse is efficient and smooth in terms of delivering downstream signals. However, the effective immune synapse formation in T cell declines with increasing age (Marko et al. 2007). It has been shown that the expressions of lymphocyte adhesion molecules are altered on aged cells. Memory cells are found in higher numbers with the increase in age and shown to express a high level of LFA-1.

Interestingly, their response (i.e., of T cells) to stimulant like PMA (phorbol 12-myristrate 13-acetate), which skips the TCR and acts on PKC, are equal in young as well as elderly (Powers, Morley, and Flood 1992). However, aged T cells show reduced proliferation response to mitogen than that of their young counterpart. Moreover, the increased functional avidity offered by co-receptor and adhesion molecule is still not sufficient to fully activate the aged T cell. This raises a question that whether the defect in aged cells lies at TCR level and/or in synapse.

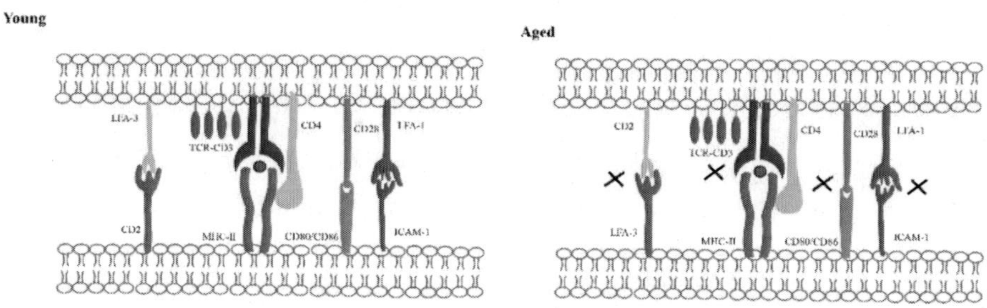

Figure 2. Effect of ageing on immunological synapse during T-cell activation. Antigen-presenting cells (APCs) and T cells pairing is a prerequisite and considered the first step towards T cell activation. Apart from the core interaction i.e., MHC-peptide-TCR, other interactions such as costimulatory molecules [CD28 and CD80/86] and accessory molecules [LFA3 and CD2, LFA-1 and ICAM-1] help in establishing a strong and effective immunological synapse between T cell-macrophage. The effectiveness of this synapse is compromised in aged as compared to young and the reason could be a low grade inflammation, poor expressions of MHC and other molecules resulting in the formation of the poor immune synapse.

4. Expression of Costimulatory Molecules

Costimulatory signals are required for optimal T cell activation and CD28 is one of the important of all costimulatory molecules. It binds to two distinct ligands of B7 family of proteins i.e., CD80 (B7-1) and CD86 (B7-2). These are the members of immunoglobulin superfamily and are expressed only by the professional APCs. Besides CD28, other molecules also provide costimulatory signals during T cell activation. One of such costimulatory molecules i.e., ICOS provides positive co-stimulation during the process of T cell activation. However, similar to CD28, ICOS binds to another member of B7 family i.e., ICOS ligand (ICOS-L), which is expressed on a subset of activated APCs. Unlike CD28, ICOS is not expressed on naïve T cells rather it is expressed on memory and effector T cells. It has been suggested that CD28 play a key costimulatory role during the initiation of activation and ICOS maintains the activity of already differentiated effector and memory T cells at a later stage (Esensten et al. 2016). Many reports suggested that the expression of CD28 molecule is declined in aged individual. Moreover, expressions of its ligands (CD80/CD86) are decreased on APCs in aged individuals and this could be one of the reasons for the occurrence of immunosenescence in such cases (Busse et al. 2015). Besides this, the expression of ICOS is impaired in aged T cells after allogeneic stimulation (Tesar, Asea, and Goldstein 2005). Importantly, ICOS expression is increased on Treg cells and contributes to its maintenance in the elderly (Raynor et al. 2015). However, expression of its ligand i.e., ICOS-L is not yet attempted in the elderly.

CTLA-4 is the second member of the CD28 family to be identified and well researched. However, it did not act as a positive costimulatory molecule, as it antagonizes the T cell activating signals and is now referred to as a negative costimulatory receptor (Walunas, Bakker, and Bluestone 1996). CTLA-4 is not constitutively expressed on resting T cells, rather it is induced within 24 hours after activation on a naïve T cell and its expression get heightened within 2 to 3-days of stimulation. However, the expression of CD28 is higher in the early part of activation (i.e., within 1-2 days) followed by the expression of CTLA-4 in the later part (Jago et al.

2004). This must be noted that the level of peak expression of CTLA-4 is quantitatively lower than the peak expression level of CD28, but the CTLA-4's affinity to CD80 and CD86 is higher in comparison to that of CD28. This is also suggested that the CTLA-4 puts the break on TCR-CD28 engagement and thus reduces the activation of T cells (Linsley and Golstein 1996). This has been observed that the expression of CTLA-4 is increased in aged T cells upon activation in comparison to their young counterpart (Canaday et al. 2013).

Program Death-1 (PD-1) is also a negative costimulatory receptor and inhibit TCR mediated T cell activation. PD-1 is expressed by B as well as T cells and binds to two ligands PD-L1 (B7-H1) and PD-L2 (B7-DC), which are also members of the B7superfamily. PD-L2 is expressed predominately on APC and PD-L1 is expressed on almost all types of lympho-hematopoietic cells at varying levels. It is constitutively expressed on T cells, B cells, macrophage and dendritic cells (DCs) (Shi et al. 2013). PD-1 may contribute to age associated T cell dysfunction. Studies suggest that the number of PD-1-expressing T cells and its expression *per cell* were increased. The expression levels of its ligands were also increased on DC subsets and T cells. Therefore, it can be said that the inhibitory costimulatory molecules are more expressed in aged individual (Lages et al. 2010).

5. Expression of Cytokine for T Cell Activation

Summarily, naïve T cells will initiate the process of activation, when they are engaged with APC expressing both MHC-peptide complex as well as costimulatory ligands. However, the consequences and extent of T cell activation are also critically shaped by the soluble cytokine (s) present in the milieu. These are either produced by APC and/or T cells. The activation as well as functional differentiation of T cell is driven by the type and the level of cytokines. The interaction between cytokines and their receptors provide a signal that is necessary to execute the final step of activation process. Cytokine binds their receptor expressed on the surface of the cells and stimulates a cascade of intracellular signals that can enhance proliferation and survival. One of the well studied cytokines, IL-2 is involved in T cells activation and plays a key role in optimal T cell proliferation. Its presence becomes more significant when antigen and costimulatory ligands are limiting. CD28 costimulation induces the expression of both the IL-2 and its high affinity IL-2 receptor (CD25) (Ross and Cantrell 2018). The addition of IL-2 activates and induces the naïve T cells to proliferate vigorously. IL-2 not only promotes the proliferation of T cell, but it also maintains the growth and function of number of the immune cells (e.g., B cells, cytotoxic T cells, natural killer cells lymphokine-activated killer cells) (Bachmann and Oxenius 2007). Several laboratories have investigated the levels of IL-2 expression in aged cases and found that the induction of IL-2 activity decreased with age in mice, rat and human (Pahlavani, Harris, and Richardson 1995).

Decrease in the production of mitogenic cytokine like IL-2 and an increase in other cytokines such as IL-6 (Myśliwska et al. 1998) with age is well documented. Besides the production of cytokines, their receptor expression is also modulated and affects the T cell response in the elderly. This was further confirmed when T cells from aged mice fail to proliferate when subjected to proliferative cytokines like IL-2, IL-4, IFNγ, IL-1a, or IL6 (Bernstein and Murasko 1998). Similarly, splenic T cells from aged mice carrying low levels of IL-2 receptor show a relatively poor response to IL-2 cytokine as compared to their young counterpart (Hara et al. 1988). Besides this, an increase in the soluble form of cytokine receptor like serum sIL-6R could lead to the development of autoimmune diseases in aged mice (Robak et al. 1998).

A phenomenon called 'Inflammaging' is well evident in the elderly i.e., dysregulated functioning of pro as well as anti-inflammatory cytokines. The main contributors to this phenomenon are IL-6, TNF-α, and IL-1α (Franceschi et al. 2000). The IL-1 family cytokines include IL-1α and IL-1β; their binding to respective IL-1R leads to stress induced inflammatory cascade (Sims and Smith 2010). However, IL-1Rα an antagonist to IL-1R blocks this signaling. Evidence suggest that an increase in IL-1α with age has been found to be associated with increased morbidity and mortality (Sansoni et al. 2008). IL-6 a bi-functional cytokine also called 'Gerentologist's Cytokine' plays a crucial role in modulating acute inflammatory response either by producing IL-1Rα to inhibit IL-1 induced signaling or by producing soluble tumor necrosis factor (sTNF-R55) to suppress TNF-α cascade (Ershler 1993). An increase in IL-6 with age has been found to be associated with increased mortality and age related muscle loss (Puzianowska-Kuźnicka et al. 2016). TNF-α, another important pro-inflammatory cytokine with an increased concentration is found to be associated with ageing and age related diseases. Allelic variations in TNF-α are associated with increased risk of age related diseases like Myocardial Infraction (Ridker et al. 2000).

Studies in elderly have displayed a low level of IL-17 with a decrease in frequency of IL-17 producing memory cells (Lee et al. 2011). IL-17 serves as an inducer in the production of IL-6, TNF-α and C-reactive protein (Gaffen 2009). On the other hand, anti-inflammatory cytokines play a crucial role in maintaining the inflammatory homeostasis either by blocking the secretion of pro-inflammatory cytokines or by modulating the release of other immunomodulatory molecules. As ageing is predominantly associated with the increase in pro-inflammatory cytokines, it indicates the compromised state of anti-inflammatory branch. Reports on the elderly have shown an increased serum IL-10 along with high production by both monocyte and lymphocyte cells (Rink, Cakman, and Kirchner 1998). IL-10 one of the major anti-inflammatory cytokines serves as a negative regulator to TNF-α, IL-6 and IL-8 signaling (Commins, Steinke, and Borish 2008). Studies about another anti-inflammatory cytokine, show discordant expressions of TGF-β in elderly, few of them have reported an increase in TGF-β with age and have found significant association with age related diseases (Krieglstein et al. 2012). Another report has found levels of TGF-β to be associated with longevity (Carrieri et al. 2004). However, the exact role of TGF-β is not clear. The paradoxical balance between pro and anti-inflammatory cytokines in ageing is not clearly understood. On one hand, there is an increase in pro-inflammatory cytokines suggesting a low level of anti-inflammatory response. Contrary to our expectation, an increase in anti-inflammatory cytokines has also been reported, supposedly balance the enhanced low grade chronic inflammation in ageing. However, it needs to be further investigated.

6. TCR Signaling in T Cell Activation

In general term, cell activation is a group of signaling events that leads to positive cell response such as cell survival, proliferation, cytoskeleton rearrangement, changes in gene expression, and increased metabolic activity. Activation means a way of responding to a stimulus by ignoring the unresponsiveness or apoptosis. The molecular mechanism underlying the decline in T cell activation during ageing depends on the signaling pathways that normally contribute to T cell responsiveness. An impaired signaling pathway in aged individuals may lead to compromised activation of T cells, which was otherwise normal in their young counterpart. These signals may be positive and negative in nature. Positive signals are actually accompanied by negative signals possibly at later stage that help to maintain homeostasis (Heissmeyer et al. 2004).

Cell activation begins with the phosphorylation of immunoreceptor tyrosine activation motifs (ITAMs) located in the cytoplasmic tails of the CD3 and zeta chain of the TCR and some coreceptor molecules. This phosphorylation results in the clustering of enzymes and adaptor molecules in the proximity of the plasma membrane near the cytoplasmic tail of receptors forming the 'signalosome.' Many proteins of TCR dependent signaling pathway include tyrosine kinase, serine-threonine kinase, small GTPase, phosphatases, adaptor protein and transcription factors etc. (Gorentla and Zhong 2012). Interestingly, the age-dependent decline in both baseline and activation induced zeta phosphorylation contribute to downstream defect in signal transduction of T cells from old mice (Garcia and Miller 1997). Although, it is also reported that T cells stimulated with anti-CD3 monoclonal antibodies (mAb) show age-related reduction in tyrosine phosphorylation of cellular protein (Whisler et al. 1997).

The Src kinases (lck and fyn) phosphorylates ITAMs, which are the docking site for tyrosine kinase SAP-70 and Syk, both of which contain

SH2 domain (Kanda et al. 1999). The levels of fyn activation in anti-CD3 stimulated peripheral blood T cell from elderly human were reduced compared to that of from young individuals (Whisler et al. 1997). These enzymes phosphorylate adaptor proteins which recruit other signaling molecules to the proximity of TCR. Linker for activation of T cell (LAT) protein is phosphorylated early by ZAP-70 and act as a link to downstream signal transduction events by recruiting PLCγ, Gads, SLP-76 etc. (Balagopalan et al. 2015). PLCγ is also directly phosphorylated by ZAP-70. Interestingly, decreased ZAP-70 phosphorylation in aged T cells compared to that from young counterpart is reported. Furthermore, age-related impairment of ZAP-70 activation in CD3-stimulated T cells was accompanied by decreased tyrosine phosphorylation of ζ-chain and autophosphorylation of PTKs $p56^{lck}/p59^{fyn}$ (Whisler et al. 1999).

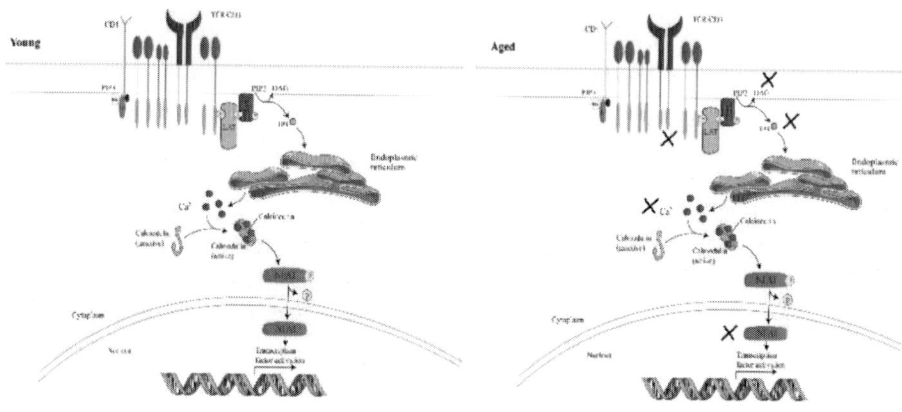

Figure 3. Ca^{2+} mediated NFAT nuclear localization and cytokine expression. TCR/CD3 induced activation results in the activation of other adaptor molecule like LAT, which is present near to the cytoplasmic Zeta chain of TCR. Phosphorylated LAT recruits and phosphorylates PLCγ, this PLCγ breaks membrane bound PIP_2 into DAG and IP_3. IP3 binds to IP3R present on ER membrane and causes the release of Ca^{2+} into the cytoplasm. Increased cytoplasmic Ca^{2+} from extracellular mileu leads to the activation of calcineurin. Further, activated calcineurin dephosphorylates NFAT and facilitates its entry to the nucleus, which activates the expression of cytokine genes. Contrary, ageing diminishes the level of activation of these molecules followed by a low efflux of Ca^{2+} from ER and decreased NFAT nuclear localization.

LAT-PLCγ-1-Gads-SLP76 further phosphorylates phospholipase C, which initiates two other signaling pathways, i.e., diacylglycerol (DAG) and inositol triphosphate (IP-3). DAG is produced through the activation of Phospholipase Cγ1 (PLCγ1), which hydrolyzes membrane phosphatidyl-inositol bisphosphate (PIP2) to DAG and IP3 (Figure 3). DAG recruits PKCθ to the plasma membrane and the activation of PKCθ leads to TCR-mediated NF-κB activation in T cells. This must be noted here that the production of DAG is also decreased with age (de Boland et al. 1996).

On other hand, IP3 binds with IP3 receptor and open the calcium channels of endoplasmic reticulum, results in the release of Ca^{2+} from the ER lumen to the cytoplasm (Koretzky 2003, Krogsgaard and Davis 2005). The presence of Ca^{2+} in cytoplasm further opens the ion channels present in the membrane resulting in its increased concentration in the cytoplasm. The increase in cytosolic Ca^{2+} activates mitogen activation kinase (MAPK), calmodulin dependent kinase (CamK) and calcineurin i.e a phosphatase (Berridge 1997). Calcineurin dephosphorylated NFAT (Nuclear factor of activated transcription factors) allowing translocation of NFAT to the nucleus, where it induces cytokine gene expression- including that of IL-2 (Figure 3) (Hogan et al. 2003). Age associated defect in the generation of IP-3 is also reported, which indicates an impaired signaling events leading to compromised mitogen induced IL-2 production in aged T cells (Proust et al. 1987). Conclusively, ConA stimulated T cells from aged mice showed decreased influx of Ca^{2+} in the first few minutes after activation as compared to its young counterpart (Miller et al. 1987). The finding of impaired IP-3 pathway in aged T cells is further corroborated by the findings an interesting experiment, where ability of nuclear extract isolated from T cells of aged mice to bind with oligonucleotide (NFAT binding site) is decreased by 50 to 60% compared to their young counterpart (Pahlavani, Harris, and Richardson 1995).

The important serine-threonine kinases involved in TCR signaling are the MAPKs, PKCs, and PKB (Bauer and Baier 2002, Matsuda and Koyasu 2002). In MAPKs, p38, ERK (extracellular signal-regulated kinase) and JUNK (or JNK; c/jun NH2/terminal kinase) control phosphorylation of transcription factor and chromatin remodeling process leading to important biological responses. The ERK pathway primarily mediates cell growth, differentiation, and survival, while p38 and JUNK pathways control the synthesis of cytokines leading to proinflammatory response, cell differentiation. In some cases, proapoptotic and growth inhibitory signals are also regulated by p38 (Matsuda and Koyasu 2002). It is reported that ageing compromises the anti-CD3 mab mediated induction of ERK by two folds (Gorgas et al. 1997). As shown in Figure 4, these MAPKs are activated by another set of kinases i.e., mitogen-activated protein kinase kinases [MAPKKs or MAP/ERK kinases (MEK)]. These upstream signaling molecules are ERK kinase (ERK1 and ERK2 by MEK1/MKK1 and MEK2/MKK2 respectively), p38 MAPKK (MKK3, MKK4 and MKK6), and JUNKK (MKK4 and MKK7). It is observed that ageing compromises the anti-CD3 mab mediated induction of MEK by two folds. Besides this, both naïve and memory T cells from young mice showed an equal level of MEK induction. Thus, age-related decline in MEK induction is unlikely to result from a skewed accumulation of memory T cells in old age, suggesting a selective inhibition of MEK in aged T cells (Gorgas et al. 1997). These MKKs are in turn activated by MAPKK kinase (MAPKKK; MAPKKK→MAPKK→MAPK) (Figure 4). The MAPKKKs activating ERK pathway are Raf kinases, Mos and Tpl2. While those activating JNK and p38 are mixed lineage kinase (MLKs), MEKK kinase, Tak1, Ask1 and 2 and Tip-2. Diminished ERK2 and JNK catalytic activity have been detected in T cells from elderly humans stimulated with anti-CD3 mAb OKT3 and PMA. The impaired ERK activity could be attributed to decreased Raf-1 kinase activation (Liu, Carle, and Whisler 1997). The extensive MAP kinase network and multiplicity of regulators along with tightly associated specificities permit the wide cellular response to the stimuli encountered (Johnson, Dohlman, and Graves 2005, Uhlik et al. 2004). A detailed study is required to unravel their activity in aged T cells.

The relocation of signaling molecules to the specific area of the plasma membrane where receptors are clustered is important for their activity. Upstream to the MAPKKK are small G protein of the Ras and Rho families whose controlling protein associates with adaptor proteins in the signalosome. Vav and SOS are among the best known small GTPase activator associated with adaptor protein in the early signalosome that activates Ras and Rho GTPase respectively (Gallucci and Matzinger 2001, Tybulewicz 2005). However, reports show that there is no significant change in the expression of sos with ageing (Garcia and Miller 2009) but vav phosphorylation on the other hand is found to be increased in aged mouse models (Garcia and Miller 2009).

PKC activation leads to the induction of MAPK pathway and also to the activation of inhibitory kappa kinase (IKK) (Figure 5). IKK is a complex of two kinases subunits IKK1/α as well as IKK2/β and one regulatory subunit NEMO/IKKγ. Phosphorylation of IκB (Inhibitor of kappa B) protein by IKKα and β marks them for ubiquitinylation and further degradation, allowing NF-κB to migrate to the nucleus and activate the expression of cytokine and survival gene. Actually, IκB binds with the nuclear localization signal of NF-κB protein, which does not allow their transport to the nucleus for transcription of relevant genes. Degradation of IκB unleashes the NF-κB for their nuclear transport. This is reported that NF-κB induction in activated T cells from old individual is reduced as compared to their young counterpart (Trebilcock and Ponnappan 1996).

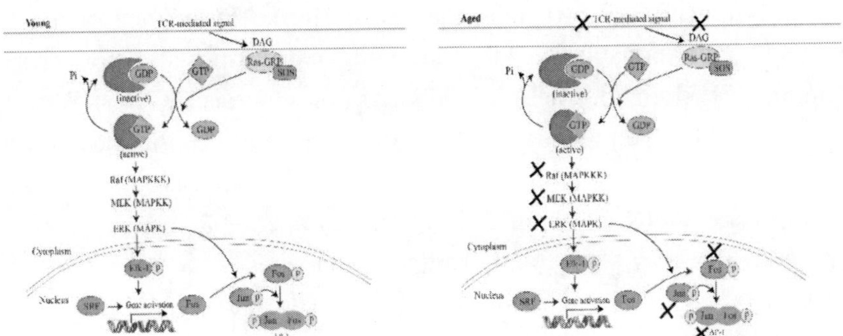

Figure 4. Effect of ageing on Raspathway. TCR mediated activation of PLCγ generates DAG followed by the recruitment of Ras-GRP and SOS complex. SOS catalyses the formation of Ras-GTP, and then the activated Ras-GTP facilitates downstream cascade by recruiting Raf, MEK and ERK. Activated ERK localizes to the nucleus and promotes gene activation via SRF or via Jun-Fos activation. Contrary, in aged as compared to young, this cascade is compromised at multiple steps starting from the week TCR signal, reduced ERK phosphorylation and localization, along with the diminished activation of regulatory genes by Jun-Fos complex.

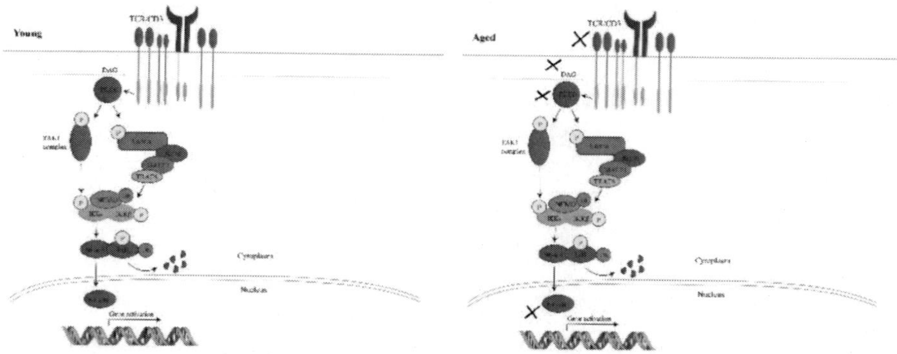

Figure 5. Effect of ageing on NFκB translocation to the nucleus. TCR/CD3 mediated activation of adaptor molecules leads to the formation of DAG followed by activation of PKC. PKC mediates the activation of IKK1/α, IKK2/β and NEMO/IKKγ complex (IKK-complexes) via the phosphorylation of TAK1 complex. IKKα and IKKβ phosphorylate IκB and markes them for ubiquitinylation and further degradation. IκB is an inhibitory protein that blocks NFκB localization to the nucleus. After IκB degradation, NFκB localizes to the nucleus and facilitates the gene expression. Opposite to their young counterpart, in aged T-cells, poor TCR stimulation followed by compromised activity of PKC leads to diminished NFκBnuclear localization.

As summarized above, T cells are activated through TCR and CD28, which in turn activates PI3K resulting in the formation of phosphatidylinositol 3,4,5-triphosphate at the intracellular face of the cell membrane. This constitutes the intracellular docking site for protein containing a PH domain. The most important of which is PKB. PKB is also activated by PI3K mediated phosphorylation and it phosphorylates several targets in T cells leading to an increase in cell proliferation coupled with a decrease in apoptosis (Fruman 2004). This is accompanied by increased cell growth, together with parallel changes in rates of protein synthesis, general metabolism and glucose transport (Plas and Thompson 2005). However, the extent of cell cycle and basal metabolism is constrained by inhibitory factors in naïve cells. The overall role of PKB activation is to stimulate cellular activity by counteracting these negative regulators (Song et al. 2004). Degradation of PKB phosphorylated tuberin complex TSC1-TSC2 leads to activation of mammalian target of rapamycin (mTOR), which in turn activates the S6 kinase. S6 kinase important for ribosomal function and activation of translation machinery. Furthermore, inhibition of 4E-BPI by mTOR leads to cell cycle initiation and progression. Another inhibitory target of PKB is glycogen synthase kinase/3 (GSK3) which is involved in nuclear export of Nuclear Factor of Activated T-Cells (NFAT) and β-catenin. Inactivation of O subgroup of Forkhead Box transcription factor (FOXO) by PKB helps the cell in escaping cell cycle arrest. In addition, activation of MAPKKK Tpl2 by PKB followed by activation of IKK and NF-κB further supports cell proliferation (Fruman 2004). The role of PKB in ageing is partly understood however age related increase in PKB activity has been observed in skeletal muscle of aged mice model (Gaugler et al. 2011). The effect of mTOR activity on lifespan is well studied. Studies show inhibition of mTOR repressor and mTOR activator leads to decreased and increased lifespan respectively in different ageing study models (Antikainen et al. 2017). Similarly, another important player in ageing PI3K shows increased activity in aged as compared to young and contributes towards dysregulates inflammation (Fallah et al. 2011).

T cell activation is stupendously controlled by an integrated series of negative regulators at every step. These include phosphatases reversing the activity of kinases, inhibitory adaptors, capturing signaling molecule like the csk inhibitory tyrosine kinase and protecting the inhibitory site of Src Kinase and ubiquitin ligase from getting phosphorylated. Inhibitory receptors like MHC recognizing receptor and the co-receptor CTLA-4 help in establishing the threshold necessary for positive signal to surpass the negative regulatory signal in lymphocyte activation (Carter and Carreno 2003, Krebs and Hilton 2001, Rao, Dodge, and Band 2002, Singer and Koretzky 2002). Once activated, cells secrete cytokines followed by upregulation of cytokine receptors which leads to enhanced expression of activated clones and their differentiation into effector cells. Cytokine secreted by APC determine the outcome of activation (Th1 or Th2). Qibin Leng et al. demonstrated that such negative regulators (i.e., CTLA-4 etc.) are upregulated during ageing (Leng, Bentwich, and Borkow 2002).

7. PROLIFERATION

Cell proliferation and cell death are two inseparable physiological phenomena. Ageing is characterized as the loss of cell proliferation potency, involution of tissues and organs with successive cell loss and reduced potential to maintain hemostasis in stressful conditions (Franceschi 1989). An aecrease in the proliferative response of T cells with ageing is well documented in both humans and rodents (Kanno et al. 1997). It has been found that the crucial immunological changes in T cell activation leads to reduced proliferative capacity of T cells after antigen stimuli (Cristofalo and Pignolo 1993). The limited number of replication cycle (hayflick phenomenon) could be the cause of loss of proliferation potential (Cossarizza et al. 1997). The mechanism that underlies this event and its *in-vivo* physiologic relevance is poorly understood. Clonal expansion of immune cells is majorly dependent on the effective antigen-specific response, but in the aged individual insufficient thymic output of naive cells limits the process of clonal expansion (Pawelec et al. 1997). Having shorter telomere length in CD28- cells than that of $CD28^+$ cells from the same donor, implies that the former has undertaken additional rounds of cell division than the later (Effros 1996). There are situations where T cell proliferative senescence plays a crucial role in modulating immune response which is independent of the age (viral diseases, for example, AIDS, CLL, rheumatoid arthritis, and Crohn's disease) (Kämmerer et al. 1996, Posnett et al. 1994, Roman et al. 1996, Rossi et al. 1996, Schmidt, Goronzy, and Weyand 1996). The effects of this kind of "clonal exhaustion" in elderly are more obvious than in the young and the reason behind could be the lack of effective generation of naïve T cells due to thymic involution. This may also be interpreted that the T cells in elderly have undergone many rounds of cell division (Pawelec et al. 1997). However, we may observe varying pattern in different cell subsets. Hence, studying specific cell types in elderly is essential to conclude.

8. T Cell Activation vs T Cell Effector Response

The two major pillars of protective immune response are circulatory antibody and antigen specific CD8 T cells produced as a result of prior infection or vaccination. Evidences suggest that the antibody response generated at young age before the commencement of immune senescence persist and function well till old age. It was shown that during the epidemic of 1918 influenza infection, the cure was protective antibodies from survivors (Yu et al. 2008). Similarly, it has been found that memory T cells (both CD4 and CD8) generated at a young age largely function well in elderly as compared to those generated in the elderly (Haynes et al. 2003). Therefore, an impaired immune response against vaccines, tumors, or pathogens in the elderly is substantially a consequence of impaired T cell activation in the elderly. Additionally, other changes that could contribute to this impairment are increase in regulatory T cell population, clonal expansion of T cells and change in T cell receptor (TCR) repertoire. Recent advances in understanding of T cell function provide a novel insight about the effect of T cells on ageing and immune function.

9. Altered Function of Aged $CD4^+$ T Cells

In the elderly, stimulation of naïve $CD4^+$ T cells with peptide loaded APCs has shown to form a weaker immunological synapse resulting in the generation of less intense signaling cascade than that in young T cells (Garcia and Miller 2002). Ultimately as a result of this week interaction, aged naïve CD4 T cells do not expand. Neither they produce cytokine with the same efficiency nor differentiate from that of their young counterpart. Further, the inability of aged naïve T cells to produce a significant amount of IL-2 upon TCR stimulation leads to biased as well as poor generation of T helper cell subset (Th1 and Th2) (Haynes et al. 1999). This age-related biasness in CD4 T cell differentiation results in the generation of Th cells with reduced B cell helper activity (Eaton et al. 2004). In a set of experiments, when transferred to the young immunized host, naïve $CD4^+$ T cells from both young and aged mice were found to localize in B cell follicle and germinal center and there was no difference in terms of their trafficking behavior. However, this localization could not help aged CD4 T cells in generating a robust humoral response. Subsequently, the antibody response generated by aged CD4 T cells was poor in terms of reduced IgG titers. Furthermore, the rates of somatic hypermutation in the immunoglobulin heavy chain gene were reduced (Maue et al. 2009). This ultimately results in the generation of a week and less protective antibody response as described in studies where vaccination response was investigated in the elderly (Lord 2013). Although, aged naïve $CD4^+$ T cells show a biased Th1 and Th2 effector subset differentiation. Recently it has been found that they retain the ability to generate functional Th17 effector cells and are readily available in older individuals. As a support to this observation, naïve CD4+ T cells from the elderly differentiate more readily into Th17 phenotype in presence of required cytokines (Huang et al. 2008), this skewness towards Th17 subsets appears to be an inherent property of the aged naïve $CD4^+$ T cells. These aged Th17 effector cells produce a high level of cytokines of IL-17 family (IL-17, IL-21, and IL-22) and they also play a role in potentiating helper T cells which leads to widespread antigen-specific B cell expansion and germinal center formation (Maue et al. 2009). In contrast, cells do lose their responsiveness towards IL-12 and IL-4 with ageing, but these naïve $CD4^+$ T cells in elderly do respond well to IL-1, IL-6, TGF β, and IL-23 to generate Th17 effector cells.

10. Altered Function of Aged $CD8^+$ T Cells

$CD8^+$ T cells are major effector cells against intracellular infections including viral diseases. A highly diverse TCR repertoire (both CD4 and CD8) is critical for protection from viral infection. A decrease in the TCR repertoire of $CD8^+$ cells, but not of $CD4^+$ T cells, is evident in the elderly. However, more studies are required to support the finding of unaltered TCR repertoire in aged $CD4^+$ T cells. A recent study by Yager et. al.

demonstrated that usage of available TCR repertoire in $CD8^+$ T cells are dramatically decreased in response to influenza infection in older mice (Yager et al. 2008). Besides this, a shift in naïve $CD8^+$ T cell frequency was observed. This shift can make the animal more susceptible to severing intracellular infections. One possible cause of this shift in TCR repertoire usage is thymic involution followed by the absence of new thymic emigrants, leading towards generation of CD8TCE. TCE are T cells expressing a particular combination of TCR-Vβ (Callahan, Kappler, and Marrack 1993). These TCE occupy the $CD8^+$ T cell compartment and their clonal expansion also have been shown to negatively affect the usage of TCR repertoire in response to both herpes simplex virus (HSV)-1 infection and influenza infection (Messaoudi et al. 2004). Thus, TCE developed with ageing functionally impairs the efficacy of antiviral CD8 T cell responses and are potent contributors' in age related immunodeficiency. Additionally, influenza vaccination studies in the elderly also showed a poor humoral response suggesting a wide impact of TCE on the aged immune system (Saurwein-Teissl et al. 2002).

11. Altered Function of Aged Regulatory T Cells

Regulatory T (Treg) cells are crucial in maintaining homeostasis; they do so by limiting the autoimmune response. Contrary to what they are meant for, Treg cells act as a limiting factor in response to infectious agents and tumors. Recent findings have shown an increase in Treg cell population in aged mice (Nishioka et al. 2006). Briefly, it has been documented that Treg cell (defined by expression of CD4, CD25 and FoxP3) mediated suppression inhibits the function (s) of effector T cells via contact dependent (PD-PDL; mTGF-bβ, CTLA-4 etc.) or contact independent (secretion of regulatory cytokines/factor; IL-10, adenosine etc.) methods. Furthermore, the number of Treg cells in the elderly is increased as compared to their young counterpart, which is well correlated with the level of suppression (Lages et al. 2008). The increase in Treg cells has been shown to impair the rejection of transplanted tumors in aged mice

(Ruby and Weinberg 2009, Sharma, Dominguez, and Lustgarten 2006). In these studies, the consequences of antitumor immunotherapies were examined in the elderly, who exhibit an increase incidence of tumors. While young mice survive and develop robust antitumor responses, aged mice succumb and develop few tumor-specific cytolytic CD8+ T cells. Furthermore, depletion of Treg cells with an anti-CD25 monoclonal antibody could restore antitumor responses to the level which is found in young mice.

12. Cytolytic Response

$CD8^+$ T cells subset from old subjects show decreased cytolytic activity (Mariani et al. 1990, Vitale et al. 1992). T cell-mediated cytotoxic response starts with the recognition and binding of the effector cell to its target followed by conjugate formation and lysis of target cells and finally recycling of the effector cell takes place to start another cycle of target lysis. Fas-FasL interaction and induction of programmed cell death in the target cells as well as the release of cytolytic molecules like perforins, granzymes etc. are the two important cytocidal mechanisms employed by cytotoxic T cell (Dupuis et al. 1993, Masson and Tschopp 1987, Tschopp and Nabholz 1990, Young and Cohn 1987). These molecules, expressed/released by the effector cell, are employed onto the target cell at the site of contact (Berke 1994). However, perforins are the major component of cytolytic granules which are essential for the initiation of target cell lysis (Podack, Young and Cohn 1987). In a conclusive manner, a study showed an increase in the number of perforin expressing cytolytic cells in the elderly. However, they had a diminished lytic response towards infection (Mariani et al. 1996). Further studies are required to corroborate these findings.

13. Failure of Activation in Aged T Cells

Several age-related defects have been reported which affect the T cell activation. One of the defect is decreased expression of lymphocyte adhesion molecules which participate in T cell/APC interaction (Powers, Morley, and Flood 1992). Therefore, T cells show reduced ability to form a strong and functional immunological synapse with APCs upon stimulation with antigen. As a consequence, the initial signaling cascade generated in aged T cells is less intense than that of young. Moreover, activation of T cell requires a primary signal by TCR-MHC interaction (TCR) and secondary signal by costimulatory molecules like CD28, ICOS etc. As we discussed earlier, the expression of CD28 molecule declines with age and expression of CD28 ligands (CD80/CD86) is also altered on APCs. The decline in CD28 expression may be one of the reasons for impaired T cell activation in the elderly. Other negative costimulatory molecules like CTLA-4 are shown to be upregulated in aged individuals after activation (Linsley and Golstein 1996). Efficient T cell activation depends on both the co-stimulation and the durability of immunological synapse led by TCR-MHC complex (Williams and Bevan 2007). The effect of ageing on TCR signaling is so broad that most of the TCR mediated signaling pathways including calcium mobilization, protein tyrosine phosphorylation, translocation of PKC to plasma membrane (Larbi et al. 2004, Pahlavani 1998), activity of transcription factors particularly NF-κB and NF-AT gets altered at certain point (Fulop et al. 2012). As a part of the regulatory signaling pathway, Lck pathway has been found crucial in controlling T cell signaling (Acuto, Di Bartolo, and Michel 2008). Lck activity is controlled by two-point phosphorylation at Tyr394 and Tyr505 which stabilizes open and closed conformations respectively leading to increased and decreased kinase activities respectively. Failure of any of the events could diminish the functionality of Lck and their phosphorylated state is said to determine the enzymatic activity of Lck in T cells (Brownlie and Zamoyska 2013). However, in elderly, phosphorylation at both residues have been observed, but it does not indicate the impaired activation of T cells. Other finding prioritizes the availability of active Lck locally over their phosphorylated state (Garcia and Miller 2009). Similarly, ZAP-70, an important downstream molecule of TCR signaling, needs to be investigated for failure of T cell activation. In activated T cells from elderly, phosphorylation of ZAP-70 has been decreased. Accordingly, the level of IL-2 release in elderly is also decreased as compared to their young counterpart (Thoman and Weigle 1981).

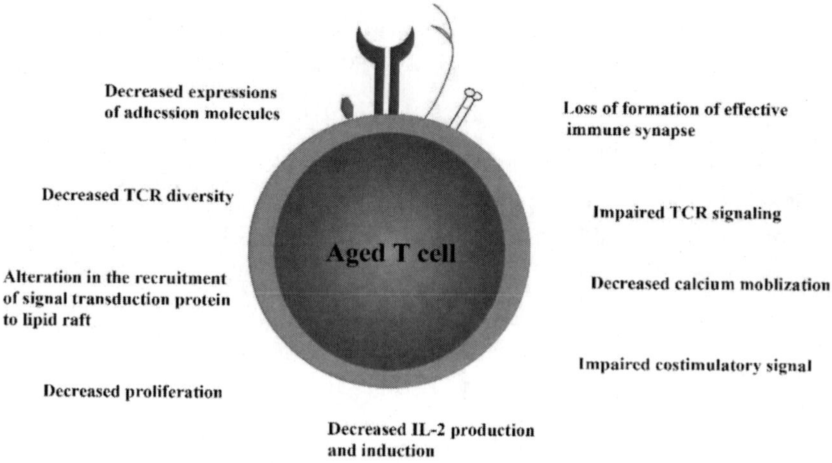

Figure 6. Impaired functions of aged T cell. Ageing is a multifactorial and multifaceted phenomenon. Various features and functions of T cells are compromised. Many of these functions are schematically represented here.

14. OUTCOME OF IMPAIRED T CELL ACTIVATION IN AGED T CELLS

14.1. Immune Response to Vaccine

Vaccination in the elderly could be one of the most paramount ways to restore immune response to a pathogen. However, the role and efficacy of vaccination in the elderly are poorly understood and often doubtful. In aged individual, a decline in the innate and adaptive immunity results in dramatically reduced vaccine response and efficacy. Neutrophils and macrophage show reduced phagocytic activity in the elderly person. In addition, expression of MHC class II is impaired in old macrophage. Phagocytic cells recognize pathogen via toll-like receptor (TLRs), TLRs signaling activate an efficient innate immune response (Van Duin and Shaw 2007). Defect in the expression of TLRs have been shown in macrophage of elderly person, suggesting poor innate immune response as well (Renshaw et al. 2002). Expressions of MHC class 1 and II and thus antigen presentation are reduced in dendritic cells from old mice (Grewe 2001). This age-related impairments of innate immune response can decrease uptake of antigen at the site of infection resulting from reduced phagocytosis. The decreased number of naive T cells in aged persons is accompanied by the accumulation of highly differentiated effector T cells. These differentiated effector T cells have short telomeres; possess highly restricted T cell receptor repertoire; shows impaired capacity to migrate to lymph nodes; display decreased ability to be stimulated by APCs and loss of the costimulatory molecules CD28 and CD27 on their surface (Appay et al. 2002). Summarily, these effector cells represent exhausted, but not unresponsive cells. To support our argument, $CD28^-$ effector T cells also produce high amounts of the pro-inflammatory cytokine IFN-γ, which contributes to a pro-inflammatory background typical of old age (Almanzar et al. 2004), supporting the development and progression of age-related diseases (i.e., osteoporosis, atherosclerosis, and neuro-degeneration). The question arises whether this pro-inflammatory milieu mounts sufficient immune response; then answer seems to be no. The accumulation of $CD28^-$ effector T cells has also been shown to be correlated with impaired humoral responses to influenza vaccination (i.e., seemingly unresponsiveness) (Goronzy et al. 2001).

It is suggested that memory T cells have characteristics of replicative senescence in aged individual. This age-related decline in immune regulation potentiates the risk of other infection in aged individuals and leads to a phase of compromised vaccination response. In spite of this diminished response vaccination could provide effective protection against diseases like influenza (McElhaney 2003). Moreover, influenza vaccination has been proven to be effective in preventing other complications like pneumonia and other cardiovascular diseases in the elderly (Meyers 2003). Several pharmacoeconomic studies have highlighted the benefit of influenza vaccines in terms of socio-economic status of the participants linked to reduced morbidity and mortality. Moreover, failure of vaccination is associated with mortality due to additional infections and its complications. Live attenuated vaccination in case of Herpes zoster infection in older age group and conjugated pneumococcal vaccine in subjects ≥75-year-old have been found to be efficient at a significant level. In addition to conventional vaccines virosomal vaccines, DNA vaccine, high dose vaccine and adjuvanted vaccines are under consideration for providing more effective immune protection in elderly. Adjuvanted influenza vaccine has shown to produce the more effective and strong serological response in the elderly as compared to conventional ones (Del Giudice et al. 2006).

14.2. Compromised Response to Infections

A compromised state of the immune system in the elderly could affect the severity and susceptibility of late stage infections. Reports have suggested that the aged individuals are more prone to infection from respiratory pathogen and gram-negative bacteria (Myerowitz, Medeiros, and O'Brien 1971, Phair, Kauffman, and Bjornson 1978) as compared to young. The reason could be the increased presence of pharyngeal gram-negative bacilli and *Staphylococcus aureus* with age. Older individuals are often reported with a wide range of infections including tuberculosis, salmonellosis, hepatitis, bacterial endocarditis and meningitis due to *Streptococcus pneumonia* as compared to their young counterparts. The occurrence of asymptomatic bacteremia and bacteriuria increases steadily with age. The mortality due to bacteremia rises progressively in people of age older than 40 years. Similarly, a high frequency of bacteriuria in elderly females leads to acute urinary tract infection. Besides this, skin and mucosal infections are also common and spread more rapidly in aged individuals (Bendall 1984). Mortality in the older age group along with the reactivation of latent infection has been increased in recent years.

14.3. Occurrence of Solid Tumors and Hematological Malignancies

Cellular senescence is one of the prominent characteristics achieved by the ageing cell. Senescence has shown to produce anticancer effect by inhibiting the proliferation of cancer cells and limiting the expression of oncogenes (Coppé et al. 2010). However, senescent cells can produce tumor promoting effect as they still have the ability to secrete proliferative cytokines and growth factor known as senescence associated secretory phenotype (SASPs) (Aunan et al. 2016, Falandry et al. 2014). Accumulation of these cells is also evident in the elderly (Aunan et al. 2016). Similarly, confounding results in the progression of the tumor in old individuals have also been produced by researchers. The rate of tumor growth and metastasis in older animals under experimental conditions is found to be slow. Contrary to that, certain tumors like 3-methylcholan-threne-induced fibrosarcomas and UV -induced sarcomas grow more rapidly in the elderly as compared to young animals (Flood et al. 1981, Urban and Schreiber 1984).

Besides the higher occurrence of the solid tumor, the majority of myeloid and lymphoid malignancies are also widely noted in patients of age for more than 70 years. The precursor B-cell and T-cell lymphoblastic leukemia tend to occur at a very early age (~1-14 years). However, in adulthood, most acute myeloid malignancy subtypes increase with advanced age (>70 years) (Dores et al. 2012). Besides this, the total number of lymphoid neoplasms increases unilaterally with age in all ethnic and sex subgroups. For instance, occurrence of Burkitt lymphoma/ leukemia and mixed cellularity/lymphocyte-depleted Hodgkin lymphoma increase more gradually with age (Dores et al. 2012, Smith et al. 2011). As shown in other studies, B-cell and T-cell lymphoblastic lymphoma/ leukemia are diagnosed predominantly in children. Moreover, nodular lymphocyte-predominant Hodgkin lymphomas were diagnosed predominantly in persons aged 15–34 and 15–64 years, respectively (Morton et al. 2006).

15. Approaches to Overcome The Failed T Cell Activation in Aged T Cells

Restoration of T cell activation is somehow possible if the stimulatory function of various cytokines and other immune molecules is restored either by genetic means or by implicating these externally. Evidence suggest that if we treat spleen cells in culture with mitogens and recombinant cytokines, cytokine production is enhanced as compared to mitogen only treatment (Frasca et al. 1997). This conclusion applies to IL 2 and IFN-γ production as protein and mRNA. Enhanced production of IL-2 upon addition of recombinant IL-12 and IL-4 is well documented (Frasca et al. 1997). Similarly, IL-4 can also induce amplification in Th2 cells leading towards increased release of IL-6. IL-6 works as a multidirectional cytokine as its effect on lymphocytes and accessory cells are wide. IL-6 release also activates macrophages followed by the release of cytokines like IL-12 and IL-1 involved in Th1 cell maturation and differentiation in a bidirectional manner (Rincón et al. 1997). This bidirectional control of Th1 cell activity by IL-6 could possibly explain the Th1 to Th2 shift in aged individuals with the increase of IL-6 production in the elderly. Another report suggests that IL-2 specific mRNA in spleen cells of older mice is effectively up regulated but with a lesser extent upon recombinant cytokine treatment as compared to young questioning the role of impaired posttranscriptional machinery in ageing. Also when CD4+ cells are activated with anti –CD3 and anti-CD28 mAbs they show an increase in the half-life of produced IL-2 specific mRNA. Cytokine dependent increase in the production of IFN-γ- specific mRNA and IFN-γ protein follows almost the similar pattern as IL-2 except at posttranscriptional level (Frasca et al. 1997). In case of IL-4 it has been found that production of this Th2 type cytokine can be enhanced with the help of recombinant cytokine in older individuals however, a difference at posttranscriptional regulatory phase has also been noted suggesting alterations in translational kinetics (Frasca et al. 1997) These findings altogether provides an insight towards the use of recombinant cytokines as immunomodulators in clinical practices.

Genetic remodeling of immune components could possibly have a favorable effect on immune response restoration. Genetic modification could drive the immune response in a positive direction. An evidence for the same shows the presence of viral IL-10 moiety in CMV and EBV which contributes to the immunological remodeling in the case of CMV infection (Kotenko et al. 2000). In a kind of study using Gene therapeutic approach targeted disruption of STAT6 has shown to deregulate IL-4 driven Th2 response (Wang et al. 2000). Even after losing the activity of IL-2 secretion T cells retains the capability to secrete other cytokines like GM-CSF in response to antigen stimulation via TCR however these semi functional T cells do not respond to GM-CSF a cytokine crucial in cell proliferation. In vitro studies where T cell transduced with chimeric GM-CSF/IL-R gene have shown to respond well to GM-CSF in the absence of exogenous cytokines (Evans et al. 1999). This can be considered as a crucial milestone in T cell function restoration in elderly because even young T cells need exogenous factors for proliferation as they lack sufficient autocrine function (Barton-Davis et al. 1998).

Chronic low-grade inflammation with age promotes expansion of suppressive myeloid cells followed by diminished T-cell activity; as a result, T-cells with marginal anti-tumor activity grow and outnumber the other cells. Targeting innate immune cells including macrophages, dendritic cells and other myeloid lineage suppressor cells can be of potential benefit in the elderly. APCs including DC and Macrophage show a promising candidature to fight against cancer in aged individuals. The level of circulating dysfunctional DC increases in tumor environment (Curiel et al. 2003) as well as circulating DC precursor also decreases with ageing which could hamper anti-tumor response. This age related decline in DC activity could contribute to the cancer risk in the elderly.

Augmenting the antigen presenting function of DC by boosting CD40L activity in elderly cancer patients have shown promising results (Tang et al. 2009). Myelopoeisis increases with age as contrary to reduced lymphopoiesis (Geiger and Rudolph 2009). Tumor associated macrophages have been found to produce increased level of suppressive cytokine TGF-β as correlated with M2 phenotype thus promoting pro-tumorigenic environment (Watkins et al. 2007) IL-12 driven conversion of M2 type mφ to M1 typemφ creates an anti-tumor inflammatory environment in aged cancer patients. Apart from innate cells, targeting other immune regulatory molecules like PD-L1, PD-1, mTOR, CTLA-4 etc could possibly restore the skewed immune balance in elderly.

REFERENCES

Acuto, Oreste, Vincenzo Di Bartolo, and Frédérique Michel. 2008. "Tailoring T-cell receptor signals by proximal negative feedback mechanisms." *Nature Reviews Immunology* 8 (9):699.

Almanzar, Giovanni, Susanne Schwaiger, Brigitte Jenewein, Michael Keller, Beatrix Grubeck-Loebenstein, Reinhard WüRZNER, and Dietmar Schönitzer. 2004. "IFN-gamma production by CMV-specific CD8+ T cells is high in elderly donors." *Experimental gerontology* 39 (5):863.

Antikainen, Henri, Monica Driscoll, Gal Haspel, and Radek Dobrowolski. 2017. "TOR-mediated regulation of metabolism in aging." *Aging cell* 16 (6):1219-1233.

Appay, Victor, P Rod Dunbar, Margaret Callan, Paul Klenerman, Geraldine MA Gillespie, Laura Papagno, Graham S Ogg, Abigail King, Franziska Lechner, and Celsa A Spina. 2002. "Memory CD8+ T cells vary in differentiation phenotype in different persistent virus infections." *Nature medicine* 8 (4):379.

Aunan, JR, MM Watson, HR Hagland, and K Søreide. 2016. "Molecular and biological hallmarks of ageing." *British Journal of Surgery* 103 (2):e29-e46.

Bachmann, Martin F, and Annette Oxenius. 2007. "Interleukin 2: from immunostimulation to immunoregulation and back again." *EMBO reports* 8 (12):1142-1148.

Balagopalan, Lakshmi, Robert L Kortum, Nathan P Coussens, Valarie A Barr, and Lawrence E Samelson. 2015. "The linker for activation of T cells (LAT) signaling hub: from signaling complexes to micro-clusters." *Journal of Biological Chemistry* 290 (44):26422-26429.

Barton-Davis, Elisabeth R, Daria I Shoturma, Antonio Musaro, Nadia Rosenthal, and H Lee Sweeney. 1998. "Viral mediated expression of insulin-like growth factor I blocks the aging-related loss of skeletal muscle function." *Proceedings of the national academy of sciences* 95 (26):15603-15607.

Bauer, Birgit, and Gottfried Baier. 2002. "Protein kinase C and AKT/protein kinase B in CD4+ T-lymphocytes: new partners in TCR/CD28 signal integration." *Molecular immunology* 38 (15):1087-1099.

Bendall, MJ. 1984. "A review of urinary tract infection in the elderly." *Journal of Antimicrobial Chemotherapy* 13 (suppl_B):69-78.

Berke, G. 1994. "The binding and lysis of target cells by cytotoxic lymphocytes: molecular and cellular aspects." *Annual review of immunology* 12 (1):735-773.

Bernstein, Erica D, and Donna M Murasko. 1998. "Effect of age on cytokine production in humans." *Age* 21 (4):137-151.

Berridge, Michael J. 1997. "The AM and FM of calcium signalling." *Nature* 386:759-760.

Brownlie, Rebecca J, and Rose Zamoyska. 2013. "T cell receptor signalling networks: branched, diversified and bounded." *Nature Reviews Immunology* 13 (4):257.

Busse, Stefan, Johann Steiner, Juliane Alter, Henrik Dobrowolny, Christian Mawrin, Bernhard Bogerts, Roland Hartig, and Mandy Busse. 2015. "Expression of HLA-DR, CD80, and CD86 in healthy aging and Alzheimer's disease." *Journal of Alzheimer's Disease* 47 (1):177-184.

Callahan, Jill E, John W Kappler, and Philippa Marrack. 1993. "Unexpected expansions of CD8-bearing cells in old mice." *The Journal of Immunology* 151 (12):6657-6669.

Canaday, David H, Karen E Parker, Htin Aung, Hui Emily Chen, Dariana Nunez-Medina, and Christopher J Burant. 2013. "Age-dependent changes in the expression of regulatory cell surface ligands in activated human T-cells." *BMC immunology* 14 (1):45.

Carrieri, Giuseppina, Erika Marzi, Fabiola Olivieri, Francesca Marchegiani, Luca Cavallone, Maurizio Cardelli, Simona Giovagnetti, Rosalia Stecconi, Cinzia Molendini, and Chiara Trapassi. 2004. "The G/C915 polymorphism of transforming growth factor β1 is associated with human longevity: a study in Italian centenarians." *Aging cell* 3 (6):443-448.

Carter, Laura L, and Beatriz M Carreno. 2003. "Cytotoxic T-lymphocyte antigen-4 and programmed death-1 function as negative regulators of lymphocyte activation." *Immunologic research* 28 (1):49-59.

Coffman, Frederick D, and Stanley Cohen. 1989. "Aging and deffective lymphoid cell activation." *Experimental gerontology* 24 (5-6):437-449.

Commins, Scott, John W Steinke, and Larry Borish. 2008. "The extended IL-10 superfamily: IL-10, IL-19, IL-20, IL-22, IL-24, IL-26, IL-28, and IL-29." *Journal of Allergy and Clinical Immunology* 121 (5):1108-1111.

Coppé, Jean-Philippe, Pierre-Yves Desprez, Ana Krtolica, and Judith Campisi. 2010. "The senescence-associated secretory phenotype: the dark side of tumor suppression." *Annual Review of Pathological Mechanical Disease* 5:99-118.

Cossarizza, Andrea, Claudio Ortolani, Daniela Monti, and Claudio Franceschi. 1997. "Cytometric analysis of immunosenescence." *Cytometry: The Journal of the International Society for Analytical Cytology* 27 (4):297-313.

Cristofalo, Vincent J, and Robert J Pignolo. 1993. "Replicative senescence of human fibroblast-like cells in culture." *Physiological reviews* 73 (3):617-638.

Curiel, Tyler J, Shuang Wei, Haidong Dong, Xavier Alvarez, Pui Cheng, Peter Mottram, Roman Krzysiek, Keith L Knutson, Ben Daniel, and Maria Carla Zimmermann. 2003. "Blockade of B7-H1 improves myeloid dendritic cell–mediated antitumor immunity." *Nature medicine* 9 (5):562.

de Boland, Ana R, Maria M Facchinetti, Gabriela Balogh, Virginia Massheimer, and Ricardo L Boland. 1996. "Age-associated decrease in inositol 1, 4, 5-triphosphate and diacylglycerol generation by 1, 25 (OH) 2-vitamin D3 in rat intestine." *Cellular signalling* 8 (3):153-157.

De Grey, Aubrey DNJ. 2007. "Life span extension research and public debate: societal considerations." *Studies in Ethics, Law, and Technology* 1 (1).

Del Giudice, Giuseppe, Anne Katrin Hilbert, Roberto Bugarini, Ada Minutello, Olga Popova, Daniela Toneatto, Ines Schoendorf, Astrid Borkowski, Rino Rappuoli, and Audino Podda. 2006. "An MF59-adjuvanted inactivated influenza vaccine containing A/Panama/1999 (H3N2) induced broader serological protection against heterovariant influenza virus strain A/Fujian/2002 than a subunit and a split influenza vaccine." *Vaccine* 24 (16):3063-3065.

Dores, Graça M, Susan S Devesa, Rochelle E Curtis, Martha S Linet, and Lindsay M Morton. 2012. "Acute leukemia incidence and patient survival among children and adults in the United States, 2001-2007." *Blood* 119 (1):34-43.

Dupuis, Marc, E Schaerer, Karl-Heinz Krause, and J Tschopp. 1993. "The calcium-binding protein calreticulin is a major constituent of lytic granules in cytolytic T lymphocytes." *Journal of Experimental Medicine* 177 (1):1-7.

Dustin, Michael L, Arup K Chakraborty, and Andrey S Shaw. 2010. "Understanding the structure and function of the immunological synapse." *Cold Spring Harbor perspectives in biology* 2 (10):a002311.

Eaton, Sheri M, Eve M Burns, Kimberly Kusser, Troy D Randall, and Laura Haynes. 2004. "Age-related defects in CD4 T cell cognate helper function lead to reductions in humoral responses." *Journal of Experimental Medicine* 200 (12):1613-1622.

Ecological global network 2019. "world birth and death rates." accessed October 24. https://www.ecology.com/birth-death-rates/.

Effros, Rita B. 1996. "Insights on immunological aging derived from the T lymphocyte cellular senescence model." *Experimental gerontology* 31 (1-2):21-27.

Ershler, WB. 1993. "Interleukin-6: a cytokine for gerontologists." *Journal of the American Geriatrics Society* 41 (2):176-181.

Esensten, Jonathan H, Ynes A Helou, Gaurav Chopra, Arthur Weiss, and Jeffrey A Bluestone. 2016. "CD28 costimulation: from mechanism to therapy." *Immunity* 44 (5):973-988.

Evans, Lawrence S, Pamela R Witte, Andrew L Feldhaus, Brad H Nelson, Stanley R Riddell, Philip D Greenberg, Stephen D Lupton, and Lori A Jones. 1999. "Expression of chimeric granulocyte-macrophage colony-stimulating factor/interleukin 2 receptors in human cytotoxic T lymphocyte clones results in granulocyte-macrophage colony-stimulating factor-dependent growth." *Human gene therapy* 10 (12):1941-1951.

Falandry, Claire, Marc Bonnefoy, Gilles Freyer, and Eric Gilson. 2014. "Biology of cancer and aging: a complex association with cellular senescence." *Journal of Clinical Oncology* 32 (24):2604-2610.

Fallah, Mosoka P, R Lakshman Chelvarajan, Beth A Garvy, and Subbarao Bondada. 2011. "Role of phosphoinositide 3-kinase–Akt signaling pathway in the age-related cytokine dysregulation in splenic macrophages stimulated via TLR-2 or TLR-4 receptors." *Mechanisms of ageing and development* 132 (6-7):274-286.

Flood, Patrick M., Urban, James L., Kripke, Margaret L., and Schreiber, Hans. 1981. "Loss of tumor-specific and idiotype-specific immunity with age." *Journal of Experimental Medicine* 154 (2):275-290.

Fooksman, David R., Vardhana, Santosh, Vasiliver-Shamis, Gaia, Liese, Jan, Blair, David A., Waite, Janelle, Sacristán, Catarina, Victora, Gabriel D., Zanin-Zhorov, Alexandra and Dustin, Michael L. 2009. "Functional anatomy of T cell activation and synapse formation." *Annual review of immunology* 28:79-105.

Franceschi, Claudio. 1989. "Cell proliferation, cell death and aging." *Aging Clinical and Experimental Research* 1 (1):3-15.

Franceschi, Claudio, Bonafè, Massimiliano, Valensin, Silvana, Olivieri, Fabiola, Luca, Maria De, Ottaviani, Enzo and Benedictis, Giovanna De. 2000. "Inflamm-aging: an evolutionary perspective on immune-senescence." *Annals of the New York Academy of Sciences* 908 (1): 244-254.

Frasca, Daniela, Pucci, Sabina, Goso, Cristina, Barattini, Paola, Barile, Simona, Pioli, Claudio and Doria, Gino. 1997. "Regulation of cytokine production in aging: use of recombinant cytokines to upregulate mitogen-stimulated spleen cells." *Mechanisms of ageing and development* 93 (1-3):157-169.

Fruman, David A. 2004. "Phosphoinositide 3-kinase and its targets in B-cell and T-cell signaling." *Current opinion in immunology* 16 (3):314-320.

Fulop, Tamas, Page, Aurélie Le, Garneau, Hugo, Azimi, Naheed, Baehl, Sarra, Dupuis, Gilles, Pawelec, Graham and Larbi, Anis. 2012. "Aging, immunosenescence and membrane rafts: the lipid connection." *Longevity & healthspan* 1 (1):6.

Gaffen, Sarah L. 2009. "The role of interleukin-17 in the pathogenesis of rheumatoid arthritis." *Current rheumatology reports* 11 (5):365.

Gallucci, Stefania, and Matzinger, Polly. 2001. "Danger signals: SOS to the immune system." *Current opinion in immunology* 13 (1):114-119.

Garcia, Gonzalo G., and Miller, Richard A. 1997. "Differential tyrosine phosphorylation of zeta chain dimers in mouse CD4 T lymphocytes: effect of age." *Cellular immunology* 175 (1):51-57.

Garcia, Gonzalo G., and Miller, Richard A. 2002. "Age-dependent defects in TCR-triggered cytoskeletal rearrangement in CD4+ T cells." *The Journal of Immunology* 169 (9):5021-5027.

Garcia, Gonzalo G., and Miller, Richard A. 2009. "Age-related changes in lck–Vav signaling pathways in mouse CD4 T cells." *Cellular immunology* 259 (1):100-104.

Gardner, Ian D. 1980. "The effect of aging on susceptibility to infection." *Reviews of infectious diseases* 2 (5):801-810.

Gaugler, Megan, Brown, Alicia, Merrell, Erin, DiSanto-Rose, Maria, Rathmacher, John A., and Reynolds, Thomas H., 4th. 2011. "PKB signaling and atrogene expression in skeletal muscle of aged mice." *Journal of Applied Physiology* 111 (1):192-199.

Geiger, Hartmut, and Rudolph, K. Lenhard. 2009. "Aging in the lympho-hematopoietic stem cell compartment." *Trends in immunology* 30 (7):360-365.

Gorentla, Balachandra K., and Zhong, Xiao-Ping. 2012. "T cell receptor signal transduction in T lymphocytes." *Journal of clinical & cellular immunology* 2012 (Suppl 12):005.

Gorgas, Gayle, Butch, Elizabeth R., Guan, Kun-Liang, and Miller, Richard A. 1997. "Diminished activation of the MAP kinase pathway in CD3-stimulated T lymphocytes from old mice." *Mechanisms of ageing and development* 94 (1-3):71-83.

Goronzy, Jörg J., Fulbright, James W, Crowson, Cynthia S., Poland, Gregory A., O'Fallon, William M and Weyand, Cornelia M. 2001. "Value of immunological markers in predicting responsiveness to influenza vaccination in elderly individuals." *Journal of virology* 75 (24):12182-12187.

Grewe, M. 2001. "Chronological ageing and photoageing of dendritic cells." *Clinical and experimental dermatology* 26 (7):608-612.

Hara, Hideki, Tanaka, Toshio, Negoro, Shigeru, Deguchi, Yasuhiro, Nishio, Shinichi, Saiki, Osamu, and Kishimoto, Susumu. 1988. "Age-related changes of expression of IL-2 receptor subunits and kinetics of IL-2 internalization in T cells after mitogenic stimulation." *Mechanisms of ageing and development* 45 (2):167-175.

Haynes, Laura, Eaton, Sheri M., Burns, Eve M., Randall, Troy D., and Swain, Susan L. 2003. "CD4 T cell memory derived from young naive cells functions well into old age, but memory generated from aged naive cells functions poorly." *Proceedings of the National Academy of Sciences* 100 (25):15053-15058.

Haynes, Laura, Linton, Phyllis-Jean, Eaton, Sheri M., Tonkonogy, Susan L., and Swain, Susan L. 1999. "Interleukin 2, but not other common γ chain–binding cytokines, can reverse the defect in generation of CD4 effector T cells from naive T cells of aged mice." *Journal of Experimental Medicine* 190 (7):1013-1024.

Heissmeyer, Vigo, Macián, Fernando, Im, Sin-Hyeog, Varma, Rajat, Feske, Stefan, Venuprasad, K., Gu, Hua, Liu, Yun-Cai, Dustin, Michael L., and Rao, Anjana. 2004. "Calcineurin imposes T cell unresponsiveness through targeted proteolysis of signaling proteins." *Nature immunology* 5 (3):255.

Hogan, Patrick G., Chen, Lin, Nardone, Julie and Rao, Anjana. 2003. "Transcriptional regulation by calcium, calcineurin, and NFAT." *Genes & development* 17 (18):2205-2232.

Huang, Mei-Chuan, Liao, Jia-Jun, Bonasera, Stephen, Longo, Dan L., and Goetzl, Edward J. 2008. "Nuclear factor-κB-dependent reversal of aging-induced alterations in T cell cytokines." *The FASEB Journal* 22 (7):2142-2150.

Jago, C. B., Yates, J., Câmara, N Olsen Saraiva, Lechler, RI and Lombardi, G. 2004. "Differential expression of CTLA-4 among T cell subsets." *Clinical & Experimental Immunology* 136 (3):463-471.

Janick-Buckner, D., Briggs, CJ., Meyer, TE., Harvey, N., and Warner, CM. 1991. "Major histocompatibility complex antigen expression on lymphocytes from aging strain A mice." *Growth, development, and aging: GDA* 55 (1):53-62.

Johnson, Gary L, Dohlman, Henrik G and Graves, Lee M. 2005. "MAPK kinase kinases (MKKKs) as a target class for small-molecule inhibition to modulate signaling networks and gene expression." *Current opinion in chemical biology* 9 (3):325-331.

Kämmerer, R, Iten, A., Frei, P. C., and Bürgisser, P. 1996. "Expansion of T cells negative for CD28 expression in HIV infection. Relation to activation markers and cell adhesion molecules, and correlation with prognostic markers." *Medical microbiology and immunology* 185 (1):19-25.

Kanda, H, Mimura, K Hamasaki T., Yamamoto, K., Yazaki,Y., Hirai, H, and Nojima, Y. 1999. "Fyn and Lck tyrosine kinases regulate tyrosine phosphorylation of p105CasL, a member of the p130Cas docking protein family, in T-cell receptor-mediated signalling." *Immunology* 97 (1):56.

Kanno, Jun, Wakikawa, Atsuko, Utsuyama, Masanori and Hirokawa, Katsuiku. 1997. "Effect of restraint stress on immune system and experimental B16 melanoma metastasis in aged mice." *Mechanisms of ageing and development* 93 (1-3):107-117.

Koch, Ute, and Radtke, Freddy. 2011. "Mechanisms of T cell development and transformation." *Annual review of cell and developmental biology* 27:539-562.

Koretzky, Gary A. 2003. "T cell activation I: proximal events." *Immunological reviews* 191:5.

Kotenko, Sergei V., Saccani, Simona, Izotova, Lara S., Mirochnitchenko, Olga V., and Pestka, Sidney. 2000. "Human cytomegalovirus harbors its own unique IL-10 homolog (cmvIL-10)." *Proceedings of the National Academy of Sciences* 97 (4):1695-1700.

Krebs, Danielle L, and Hilton, Douglas J. 2001. "SOCS proteins: negative regulators of cytokine signaling." *Stem cells* 19 (5):378-387.

Krieglstein, K, Miyazono, K., Dijke, P Ten and Unsicker, K. 2012. TGF-β in aging and disease. Springer.

Krogsgaard, Michelle, and Davis, Mark M. 2005. "How T cells' see'antigen." *Nature immunology* 6 (3):239.

Lages, Celine S, Lewkowich, Ian, Sproles, Alyssa, Wills-Karp, Marsha and Chougnet, Claire. 2010. "Partial restoration of T-cell function in aged mice by in vitro blockade of the PD-1/PD-L1 pathway." *Aging cell* 9 (5):785-798.

Lages, Celine S, Suffia, Isabelle, Vclilla, Paula A., Huang, Bin, Warshaw, Gregg, Hildeman, David A., Belkaid, Yasmin and Chougnet, Claire. 2008. "Functional regulatory T cells accumulate in aged hosts and promote chronic infectious disease reactivation." *The Journal of Immunology* 181 (3):1835-1848.

Larbi, Anis, Douziech, Nadine, Dupuis, Gilles, Khalil, Abdelouahed, Pelletier, Hugues, Guerard, Karl-Philippe and Fülöp Jr., Tamàs. 2004. "Age-associated alterations in the recruitment of signal-transduction proteins to lipid rafts in human T lymphocytes." *Journal of leukocyte biology* 75 (2):373-381.

Lee, Jin Soo, Lee, Won-Woo, Kim, Sang Hyun, Kang, Youna, Lee, Naeun, Shin, Min Sun, Kang, Seong Wook and Kang, Insoo. 2011. "Age-associated alteration in naive and memory Th17 cell response in humans." *Clinical Immunology* 140 (1):84-91.

Leng, Qibin, Bentwich, Zvi and Borkow, Gadi. 2002. "CTLA-4 upregulation during aging." *Mechanisms of ageing and development* 123 (10):1419-1421.

Lever, Melissa, Maini, Philip K., Merwe, P Anton Van Der and Dushek, Omer. 2014. "Phenotypic models of T cell activation." *Nature Reviews Immunology* 14 (9):619.

Linsley, Peter S, and Golstein, Pierre. 1996. "Lymphocyte activation: T-cell regulation by CTLA-4." *Current Biology* 6 (4):398-400.

Liu, B, Carle, KW and Whisler, RL. 1997. "Reductions in the activation of ERK and JNK are associated with decreased IL-2 production in T cells from elderly humans stimulated by the TCR/CD3 complex and costimulatory signals." *Cellular immunology* 182 (2):79-88.

Lord, Janet M. 2013. "The effect of aging of the immune system on vaccination responses." *Human vaccines & immunotherapeutics* 9 (6):1364-1367.

Mariani, E, Roda, P., Mariani, AR., Vitale, M., Degrassi, A., Papa, S and Facchini, A. 1990. "Age-associated changes in CD8+ and CD16+ cell reactivity: clonal analysis." *Clinical & Experimental Immunology* 81 (3):479-484.

Mariani, Erminia, Sgobbi, Silvia, Meneghetti, Alessandra, Tadolini, Manuela, Tarozzi, Andrea, Sinoppi, Marco, Cattini, Luca and Facchini, Andrea. 1996. "Perforins in human cytolytic cells: the effect of age." *Mechanisms of ageing and development* 92 (2-3):195-209.

Marko, Melissa G., Ahmed, Tanvir, Bunnell, Stephen C., Wu, Dayong, Chung, Heekyung, Huber, Brigitte T., and Meydani, Simin Nikbin. 2007. "Age-associated decline in effective immune synapse formation of CD4+ T cells is reversed by vitamin E supplementation." *The Journal of Immunology* 178 (3):1443-1449.

Masson, Danièle, and Tschopp, Jürg. 1987. "A family of serine esterases in lytic granules of cytolytic T lymphocytes." *Cell* 49 (5):679-685.

Matsuda, S, and Koyasu, S. 2002. "Function of MAPK signaling pathways in the immune system." *Tanpakushitsu kakusan koso. Protein, nucleic acid, enzyme* 47 (11):1368-1378.

Maue, Alexander C, Eaton, Sheri M., Lanthier, Paula A., Sweet, Kathryn B., Blumerman, Seth L., and Haynes, Laura. 2009. "Proinflammatory adjuvants enhance the cognate helper activity of aged CD4 T cells." *The Journal of Immunology* 182 (10):6129-6135.

McElhaney, Janet E. 2003. "Overcoming the challenges of immunosenescence in the prevention of acute respiratory illness in older people." *Connecticut medicine* 67 (8):469-474.

Messaoudi, Ilhem, LeMaoult, Joël, Guevara-Patino, Jose A., Metzner, Beatrix M., and Nikolich-Žugich, Janko. 2004. "Age-related CD8 T cell clonal expansions constrict CD8 T cell repertoire and have the potential to impair immune defense." *Journal of Experimental Medicine* 200 (10):1347-1358.

Meyers, David G. 2003. "Could influenza vaccination prevent myocardial infarction, stroke and sudden cardiac death?" *American Journal of Cardiovascular Drugs* 3 (4):241-244.

Miller, Richard A, Jacobson, Bruce, Weil, Gary and Simons, Elizabeth R. 1987. "Diminished calcium influx in lectin-stimulated T cells from old mice." *Journal of cellular physiology* 132 (2):337-342.

Morton, Lindsay M., Wang, Sophia S., Devesa, Susan S., Hartge, Patricia, Weisenburger, Dennis D., and Linet, Martha S. 2006. "Lymphoma incidence patterns by WHO subtype in the United States, 1992-2001." *Blood* 107 (1):265-276.

Myerowitz, Richard L, Medeiros, Antone A., and O'Brien, Thomas F. 1971. "Recent experience with bacillemia due to gram-negative organisms." *Journal of Infectious Diseases* 124 (3):239-246.

Myśliwska, Jolanta, Bryl, Ewa, Foerster, Jerzy and Myśliwski, Andrzej. 1998. "Increase of interleukin 6 and decrease of interleukin 2 production during the ageing process are influenced by the health status." *Mechanisms of ageing and development* 100 (3):313-328.

Nikolich-Žugich, Janko. 2008. "Ageing and life-long maintenance of T-cell subsets in the face of latent persistent infections." *Nature Reviews Immunology* 8 (7):512.

Nishioka, Tomohisa, Jun Shimizu, Ryuji Iida, Sayuri Yamazaki, and Shimon Sakaguchi. 2006. "CD4+ CD25+ Foxp3+ T cells and CD4+ CD25− Foxp3+ T cells in aged mice." *The Journal of Immunology* 176 (11):6586-6593.

Pahlavani, Mohammad A. 1998. "T cell signaling: effect of age." *Front Biosci* 3 (1):D1120-1133.

Pahlavani, Mohammad A, Harris, Melissa D and Richardson, Arlan. 1995. "The age-related decline in the induction of IL-2 transcription is correlated to changes in the transcription factor NFAT." *Cellular immunology* 165 (1):84-91.

Pawelec, Graham, Adibzadeh, Mahdi, Solana, Rafaek and Beckman, Ian. 1997. "The T cell in the ageing individual." *Mechanisms of ageing and development* 93 (1-3):35-45.

Phair, J. P., Kauffman, C. A., and Bjornson, A. 1978. "Investigation of host defense mechanisms in the aged as determinants of nosocomial colonization and pneumonia." *RES Journal of the Reticuloendothelial Society* 23 (5):397-405.

Plas, David R, and Craig B Thompson. 2005. "Akt-dependent transformation: there is more to growth than just surviving." *Oncogene* 24 (50):7435.

Podack, ER. "H. Hengartner, and M. G. Lichtenheld. 1991. A central role of perforin in cytolysis." *Annu. Rev. Immunol* 9:129.

Ponnappan, Subramaniam, and Ponnappan, Usha. 2011. "Aging and immune function: molecular mechanisms to interventions." *Antioxidants & redox signaling* 14 (8):1551-1585.

Posnett, David N, Sinha, Rakhi, Kabak, Shara and Russo, Carlo. 1994. "Clonal populations of T cells in normal elderly humans: the T cell equivalent to" benign monoclonal gammapathy."" *Journal of Experimental Medicine* 179 (2):609-618.

Powers, Douglas C, Morley, John E., and Flood, James F. 1992. "Age-related changes in LFA-1 expression, cell adhesion, and PHA-induced proliferation by lymphocytes from senescence-accelerated mouse (SAM)-P/8 and SAM-R/1 substrains." *Cellular immunology* 141 (2):444-456.

Proust, J. J., Filburn, C. R., Harrison, S. A., Buchholz, M. A., and Nordin, A. A. 1987. "Age-related defect in signal transduction during lectin activation of murine T lymphocytes." *The Journal of Immunology* 139 (5):1472-1478.

Puzianowska-Kuźnicka, Monika, Owczarz, Magdalena, Wieczorowska-Tobis, Katarzyna, Nadrowski, Pawel, Chudek, Jerzy, Slusarczyk, Przemyslaw, Skalska, Anna, Jonas, Marta, Franek, Edward, and Mossakowska, Malgorzata. 2016. "Interleukin-6 and C-reactive protein, successful aging, and mortality: the PolSenior study." *Immunity & Ageing* 13 (1):21.

Rao, Navin, Dodge, Ingrid and Band, Hamid. 2002. "The Cbl family of ubiquitin ligases: critical negative regulators of tyrosine kinase signaling in the immune system." *Journal of leukocyte biology* 71 (5): 753-763.

Raynor, Jana, Karns, Rebekah, Almanan, Maha, Li, Kun-Po, Divanovic, Senad, Chougnet, Claire A., and Hildeman, David A. 2015. "IL-6 and ICOS antagonize Bim and promote regulatory T cell accrual with age." *The Journal of Immunology* 195 (3):944-952.

Renshaw, Mary, Rockwell, Julie, Engleman, Carrie, Gewirtz, Andrew, Katz, Jacqueline and Sambhara, Suryaprakash. 2002. "Cutting edge: impaired Toll-like receptor expression and function in aging." *The Journal of Immunology* 169 (9):4697-4701.

Ridker, Paul M., Rifai, Nader, Stampfer, Meir J and Hennekens, Charles H. 2000. "Plasma concentration of interleukin-6 and the risk of future myocardial infarction among apparently healthy men." *Circulation* 101 (15):1767-1772.

Rincón, Mercedes, Anguita, Juan, Nakamura, Tetsuo, Fikrig, Erol and Flavell, Richard A. 1997. "Interleukin (IL)-6 directs the differentiation of IL-4–producing CD4+ T cells." *Journal of Experimental Medicine* 185 (3):461-470.

Rink, Lothar, Cakman, Irem and Kirchner, Holger. 1998. "Altered cytokine production in the elderly." *Mechanisms of ageing and development* 102 (2-3):199-209.

Robak, T, Gladalska, A., Stępień, H., and Robak, E. 1998. "Serum levels of interleukin-6 type cytokines and soluble interleukin-6 receptor in patients with rheumatoid arthritis." *Mediators of inflammation* 7 (5): 347-353.

Roman, Luis I, Luis Manzano, Hera,Antonio De La, Abreu, Luis, Rossi, Irma and Alvarez-Mon, Melchor. 1996. "Expanded CD4+ CD45RO+ phenotype and defective proliferative response in T lymphocytes from patients with Crohn's disease." *Gastroenterology* 110 (4):1008-1019.

Ross, Sarah H., and Cantrell, Doreen A. 2018. "Signaling and function of interleukin-2 in T lymphocytes." *Annual review of immunology* 36:41 1-433.

Rossi, E, Matutes, E., Morilla, R., Owusu-Ankomah, K., Heffernan, A. M, and Catovsky, D. 1996. "Zeta chain and CD28 are poorly expressed on T lymphocytes from chronic lymphocytic leukemia." *Leukemia* 10 (3):494-497.

Ruby, Carl E., and Weinberg, Andrew D. 2009. "OX40-enhanced tumor rejection and effector T cell differentiation decreases with age." *The Journal of Immunology* 182 (3):1481-1489.

Salam, Nasir, Rane, Sanket, Das, Rituparna, Faulkner, Matthew, Gund, Rupali, Kandpal, Usha, Lewis, Virginia, Mattoo, Hamid, Prabhu, Savit, and Ranganathan, Vidya. 2013. "T cell ageing: effects of age on development, survival & function." *The Indian journal of medical research* 138 (5):595.

Sansoni, P, Vescovini, R., Fagnoni, F., Biasini, C., Zanni, F., Zanlari, L., Telera, A., Lucchini, G., Passeri, G and Monti, D. 2008. "The immune system in extreme longevity." *Experimental gerontology* 43 (2):61-65.

Saurwein-Teissl, Maria, Lung, Thomas L., Marx, Florentine, Gschösser, Claudio, Asch, Esther, Blasko, Imrich, Parson, Walther, Böck, Günther, Schönitzer, Diether and Trannoy, Emanuelle. 2002. "Lack of antibody production following immunization in old age: association with CD8+ CD28− T cell clonal expansions and an imbalance in the production of Th1 and Th2 cytokines." *The Journal of Immunology* 168 (11):5893-5899.

Schmidt, Dorle, Goronzy, Jörg J., and Weyand, Cornelia M. 1996. "CD4+ CD7-CD28-T cells are expanded in rheumatoid arthritis and are characterized by autoreactivity." *The Journal of clinical investigation* 97 (9):2027-2037.

Sharma, Sanjay, Dominguez, Ana Lucia and Lustgarten, Joseph. 2006. "High accumulation of T regulatory cells prevents the activation of immune responses in aged animals." *The Journal of Immunology* 177 (12):8348-8355.

Shi, Li, Chen, Shaohua, Yang, Lijian and Li, Yangqiu. 2013. "The role of PD-1 and PD-L1 in T-cell immune suppression in patients with hematological malignancies." *Journal of hematology & oncology* 6 (1):74.

Sims, John E., and Smith, Dirk E. 2010. "The IL-1 family: regulators of immunity." *Nature Reviews Immunology* 10 (2):89.

Singer, Andrew L., and Koretzky, Gary A. 2002. "Control of T cell function by positive and negative regulators." *Science* 296 (5573): 1639-1640.

Smith, A, D Howell, Patmore, R., Jack, A and Roman, E. 2011. "Incidence of haematological malignancy by sub-type: a report from the Haematological Malignancy Research Network." *British journal of cancer* 105 (11):1684.

Song, Jianxun, Salek-Ardakani, Shahram, Rogers, Paul R., Cheng, Mary, Parijs, Luk Van and Croft, Michael. 2004. "The costimulation-regulated duration of PKB activation controls T cell longevity." *Nature immunology* 5 (2):150.

Tang, Yu Cheng, Thoman, Marilyn, Linton, Phyllis-Jean and Deisseroth, Albert. 2009. "Use of CD40L immunoconjugates to overcome the defective immune response to vaccines for infections and cancer in the aged." *Cancer Immunology, Immunotherapy* 58 (12):1949-1957.

Tesar, B. M., Asea, A., and Goldstein D. R. 2005. "Aging leads to impaired upregulation of ICOS in response to allostimulation." *The Journal of Heart and Lung Transplantation* 24 (2):S50.

Thoman, ML., and Weigle, W. O. 1981. "Lymphokines and aging: interleukin-2 production and activity in aged animals." *The Journal of Immunology* 127 (5):2102-2106.

Trebilcock, Gina Uken, and Ponnappan, Usha. 1996. "Evidence for lowered induction of nuclear factor kappa B in activated human T lymphocytes during aging." *Gerontology* 42 (3):137-146.

Tschopp, Jürg, and Nabholz, Markus. 1990. "Perforin-mediated target cell lysis by cytolytic T lymphocytes." *Annual review of immunology* 8 (1):279-302.

Tsukamoto, Hirotake, Clise-Dwyer, Karen, Huston, Gail E., Duso, Debra K., Buck, Amanda L., Johnson, Lawrence L., Haynes, Laura and Swain, Susan L. 2009. "Age-associated increase in lifespan of naive CD4 T cells contributes to T-cell homeostasis but facilitates development of functional defects." *Proceedings of the National Academy of Sciences* 106 (43):18333-18338.

Tybulewicz, Victor, L. J. 2005. "Vav-family proteins in T-cell signalling." *Current opinion in immunology* 17 (3):267-274.

Uhlik, Mark T, Abell, Amy N., Cuevas, Bruce D., Nakamura, Kazuhiro, and Johnson, Gary L. 2004. "Wiring diagrams of MAPK regulation by MEKK1, 2, and 3." *Biochemistry and cell biology* 82 (6):658-663.

Urban, JL, and Schreiber, H. 1984. "Rescue of the tumor-specific immune response of aged mice in vitro." *The Journal of Immunology* 133 (1):527-534.

Van Duin, David, and Shaw, Albert C. 2007. "Toll-like receptors in older adults." *Journal of the American Geriatrics Society* 55 (9):1438-1444.

Vitale, M, Zamai, Loris, Neri, Luca Maria, Galanzi, A., Facchini, A., Rana, R., Cataldi, A and Papa, Stefano. 1992. "The impairment of natural killer function in the healthy aged is due to a postbinding deficient mechanism." *Cellular immunology* 145 (1):1-10.

Walunas, Theresa L., Bakker, Christina Y., and Bluestone, Jeffrey A. 1996. "CTLA-4 ligation blocks CD28-dependent T cell activation." *Journal of Experimental Medicine* 183 (6):2541-2550.

Wang, Audrey S, and Dreesen, Oliver. 2018. "Biomarkers of cellular senescence and skin aging." *Frontiers in genetics* 9.

Wang, Li Hua, Yang, Xiao Yi, Kirken, Robert A., Resau, James H., and Farrar, William L. 2000. "Targeted disruption of Stat6 DNA binding activity by an oligonucleotide decoy blocks IL-4–driven TH2 cell response." *Blood* 95 (4):1249-1257.

Watkins, Stephanie K, Egilmez, Nejat K., Suttles, Jill and Stout, Robert D. 2007. "IL-12 rapidly alters the functional profile of tumor-associated and tumor-infiltrating macrophages in vitro and in vivo." *The Journal of Immunology* 178 (3):1357-1362.

Whisler, Ronald L, Bagenstose, Scott E., Newhouse, Yvonne G., and Carle, Kristen W. 1997. "Expression and catalytic activities of protein tyrosine kinases (PTKs) Fyn and Lck in peripheral blood T cells from elderly humans stimulated through the T cell receptor (TCR)/CD3 complex." *Mechanisms of ageing and development* 98 (1):57-73.

Whisler, Ronald L, Chen, Ming, Liu, Beiqing, and Newhouse, Yvonne G. 1999. "Age-related impairments in TCR/CD3 activation of ZAP-70 are associated with reduced tyrosine phosphorylations of ζ-chains and p59fyn/p56lck in human T cells." *Mechanisms of ageing and development* 111 (1):49-66.

White, Mary C, Holman, Dawn M., Boehm, Jennifer E., Peipins, Lucy A., Grossman, Melissa and Henley, S Jane. 2014. "Age and cancer risk: a potentially modifiable relationship." *American journal of preventive medicine* 46 (3):S7-S15.

WHO, *Ageing and health*. 2018. https://www.who.int/news-room/fact-sheets/detail/ageing-and-health.

Williams, Matthew A., and Bevan, Michael J. 2007. "Effector and memory CTL differentiation." *Annu. Rev. Immunol.* 25:171-192.

Yager, Eric J, Ahmed, Mushtaq, Lanzer, Kathleen, Randall, Troy D., Woodland, David L and Blackman, Marcia A. 2008. "Age-associated decline in T cell repertoire diversity leads to holes in the repertoire and impaired immunity to influenza virus." *Journal of Experimental Medicine* 205 (3):711-723.

Young, John Ding-E, and Cohn, Zanvil A. 1987. "Cellular and humoral mechanisms of cytotoxicity: structural and functional analogies." In *Advances in immunology*, 269-332. Elsevier.

Yu, Xiaocong, Tsibane, Tshidi, McGraw, Patricia A., House, Frances S., Keefer, Christopher J., Hicar, Mark D., Tumpey, Terrence M., Pappas, Claudia, Perrone, Lucy A and Martinez, Osvaldo. 2008. "Neutralizing antibodies derived from the B cells of 1918 influenza pandemic survivors." *Nature* 455 (7212):532.

In: Current Challenges and Management … ISBN: 978-1-53617-304-8
Editor: Abhai Kumar

Chapter 3

DIABETES, NEUROPATHY IN ELDERLY POPULATION

Hamid Ashraf DM[1] and Mehdi Hayat Shahi[2]
[1]Rajiv Gandhi Centre For Diabetes & Endocrinology(RGCDE),
J.N. Medical College, A.M.U, Aligarh, Uttar Pradesh, India
[2]Interdisciplinary Brain Research Centre (IBRC),
J.N. Medical College, A.M.U.Aligarh, Uttar Pradesh, India

ABSTRACT

Population of the world is aging rapidly, by 2050 the elderly will outnumber children. This change in demography is going to have profound effect on the epidemiology of non-communicable diseases including diabetes. Number of people with diabetes is expected to rise from 425 million in 2018 to 629 million in 2045. One third of diabetic patients are aged 60 years or more. One of the major factor responsible for this rapid increase in the incidence of diabetes, is the increased life expectancy of the population. Management of diabetes in elderly requires special attention as type 2 diabetes in this subgroup of population is associated with increased mortality, a decline in the functional status, and a higher risk for hospitalization. Diabetic neuropathy is the most common chronic complication of diabetes. Risk factors for the development of diabetic neuropathy includes, the duration and degree of hyperglycaemia, dyslipidaemia, raised blood pressure, and smoking. Diabetes is most common cause of peripheral neuropathy in the world. Diabetic neuropathy is the most common cause of non-traumatic amputation of limbs in the world. Diabetic neuropathy in elderly requires special attention because of problems of instability, frailty, increased chances of fall. In this chapter, the pathogenesis, clinical presentation, types of diabetic neuropathy and management of diabetic neuropathy with special focus on elderly will be discussed.

1. INTRODUCTION

Worldwide, the 60-plus people constitute about 11.5% of the total population of 7 billion. By 2050, this fraction is projected to increase to about 22% when the elderly will outnumber children (<15 years of age). The elderly form the fastest growing age segment while the children and working age segments reduce gradually [India aging report, 2017].

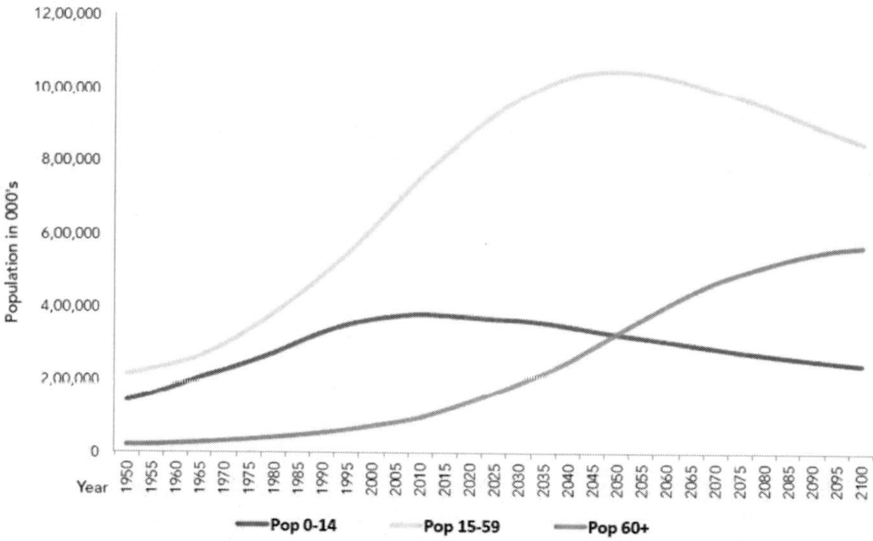

Source: United Nations (2015), World Population Prospects, 2015 Revision, Department of Economic and Social Affairs, United Nations.

Figure 1. World Population by Age Category, 1950–2100.

The changes in the demography because of aging will have a profound effect on the epidemiology of chronic, non-communicable diseases, including type 2 diabetes mellitus (T2DM).Currently, diabetes now affects > 425 million people worldwide, of which one-third are people > 65 years of age, and the number of people with diabetes is expected to rise to 629 million in 2045. Aging of the population is one of the major drivers of increased incidence of T2DM [IDF Diabetes Atlas - 8thEdition, 2017]. Diabetes in elderly individuals is associated with enhanced mortality, a decline in the functional status, and a higher risk of hospitalization. The risk of both micro and macro-vascular complication is significant in elderly individuals.

Diabetic neuropathy (DN) is one of the most common chronic complications of diabetes, affecting between 5-100% of patients of diabetes [Knuiman M. et al., 1986 & Young MJ. et al., 1993]. Distal symmetric sensory motor polyneuropathy is the commonest type of DN [Maty SC. et al., 2004]. The duration and degree of hyperglycaemia, dyslipidaemia, raised blood pressure, and smoking are key risk factors for the development of DN [Richardson JK. et al., 2004].

Both peripheral as well as autonomic nervous systems are involved in DN and lead to significant morbidity and mortality. The most frequent type of neuropathy across the world is DN, and DN related complications are responsible for more hospitalizations than all other diabetic complications combined and are the cause for 50–75% of non-traumatic amputations [Holzer SE. et al., 1998]. DN is a special problem in elderly individuals, because of problems of instability, frailty, increased chances of fall. [Richardson JK. et al., 2004].

2. Pathogenic Mechanisms

Multiple pathogenic mechanism such as metabolic, vascular, autoimmune, oxidative and nitrosative stress, and neurohormonal growth-factor deficiency has been implicated in the development of DN.

2.1. Polyol Pathway Hyperactivity and Oxidative Stress

Hyperglycemia in diabetes leads to enhancement in the polyol pathway activity. Sorbitol is formed from glucose with the help of rate-limiting first enzyme of this pathway aldose reductase, with the oxidation of nicotinamide adenine dinucleotide phosphate (NADPH) to $NADP^+$. Sorbitol is further converted to fructose by fructose by sorbitol dehydrogenase, which is coupled with the reduction of nicotinamide adenine dinucleotide (NAD^+) to NADH. It is been postulated that hyperglycemialeads to higher affinity of aldose reductase for glucose, creating intracellular osmotic stress due to increased levels of sorbitol, as sorbitol can't cross cell membranes. Few studies have reported very low levels of sorbitol in the nerves of diabetic patients [Holzer SE. et al., 1998, Baynes JW. et al., 1999& Oates PJ. 2002]. Though, the present hypothesis states that the enhanced activity of polyol pathway leads to high turnover of cofactors such as NADPH and NAD^+, which causes depletion in the reduction and regeneration of glutathione, as well as enhanced generation of advanced glycation end products (AGEs), and activation of diacylglycerol and protein kinase C (PKC) isoforms. Decreased levels of glutathione might be the primary cause of oxidative stress and subsequent accumulation of toxic species [Oates PJ. 2002].Oxidative and nitrosative stress induced by polyol pathway activation may be the primary cause of oxidative stress associated with diabetes. But autoxidation of glucose and their products, enhanced production of intracellular AGEs, augmented expression of the receptor for AGEs, mitochondrial and endoplasmic reticulum stress, stimulation of PKC isoforms and increased activity of the hexosamine pathway can also induce the oxidative stress [Brownlee M. et al., 2010 & Baynes JW. 1991]. Additional evidence also points that oxidative stress is triggered by heightened free radical formation due to glucose metabolism itself and/or insufficiencies in antioxidant defense and it may play a major role among the putative pathogenic mechanisms of diabetic neuropathy. Along with oxidative stress, reactive nitrogen species, especially the peroxynitrite also has a significant role in the development of diabetes and its complications [Obrosova IG. et al., 2005Drel VR. et al.,

2007&Vareniuk I. et al., 2007]. Even though animal models of diabetes is suggestive of significant changes in oxidative status, tissue concentrations of known carbonyl compounds are nearly negligible and plasma ET-1, nitric oxide, catalase and glutathione levels did not differ in neuropathic diabetic patients when compared to non-neuropathic diabetic ones [Cunha JM. et al., 2008 & Ozkul A. et al., 2010]. Clinical observations are also having discriminant results for antioxidants agents such as alpha lipoic acid, ranging from little benefit to interesting advantages [Ziegler D. et al., 2011, Mijnhout GS. et al., 2010, Ruessmann HJ, 2009 &Tang J. et al., 2007].

2.2. Microvascular Changes

DPN is frequently associated with impairment in the peripheral circulation, in both the neurons and in the skin [Cameron NE. et al., 2001, Tuck RR. et al., 1984 & Jin HY.et al., 2012]. Neuronal ischemia occurs, secondary to increased wall thickness and hyalinization of the basal lamina of vessels that nurture peripheral nerves along with luminal reduction [Malik RA. et al., 1993]. These changes are secondary to plasma protein scape of capillary membrane to endoneurium, leading to swelling and amplified interstitial pressure in the neurons, associated with increased capillary pressure, deposition of fibrin and thrombus development [Czyzyk A. 1986]. Hyperglycemia itself can induce neuronal hypoxia, especially in sensory nerves, changing their electrical stability [Fuchs D. et al., 2010].There is progressive loss of neurons secondary to neuronal ischemia in diabetic patients and diabetic animals [Shun CT. et al., 2004], leading to decline in the intraepidermal nerve fibre density. Endothelial dysfunction also plays an important role in the development of DPN. There is alteration in both vasodilatation induced by acetylcholine and vasoconstriction mediated by the sympathetic system [Quattrini C. et al., 2007]. One of the causes of microvascular changes is oxidative stress, as the treatment with antioxidant agents can preserve regular perfusion, re-establishing sensory transmission in type 1 diabetes model [Inkster ME. et al., 2007].

2.3. Channels Sprouting

Pain in the patients of DPN can be traced to the damaged nerve endings. The erratic action potentials arising from the damaged nerve endingsare interpreted by central nervous system (CNS) as pain or dysesthesias [Said G. et al., 1983]. Injury to the neurons can also lead to changes in ion channel expression in peripheral nerves, leading to hyperexcitability [Stewart JD. et al., 1992]. Increased expression of the voltage-gated sodium channels (Nav) has been established in neuropathic pain models [Black JA. et al., 1999]. Nav channels are required in the generation and transmission of action potential, and can be divided into sensitive (TTX-S) or resistant (TTX-R) to tetrodotoxin [Roy ML. et al., 1992]. Few studies have shown that the TTX-S channels Nav1.3 and Nav 1.7 are up-regulated in the dorsal root ganglion (DRG) in the animal models of diabetes [Hong S. et al., 2004& Cheng KI. et al., 2014]. Diabetic rats presenting with allodynia have shown enhanced Nav1.3 expression in small and large diameter DRG neurons [Craner MJ. et al., 2002]. The abnormal expression and function of both TTX-R and TTX-S sodium channels can lead to alteration in the activity of nociceptive fibres [Hong S. et al., 2004]. Increased expression of nodal Na+ currents has been described in patients with painful DPN when compared to patients without diabetic neuropathy [Misawa S. et al., 2009].

2.4. Microglial Activation

Glial cells play an important role in the pathogenesis of various conditions affecting the nervous system, including chronic pain states [Mika J. et al., 2013]. Glial cells are required for the maintenance of homeostasis, it forms form myelin, and offer support and protection for neurons from both central and peripheral nervous system [Mika J. et al., 2013]. Microglial cells are activated in response to neuronal injury which lasts for around three months and leads to pro-inflammatory milieu [Vydyanathan A. et al., 2005]. Persistent microglial activation has been demonstrated in the spinal cord of streptozocin induced diabetic rats [Toth CC. et al., 2010].

The microglial activation is associated with enhanced expression of Nav1.3 sodium channels in the DRG, probably via p38 mitogen activated protein kinase dependent mechanism [Crown ED. 2012].

2.5. Central Sensitization

DPN is characterized by the involvement of both peripheral and central nervous system [Aslam A. et al., 2014]. Enhanced sensitivity of primary afferents neurons and neuroplastic changes in central sensory neurons has been described in patients with DPN. The presence of allodynia in DPN suggests that the pain processing in the CNS is altered [Chen SR. et al., 2002]. Increased activity of glutaminergic neurons and enhanced activity of N-Methyl-D-aspartate (NMDA) receptor has been described in DPN [Bai HP. et al., 2014]. This might be responsible for augmented and repeated excitatory post synaptic currents in the lamina [Wang XL. et al., 2007]. Thus, it is plausible that augmented NMDA expression and glutamate release might contribute to spinal cord hyperactivity. On the other hand, GABAB receptors seem to be down regulated in the spinal cord in diabetic neuropathy [Bai HP. et al., 2014].

2.6. Inflammation

Inflammation plays a central role in specific inflammatory neuropathies such as vasculitic and granulomatous disease than in diabetic neuropathy per se [Lindenlaub T. et al., 2003]. Microvasular changes in the endoneurial vessels leading to alteration in the blood flow play a crucial role in the development of diabetic neuropathy. Metabolic alteration secondary to hyperglycaemia in a genetically predisposed individual leads to reduced nerve perfusion. Oxidative stress secondary to elevated free radicals are also responsible for the vasculardys function, and subsequent vasoconstriction [Jude EB. et al., 1998].

3. Clinical Presentation

3.1. Focal Mononeuropathies

The incidence of cranial mononeuropathiesis higher in patients with diabetes. Usually, they have sudden onset, often associated with pain, and are self-limited. Vascular obstruction and ischemia are the major underlying pathology. Classically involves the III, VI, and VII cranial nerves. Entrapment neuropathies are also more frequent in diabetic patients and they differ from mononeuropathies that they have slower onset, usually progressive and they are persistent in absence of intervention. Commonly involved nerves include the median, ulnar, peroneal, lateral cutaneous nerve of the thigh [Vinik A. et al., 2004]. Carpal tunnel syndrome is the most common entrapment syndrome occurring in diabetics, affecting 8.7-20% [Wilbourn AJ. 1999]. It occurs three times more frequently in patients with diabetes compared with the normal healthy population [Kapritskaya Y. et al., 2002]. These entrapment neuropathies are usually treated by surgical means. The clinical features of mononeuropathy and entrapment syndromes have been described in Table 1.

Table 1. Comparison of features of mononeuropathy and entrapment syndromes

Clinical Feature	Mononeuropathies	Entrapment syndrome
Onset	Acute	Subacute
Incidence	Less common	Common
Involvement	Usually single nerve	Single nerves exposed to trauma
Commonly involved nerve	Cranial III, IV, VI, VII, peroneal, sural, sciatic, femoral, ulnar, median	Median, ulnar, peroneal, lateral cutaneous of the thigh, tibial
Progression	Not progressive, resolve spontaneously	Progressive
Treatment	Symptomatic	Rest, splints, diuretics, steroid injections, surgery for weakness

3.2. Diffuse Neuropathies

3.2.1. Proximal Motor Neuropathies/Diabetic Amyotrophy

Proximal motor neuropathy typically involves the lumbosacral region, clinically it presents with pain in the affected limb, proximal muscle weakness and muscle wasting which can be symmetrical or asymmetrical. It primarily affects elderly patients [Leedman PJ. et al., 1988 & Barohn R. et al., 1991]. There is difficulty in rise from sitting position (Gower sign). The onset is acute or subacute, pain can be severe and persistent, begins asymmetrically, involve proximal more frequently. As the pain subsides weakness becomes more apparent. Coexistent distal symmetric polyneuropathy, autonomic neuropathy, spontaneous muscle fasciculation might be present. Muscle fasciculation can be triggered bypercussion. Significant weight loss is also a common finding. The natural history is of slow but incomplete improvement. Significant improvement in pain occurs earlier than improvement in the weakness [Barohn R. et al., 1991].

Proximal motor neuropathy accompanies a wide range of disorders unrelated to diabetes, such as chronic inflammatory demyelinatingpoly-neuropathy (CIDP), monoclonal gammopathy of undetermined significance (MGUS), circulating GM1 antibodies and antibodies to neuronal cells, and inflammatory vasculitis [Vinik AI. et al., 1998 & Steck AJ. et al., 1994]. A study of more than 1000 patients with neurologic disorders revealed that CIDP was 11 times more common in patients with diabetes [Sharma K. et al., 2002]. If demyelination predominates and weakness affects both proximal and distal groups of muscles, the diagnosis of CIDP should be considered. It is important to differentiate proximal motor neuropathy from CIDP, as CIDP responds dramatically to various interventions, while proximal motor neuropathy needs symptomatic treatment. Another important differential diagnosis is spinal stenosis syndromes. In spinal stenosis, there is impingement and compression of nerve roots secondary to osteophytes. Aging is also associated with hypertrophy of the ligamentum flavumand disk desiccation. If there is associated compression of vascular system, claudication on walking downhill might occur, and it is typically relieved by leaning forward

[Nadeau M. 2013]. Diagnosis is important as management is different, which can be modest physical therapy to surgical decompression if symptoms are severe or there is motor weakness [Vinik AI et al. 1992].

The exact pathophysiology is not known, but ischemia from microvasculitis is thought to play an important role. This hypothesis can explain both the axonal degeneration and patchy demyelination found on histopathology. Alteration in the immunity secondary to diabetes might be responsible for the microvasculitis [Vinik AI. et al., 1992].

3.2.2. Diabetes Autonomic Neuropathy

Autonomicneuropathy is common in patients with diabetic neuropathy, it can involve cardiovascular, genitourinary or gastrointestinal system leading to a variety of symptoms and signs. Erectile dysfunction, resting tachycardia, postural hypotension, gastroparesis and urinary bladder dysfunction are important manifestation of autonomic neuropathy in patients with diabetes. Sudomotor dysfunction can lead to anhydrosis in length dependent fashion, it can progress to global anhydrosis, compensatory hyperhidrosis over trunks can also occur in combination with anhydrosis over extremities. Anhydrosis of foot predisposes heel to fissures and cracks, increasing the risk of infection and diabetic foot development [Zola BE. et al., 1992, & Vinik AI. et al., 1992].

Delayed gastric emptying can occur in absence of any physical obstruction, leading to postprandial fullness, early satiety, nausea, vomiting, bloating. Gastroparesis can also lead to erratic glucose levels secondary to erratic absorption of glucose. It has important effect on quality of life [Melga P. et al., 1997, & Stacher G. et al., 1999].

Involvement of genitourinary system is common in diabetic patients as it is richly innervated by the autonomic fibres. Impaired bladder sensation leading to elevated threshold for initiation of the micturition and retention can occur. Voiding difficulties in the form of hesitancy, poor stream, dribbling can occur secondary to weekend detrusor activity. Incomplete bladder emptying, increased post voidal urine volume, bladder over distension and urinary retention lead to stasis in flow of urine, increasing the chances of urinary tract infection. Another very important presentation of autonomic neuropathy is erectile dysfunction, might be present in 50% of male patients within 10 years of the diagnosis of diabetes. Early morning erections are diminished or lost, there is impotence and retrograde ejaculation might be present [Vinik AI. 1998 &Vinik AI. 1997].

Cardiovascular autonomic neuropathy is an important source of morbidity and mortality in patients of diabetes. The duration of diabetes and degree of glycaemic control are important risk factors for the autonomic neuropathy. Initially, it may present with resting tachycardia, progressing to diminished heart rate variability and postural hypotension. 30% mortality at 5 years has been described in individuals with established autonomic neuropathy [Zola BE. et al. 1992, Valensi P. 1998 & Ziegler D. et al., 2008]. Clinical features of autonomic neuropathy have been described in Table 2.

3.2.3. Distal Sensorimotor Polyneuropathy (DPN)

Chronic distal sensorimotor polyneuropathy (DPN) is the most common form of diabetic neuropathy. It has got an insidious onset, might be gradually progressive. It can involve either sensory or motor, and it affects small fibers, large fibres, or both [Vinik AI, et al. 1995]. Most patients with DPN have a combination of both largeand small nerve fibreinvolvements.

Table 2. Clinical features of diabetic autonomic neuropathy

System	Clinical feature
Cardiovsacular	Resting tachycardia Exercise intolerance Postural hypotension Painless myocardial infarction
Sudomotor	Anhydrosis Heat intolerance Gustatory sweating Compensatory hyperhidrosis over trunk
Genitourinary	Erectile dysfunction Bladder dysfunction Retrograde ejaculation
Metabolic	Hypoglycaemic unawareness Hypoglycaemia associated autonomic failure

3.2.3.1. Large Fibre Neuropathies

Large fibre neuropathy is common in elderly diabetic patients, it affects both motor and sensory system and clinically presents as "glove and stocking" distribution of sensory loss [Yu RK. et al., 1990]. Involvement of large fibres leads to a number of signs but few symptoms. There is reduction in the vibration perception, reduced position sense, weakness, muscle wasting and suppressed tendon reflexes. Early in the course of the neuropathic process, multifocal sensory loss might also be found. The classical symptoms of large fibre neuropathy are sensation of walking on cotton, floors feeling "strange", incapability to turn the pages of a book, or inability to differentiate among coins [Vinik AI, et al. 1995].

The role of age related decline in the peripheral nervous system and loss of muscle mass (sarcopenia) is still not clear in patients with DPN. Elderly individuals with large fibre neuropathies have instability while walking on irregular surfaces, with concomitant impairment in reaction time and balance [Menz HB. et al., 2004].This decline in the peripheral sensory input enhances the risk of falls and subsequent fractures in these patients. In diabetic population the difficulty in performing activities of daily living such as 14 of 15 daily tasks which included walking 2–3 blocks, lifting 10 pounds, using a telephone, and bathing is more than non-diabetic population [Maty SC. et al., 2004]. The inability to carry out basic activities of daily living, frequently compromise an individual's freedom and quality of life, which enhances the mortality and morbidity in this vulnerable population [Vinik EJ. et al., 2005].

Epidemiologic studies have revealed that elderly individuals with peripheral neuropathy have poorer physical performance, balance, muscle strength and bone density [Resnick HE. et al., 2002, Strotmeyer ES. et al., 2006 & Lauretani F. 2006], and these declines were independent of the diabetes status of the patient. In a study conducted in individuals with ≥70 years of age, those with sensory deficit had a 2.5 times greater risk of falls and subsequent fractures, joint dislocations, lacerations requiring sutures, and intracranial injuries [Koski K. et al., 1998]. Clinical features of large fibre neuropathy have been described in Table 3.

Table 3. Clinical features of DPN

Large fibre neuropathies	Small fibre neuropathies
Deep-seated pain Wasting and weakness Numbness, pins and needles, tingling, ataxia Impaired vibration perception Loss of position sense Loss of reflexes Impaired nerve conduction velocity Interferes with normal life Risk of falling and fractures	Superficial pain Electric shock, burning, allodynia Autonomic dysfunction Thermal imperception Normal strength and reflexes Electrophysiogically silent Quantitative sensory testing and skin biopsies Produces symptoms Leads to morbidity and death

DPN; Distal sensorimotor polyneuropathy

3.2.3.2. Small Fibre Neuropathies

Involvement of small nerve fibre is a disease of symptoms rather than signs; often it is present without objective signs or electrophysiologic signs of nerve injury [Vinik AI. et al., 1995]. First it appears in the lower limbs with symptoms of pain, burning sensations, and hyperalgesia, followed by a loss of thermal sensation and reduced light-touch and pinprick sensation [Zhuang HX. Et al., 1996]. Small unmyelinated C-fibres are responsible for pain sensation, warm thermal perception and autonomic function.

A diabetic individual with involvement of these nerves clinically presents with burning, dysesthetic pain, often accompanied by hyperalgesia, and allodynia. This pain is different from that of large fibre neuropathy, where the pain is usually described as deep seated and "gnawing."

3.3. Charcot Neuroarthropathy

One of the devastating complications of DPN, is the development of Charcotfoot (CF) or Charcot neuropathic osteoarthropathy. CF is named after the famous French neurologist Jean-Martin Charcot, who in 1868first described neuroarthropathic changes in patients with tertiary syphilis [Charcot JM. 1868].William Riley Jordan in 1936, first described the link between DM and painless neuropathic arthropathy of ankle [Jordan WR. 1936].It is a rare disorder that is characterized by destruction of bones and joints leading to fractures, dislocations, deformities and amputation. CF is commonly associated with DM, alcoholic peripheral neuropathy, tertiary syphilis, leprosy, spinal cord injury, Charcot-Marie-Tooth disease and idiopathic neuropathy. Presently, the number of patients with diabetes is increasing throughout the world, and with improvement in the diabetes care these patients are living longer. This has led to a situation where DM is the most common cause of CN and the numbers of patients with CN are expected to increase. The reported incidence of CF varies widely in literature from 0.1–7.5%, because of different diagnostic criteria used, different inclusion criteria and different duration of diabetes [Rajbhandari SM. et al., 2002]. Recently, a study from India revealed a high prevalence of CA (9.8%) in patients of type 2 DM with DPN [Salini D. et al., 2018].Presentation may be acute with severe pain, a warm to hot oedematous foot with increased skin blood flow, radiography may reveal osteopenia. The differential diagnosis includes cellulitis or, less commonly, deep vein thrombosis, so these conditions should be ruled out. Strict immobilization using a total contact cast is the preferred modality of treatment. There are evidences that using bisphosphonates may help in acute stages of CF. Surgery might be required along with patient education, protective footwear, and routine foot care in chronic stages of CF [Leedman PJ. et al., 1988].

4. Differential Diagnosis and Diagnosis

Diabetic neuropathy is a diagnosis of exclusion. In those patients presenting with DN the differential diagnosis includes hereditary sensory neuropathies, B12 and folate deficiency, syphilis, Lyme disease, neuropathy associated with IgM monoclonal gammopathy of undetermined significance (IgM MGUS neuropathy), other paraneoplastic conditions, autoimmune diseases, and toxic neuropathies. In patients with oneor more motor neurologic syndromes, chronic motor neuropathies, AIDP, CIDP, and IgG and IgA MGUS neuropathies should actively be sought [Rogers LC. et al., 2011].

The evaluation of DN includes a thorough history and examination, type of diabetes, degree and duration of hyperglycaemia needs to be ascertained. Poor glycaemic control and long duration are two important risk factors for DN. A history suggestive of other diabetic complications should be obtained. In general DPN is insidious in onset, while acute onset is suggestive of other type of DN.

Sensory symptoms can be divided into positive and negative symptoms, positive symptoms include paresthesia, tingling, burning and pain. Negative symptoms include numbness and loss of position and vibration senses. The smaller fibres are involved earlier than large fibres. So in absence of symptoms of small fibre involvement such as pain and burning, patient presenting with motor weakness alternate cause of neuropathy should be considered. A good history suggestive of other potential cause for neuropathy such as use of alcohol, neurotoxic drugs, nutritional deficiencies, kidney disease and neoplastic disease should be obtained [Summer CJ. et al., 2003].

Physical examination should be guided by history. Examination for postural drop, heart rate at rest is essential. General examination of skin for trophic changes and lack of hair as well as inspection of feet is necessary. The neurological examination should focus on sensation, strength, reflexes, and gait abnormalities when DPN is suspected and focus on cranial nerves when focal mononeuropathies are underlying etiology. Demonstration of ankle reflexes and examining the vibration and position sense in a patient of DN is of vital importance.10 g monofilament test should be used in a consistent manner to document the loss of protective sensation, Romberg sign needs to be elucidated [Freeman R. et al., 2011].

The examination findings can be complemented by certain investigation such as nerve conduction study (NCS). The NCS will reveal abnormality when there is involvement of large fibres. A normal NCS does not rules out DN. NCS provides information regarding the presence of neuropathy, pattern of nerve involvement, and features that may suggest a primarily axonal or demyelinating pathophysiology or a combination of both. A typical DN is characterized by axonal loss on NCS. NCS is particularly helpful in ruling out neuropathies caused by etiology other than diabetes. It is also useful in diagnosing the entrapment syndromes and radiculoplexus neuropathy [Dyck PJ. et al., 2010].

The other test which might be required in patients with DN includes quantitative sensory testing (QST), quantitative sudomotor axon reflex test (QSART), tilt table test, corneal nerve fibre density and intraepithelial nerve fibre density. QST assess both small and large fibres, QSART assess the sudomotor function [Magda P. et al., 2002]. Corneal nerve fibre density and intraepithelial nerve fibre density are emerging modality for early diagnosis of DN [Lagali NS. et al., 2017].

Other investigations like MRI, serum protein electrophoresis, vitamin B12 levels, lumbar puncture for spinal fluid analysis may be required when the suspicion of other causes of neuropathy is strong.

5. Management of Neuropathy

Many subclinical diseases are common in elderly and these are also associated with peripheral neuropathy. Early intervention for these conditions might improve the neuropathy. These include vitamin B12 deficiency, peripheral arterial disease, metabolic syndrome [Baik HW. et al., 1999].

After the diagnosis of neuropathy has been established, treatment aiming at alleviating the symptoms and preventing additional progression should be initiated. Patients with involvement of large fibre have gait instability and they have 17 times higher risk of fall than non-neuropathic patients [Cavanagh PR. et al., 1992]. Involvement of large fibre is more common in elderly individuals. It is essential to improve the strength and balance in elderly patient with large fibre neuropathy. Elderly individuals with or without neuropathy can benefit fromhigh intensity strength training by enhancing the muscle strength, improving coordination and balance, and thereby decreasing the fall and fracture risk [Nelson ME. et al., 1994 & Liu-Ambrose T. et al., 2004.]. Strategies for management of small and large fibre neuropathy have been given in Table 4.

Table 4. Strategies for management of small and large fibre neuropathy

Large fibre neuropathies	Small fibre neuropathies
• Exercise aimed at strength, gait, and balance training • Orthotic foot wear to treat and/or prevent foot deformities • Surgery for tendon lengthening for equinus • Bisphophonates for osteoporosis • Surgical reconstruction and full contact casting as necessary • Alleviation of pain	• Care of foot is utmost importance. • Management of pain • Orthotic foot wear if necessary. • Regular foot and shoe examination. Self-inspection of feet • Carefulness to prevent heat injury. • Emollient creams to take careanhydrosis leading to cracking and infection.

5.1. Targeting the Pathogenic Mechanisms

Robust evidence is available to suggest a relationship between hyperglycaemia and the development and severity of diabetic neuropathy, and substantialpositive effects of early intensive glycaemic control on prevention of neuropathy [Pirart J. 1978]. But intensive therapy for hyperglycaemia is not a routine practice in elderly. Furthermore, at this moment no epidemiologic or natural history is available to demonstrate the importance of late onset diabetes in aged populations and IFG as risk factors for the development of neuropathy in elderly individuals. Cardiovascular Health Study findings are suggestive of that impaired glucose levels is a risk factor for autonomic neuropathy in the elderly [Stein PK. et al., 2007].

Experimental models provide a conceptual outline for the cause andtreatment of diabetic neuropathy. But the imperfect translational work in human subjects continues to generate debate over the cause of human diabetic neuropathy and to date wehave no effective long-term treatment. Few studies have revealed that targeting the oxidativestress may improve peripheral and autonomic neuropathy in type 2 diabetic adults [Ziegler D. et al., 1997, Ruhnau KJ. et al., 1999 &Valensi P. et al., 2005].

Thiazolidinediones, statins and fibrates have shown some beneficial effect on the development of neuropathy in diabetic individuals [Davis t. 2007].

5.2. Therapy Aimed at Treating Symptoms in Patients with DPN

Alleviation of pain and other symptoms of DN are of utmost importance as it affects patient's quality of life. Treatment approaches include the reduction of afferent inputs, decrease the local inflammation, subdue sympathetic fortification of the stimulus, neutralize the effect of excitatory amino acids, and modify the modulation of nociceptors.

Amitriptyline has been used to treat diabetic neuropathy since long [Coppini DV. et al., 2006], but the side effect profile makes it unsuitable to use in elderly population. Anticholinergic side effects,including orthostatic hypotension, urinary retention, and possible cardiac arrhythmiasneed special attention prior to its prescription.Cardiac conduction defects, prolong QT syndrome, myocardial infarction in preceding 6 months, ventricular arrhythmias and/or frequent premature ventricular contractions are the contraindications for using amitriptyline and other tricyclic antidepressants. Patients with age > 40 years need an electrocardiogram prior to using these medications [Morello CM. et al., 1999 &Dworkin RH. et al., 2003].

Antiarrhythmics, antiepileptic drugs and local analgesic are additional commonly used drugs [Morello CM. et al., 1999]. As the evidence from the randomized clinical trials have emerged, the Fourth International Conference on the Mechanisms and Treatment of Neuropathic Pain has recommended gabapentin, 5% lidocaine patch, opioid analgesics, tramadol hydrochloride, and tricyclic anti-depressantas first line treatment of neuropathic pain [Dworkin RH. et al., 2003].

The safety and tolerability of a particular drug should be considered prior to prescribing to an elderly individual. Dosages adjustment should be based on positive response, treatment adherence, and adverse events[Dworkin RH. et al., 2003].Various anti-epileptic drugs (AEDs) have been found to be effective in the treatment of neuropathicpain since 1993 including felbamate, gabapentin, pregabalin, lamotrigine, topiramate, tiagabine, levetiracetam, oxcarbazepine, and zonisamide. Out of these the pregabalin and duloxetine have received US FDA approval for the treatment of painful diabetic neuropathy,

Table 5. Summary of medications used in the management of Diabetic neuropathy

Medication Class	Medication	Dosage	Mechanism of action	Side effects
Antidepressent TCA	Amitriptyline Nortriptyline	10-150 mg, QHS 10-150 mg QHS	Inhibition of norepinephrine and serotonin re-uptake	Dry eyes, mouth, constipation, urinary retention, confusion
	Desipramine	10-150 mg		
SNRI	Duloxetine	60-120, mg QHS	Inhibition of serotonin and norepinephrine re-uptake	Dizziness, somnolence, anorexia
	Venlafaxine	75-225 mg, QD		
Anticonvulsants	Gabapentin	300-1200 mg, TID	Inhibition of α-2-delta subunit of Ca^{2+}channel	Fatigue, dizziness, pedal edema, ataxia, somnolence,
	Carbamazepine	200 mg, QD	Inhibition of Na^{+} channel	dizziness, somnolence, leucopenia
	Pregabalin	500-200 mg, TID	Inhibition of α-2-delta subunit of Ca^{2+}channel	Fatigue, dizziness, pedal edema, ataxia, sedation
Opioids	Tramadol	50-100 mg, BID	μ-opioid receptor agonist	Nausea, constipation, headache
	Tapentadol	50-100mg, QID	Opioid spinal-supra-spinal synergy	Nausea, constipation, headache
Antioxidant	A-lipoic acid	200-1800 mg, QD	Antioxidant, anti-inflammatory	Gastrointestinal discomfort
Topical	Capsaicin cream	Topical	Activation of TRPV1channel,& depletion of substance P	Local burning

Pregabalinhas been found to be effective to reduce the pain scores within 1 week of treatment, which persisted for 6–12 weeks in four randomized controlled trials including 146–724 patientswith diabetic neuropathy [Rosenstock J. et al., 2004 &Freynhagen R. et al., 2005]. Common side effects included dose related somnolence, ataxia, confusion, peripheral edema and constipation. A freshtrial from Canada revealed that pregabalin was more cost effective when compared with gabapentin [Tarride JE. et al., 2006].

New evidence for the use of antiepileptic drugs for the treatment of DN is emerging. Failure to respond to one drug might need change to another drug with different mechanism of action [Freynhagen R. et al., 2005]. When these mechanisms are understood, it may prove beneficial to combine drugs for a synergistic effect. The summary of the medicines used in treatment of DN has been given in Table 5.

6. Special Consideration

Aged heterogeneity is an important aspect in the treatment of older adults, that they have the maximum heterogeneity among all the age groups on a wide variety of parameters such as physical, psychological, social, and functional characteristics. On one hand we have people with minimal or no medical problem and greater life expectancy and minimal age-related decline in function, this sub group require similar treatment as young people. On another hand we have people with multiple comorbidities, limited life expectancy, needs ploy pharmacy, and are functionally disabled. And a large population lies in between this two spectrum [Rowe JW. et al., 1987].

Another important consideration in treating older adultsis multimorbidity, defined as the coexistence of 2 or morediseases or conditions.Multimorbidityis common in elderly, because the incidence of chronicdiseases increases with aging. Multimorbidityaffects the treatment risks and benefits of neuropathicpainin elderly individuals [Rowe JW. et al., 1987].

One of the major goals of care in elderly population is maintenance of independent function. Neuropathic pain as well as their treatment can havecompelling negative effects onactivities of daily living.So the caregivers should monitor the status baseline and during treatment to assess the progress towardthat goal [Rowe JW. et al., 1987].

Usage of multiple medicationsor the use of superfluous medications (polypharmacy), is commonin elderly individuals and increases the risk of adverse drugreactions, non-compliance, and increased cost. Polypharmacyis also associated with enhanced risk of drug-drug interactions in general and with agents used to treat neuropathic pain specifically. Drug-related falls and injury are not so common, but this is an important consideration while prescribing drugs acting at central nervous system [Sofaer-Bennett B. et al., 2007].

Many of the agents used in treatment of neuropathic pain such as opioids, tricyclic antidepressants, gabapentin, and pregabalin, are associated with sedation, dizziness, and falls, particularly in frail or susceptible elderly patients.

Many timessigns and symptoms of an adverse drug reaction are attributed to a pre-existing, a new disease or just secondary to aging. Adverse drug events are an important differential diagnosis in almost every geriatric syndrome.This is important not only in removing the offending agent but also to avoid a vicious prescribing cycle in which another medication is used to treat the adverse drug event when it is mistakenly diagnosed as anotherdisease or condition [Rochon PA. et al., 1997].

CONCLUSION

The incidence of diabetes is increasing at a very fast pace, diabetic neuropathy being the most common chronic complication of diabetes, has enormous burden while managing these patients. The elderly individuals are also more susceptible for the development of neuropathy secondary to other causes, so it needs a careful evaluation. Treatment of diabetic neuropathy in elderly also requires special attention because of polypharmacy, multimorbidity, and decline in functional status of the patient. It is important to consider all these factors prior to prescribing treatment for diabetic neuropathy. Once on treatment this subgroup of patients requires special attention towards the adverse reaction of the prescribed agents.

REFERENCES

Aslam, A., Singh, J. & Rajbhandari, S. (2014). Pathogenesis of painful diabetic neuropathy. *Pain Res Treat*, 412041.

Bai, H. P., Liu, P., Wu, Y. M., Guo, W. Y., Guo, Y. X. & Wang, X. L. (2014). Activation of spinal GABAB receptors normalizes N-methyl-D-aspartate receptor in diabetic neuropathy. *J Neurol Sci*, *341*, 68-72.

Baik, H. W. & Russell, R. M. (1999). Vitamin B12 deficiency in the elderly. *Annu Rev Nutr*,*19*, 357–377.

Barohn, R. J., Sahenk, Z., Warmolts, J. R. & Mendell, J. R. (1991). The Bruns-Garland syndrome (Diabetic amyotrophy). *Arch Neurol*, *48*, 1130–1135.

Baynes, J. W. & Thorpe, S. R. (1999). Role of oxidative stress in diabetic complications: a new perspective on an old paradigm. *Diabetes*, *48*, 1-9.

Baynes, J. W. (1991). Role of oxidative stress in development of complications in diabetes. *Diabetes*, *40*, 405-412.

Black, J. A., Cummins, T. R., Plumpton, C., Chen, Y. H., Hormuzdiar, W., Clare, J. J. & Waxman, S. G. (1999). Upregulation of a silent sodium channel after peripheral, but not central, nerve injury in DRG neurons. *J Neurophysiol*, *82*, 2776-2785.

Brownlee, M. (2001). Biochemistry and molecular cell biology of diabetic complications. *Nature*, *414*, 813-820.

Cameron, N. E., Eaton, S. E., Cotter, M. A. &Tesfaye, S. (2001). Vascular factors and metabolic interactions in the pathogenesis of diabetic neuropathy. *Diabetologia*, *44*, 1973-1988.

Cavanagh, P. R., Derr, J. A., Ulbrecht, J. S., Maser, R. E. & Orchard, T. J. (1992). Problems with gait and posture in neuropathic patients with insulin-dependent diabetes mellitus. *Diabet Med*, *9*, 469–474.

Charcot, J. M. (1868). Sur quell quesarthropathies qui paraiised´ependre d' unel´esion du cerveauou de la mouelle ´epini`ere [*On some arthropathies which seem to depend on a lesion of the brain or the spinal cord*]. *Arch Physiol Norm Pathol,1*, 161–178.

Chen, S. R. & Pan, H. L. (2002). Hypersensitivity of spinothalamic tract neurons associated with diabetic neuropathic pain in rats. *J Neurophysiol*, *87*, 2726-2733.

Cheng, K. I., Wang, H. C., Chuang, Y. T., Chou, C. W., Tu, H. P., Yu, Y. C., Chang, L. L. & Lai, C. S. (2014). Persistent mechanical allodynia positively correlates with an increase in activated microglia and increased P-p38 mitogen-activated protein kinase activation in streptozotocin-induced diabetic rats. *Eur J Pain*, *18*, 162-173.

Coppini, D. V., Young, P. J., Weng, C., MacLeod, A. F. &Sonksen, P. H. (1998). Outcome on diabetic foot complications in relation to clinical examination and quantitative sensory testing: a case-control study. *Diabet Med*, *15*, 765–771.

Craner, M. J., Klein, J. P., Renganathan, M., Black, J. A. & Waxman, S. G. (2002). Changes of sodium channel expression in experimental painful diabetic neuropathy. *Ann Neurol*, *52*, 786-792.

Crown, E. D. (2012). The role of mitogen activated protein kinase signaling in microglia and neurons in the initiation and maintenance of chronic pain. *ExpNeurol*, *234*, 330-339.

Cunha, J. M., Jolivalt, C. G., Ramos, K. M., Gregory, J. A., Calcutt, N. A. &Mizisin, A. P. (2008). Elevated lipid peroxidation and DNA oxidation in nerve from diabetic rats: effects of aldose reductase inhibition, insulin, and neurotrophic factors. *Metabolism*, *57*, 873-881.

Czyzyk, A. (1986). Epidemiology of vascular disease in diabetes mellitus. *Pol Arch Med Wewn*, *76*, 129-136.

Davis, t. (2007). Lipid-lowering Therapy Protects Against Peripheral Sensory Neuropathy in Type 2 Diabetes. Diabetes supplement.

DCCT. (1995). Effect of intensive diabetes treatment on nerve conduction in the diabetes control and complications trial. *Ann Neurol*, *38*, 869–880.

Drel, V. R., Pacher, P., Vareniuk, I., Pavlov, I., Ilnytska, O., Lyzogubov, V. V., Tibrewala, J., Groves, J. T. & Obrosova, I. G. (2007). A peroxynitrite decomposition catalyst counteracts sensory neuropathy in streptozotocin-diabetic mice. *Eur J Pharmacol*, *569*, 48-58.

Dworkin, R. H., Backonja, M., Rowbotham, M. C., Allen, R. R., Argoff, C. R., Bennett, G. J., et al. (2003). Advances in neuropathic pain: diagnosis, mechanisms, and treatment recommendations. *Arch Neurol*, *60*, 1524–1534.

Dyck, P. J., Overland, C. J., Low, P. A., Litchy, W. J., Davis, J. L., O'Brien, P. C., et al. (2010). Signs and symptoms versus nerve conduction studies to diagnose diabetic sensorimotor poluneuropathy: CI vs. Nphys trial. *Muscle Nerve*,*42*, 157-164.

Freeman, R., Wieling, W., Axelord, F. B., Benditt, D. G., Benarroch, E., Biaggioni, I., et al. (2011). Consensus statement on the definition of orthostatic hypotension, neurally mediated syncope and postural tachycardia syndromr. *Autonomic Neurosci Basic Clin*, *161*, 46-48.

Freynhagen, R., Strojek, K., Griesing, T., Whalen, E. & Balkenohl, M. (2005). Efficacy of pregabalin in neuropathic pain evaluated in a 12-week, randomised, double-blind, multicentre, placebo-controlled trial of flexible- and fixed-dose regimens. *Pain*,*115*, 254–263.

Fuchs, D., Birklein, F., Reeh, P. W. & Sauer, S. K. (2010). Sensitized peripheral nociception in experimental diabetes of the rat. *Pain*, *151*, 496-505.

Giacco, F. & Brownlee, M. (2010). Oxidative stress and diabetic complications. *Circ Res*, *107*, 1058-1070.

Holzer, S. E., Camerota, A., Martens, L., Cuerdon, T., Crystal, P. &Zagari, M. (1998). Costs and duration of care for lower extremity ulcers in patients with diabetes. *ClinTher*,*20*, 169–181.

Hong, S., Morrow, T. J., Paulson, P. E., Isom, L. L. & Wiley, J. W. (2004). Early painful diabetic neuropathy is associated with differential changes in tetrodotoxin-sensitive and -resistant sodium channels in dorsal root ganglion neurons in the rat. *J Biol Chem*, *279*, 29341-29350.

IDF Diabetes Atlas - 8th Edition. Available from https://diabetesatlas.org/resources/2017-atlas.html [accessed on 24th March 2019].

India aging report. Available from https://india.unfpa.org/sites/default/files/pubpdf/India%20Ageing%20Report%20-%202017%20%28Final%20Version%29.pdf, [accessed on 24th March 2019].

Inkster, M. E., Cotter, M. A. & Cameron, N. E. (2007). Treatment with the xanthine oxidase inhibitor, allopurinol, improves nerve and vascular function in diabetic rats. *Eur J Pharmacol*, *561*, 63-71.

Jin, H. Y., Lee, K. A., Song, S. K., Liu, W. J., Choi, J. H., Song, C. H., Baek, H. S. & Park, T. S. (2012). Sulodexide prevents peripheral nerve damage in streptozotocin induced diabetic rats. *Eur J Pharmacol*, *674*, 217-226.

Jordan, W. R. (1936). Neuritic manifestations in diabetes mellitus. *Arch Intern Med*, *57*, 307–366

Jude, E. B., Abbott, C. A., Young, M. J., Anderson, S. G., Douglas, J. T. & Boulton, A. J. (1998). The potential role of cell adhesion molecules in the pathogens of diabetic neuropathy. *Diabetologia*, *41*, 330–336.

Kapritskaya, Y., Novak, C. & Mackinnon, S. (2002). Prevalence of smoking, obesity, diabetes mellitus and thyroid disease in patients with carpal tunnel syndrome. *Ann PlastSurg*, *48*(3), 269–279.

Knuiman, M., Welborn, T., McCann, V., Stanton, K. & Constable, I. (1986). Prevalence of diabetic complications in relation to risk factors. *Diabetes*, *35*, 1332–1339.

Koski, K., Luukinen, H., Laippala, P. &Kivela, S. L. (1998). Risk factors for major injurious falls among the homedwelling elderly by functional abilities. A prospective population-based study. *Gerontology*,*44*, 232–238.

Lagali, N. S., Allgeier, S. & Guimarães, P. (2017). Reduced corneal nerve fiber density in type 2 diabetes by wide-area mosaic analysis. *Invest Ophthalmol Vis Sci.*, *58*(14), 6318–6327.

Lauretani, F. (2006). Axonal degeneration affects muscle density in older men and women. *Neurobiology of Aging*, *27*, 1145–1154.

Leedman, P. J., Davis, S. & Harrison, L. S. (1988). Diabetic amyotrophy. Reassessment of the clinical spectrum. *Aust.N.Z.J.Med*,*18*, 768–773.

Lindenlaub, T. &Sommer, C. (2003). Cytokines in sural nerve biopsies from inflammatory and non-inflammatory neuropathies. *Acta Neuropathol*, *105*, 593–602.

Liu-Ambrose, T., Khan, K. M., Eng, J. J., Janssen, P. A., Lord, S. R. & McKay, H. A. (2004). Resistance and agility training reduce fall risk in women aged 75 to 85 with low bone mass: a 6-month randomized, controlled trial. *J Am GeriatrSoc*, *52*, 657–665.

Magda, P., Latov, N., Renard, M. V. & Sander, W. H. (2002). Quantitative sensory testing: high sensitivity in small fibre neuropathy with normal NCS/EMG. *J Peripheral NervSyst*, *7*, 225-228.

Malik, R. A., Tesfaye, S., Thompson, S. D.,Veves, A., Sharma, A. K., Boulton, A. J. & Ward, J. D. (1993). Endoneuriallocalisation of microvascular damage in human diabetic neuropathy. *Diabetologia*, *36*, 454-459.

Maty, S. C., Fried, L. P., Volpato, S., Williamson, J., Brancati, F. L. &Blaum, C. S. (2004). Patterns of disability related to diabetes mellitus in older women. *J Gerontol A BiolSci Med Sci*, *59*, 148–153.

Melga, P., Mansi, C. &Ciuchi, E. (1997). Chronic administration of levosulpiride and glycemic control in IDDM patients with gastroparesis. *Diabetes Care*, *20*, 55-58.

Menz, H. B., Lord, S. R., St George, R. & Fitzpatrick, R. C. (2004). Walking stability and sensorimotor function in older people with diabetic peripheral neuropathy. *Arch Phys Med Rehabil*, *85*, 245–252.

Mijnhout, G. S., Alkhalaf, A., Kleefstra, N. &Bilo, H. J. (2010). Alpha lipoic acid: a new treatment for neuropathic pain in patients with diabetes? *Neth J Med*, *68*, 158-162.

Mika, J., Zychowska, M., Popiolek-Barczyk, K., Rojewska, E. &Przewlocka, B. (2013). Importance of glial activation in neuropathic pain. *Eur J Pharmacol*, *716*, 106-119.

Misawa, S., Sakurai, K., Shibuya, K., Isose, S., Kanai, K., Ogino, J., Ishikawa, K. &Kuwabara, S. (2009). Neuropathic pain is associated with increased nodal persistent Na(+) currents in human diabetic neuropathy. *J PeripherNervSyst*, *14*, 279-284.

Morello, C. M., Leckband, S. G., Stoner, C. P., Moorhouse, D. F. &Sahagian, G. A. (1999). Randomized double-blind study comparing the efficacy of gabapentin with amitriptyline on diabetic peripheral neuropathy pain. *Arch Intern Med,159*, 1931–1937.

Nadeau, M., Rosas-Arellano, M. P., Gurr, K. R., Bailey, S. I., Taylor, D. C., Grewal, R., Lawlor, D. K. & Bailey, C. S. (2013). The reliability of differentiating neurogenic claudication from vascular claudication based on symptomatic presentation.*Can J Surg.*, Dec, *56*(6), 372-7.

Nelson, M. E., Fiatarone, M. A., Morganti, C. M., Trice, I., Greenberg, R. A. & Evans, W. J. (1994). Effects of high-intensity strength training on multiple risk factors for osteoporotic fractures. A randomized controlled trial. *JAMA,272*, 1909–1914.

Oates, P. J. (2002). Polyol pathway and diabetic peripheral neuropathy. *Int Rev Neurobiol*, *50*, 325-392.

Obrosova, I. G., Mabley, J. G., Zsengellér, Z., Charniauskaya, T., Abatan, O. I., Groves, J. T. &Szabó, C. (2005). Role for nitrosative stress in diabetic neuropathy: evidence from studies with a peroxynitrite decomposition catalyst. *FASEB J*, *19*, 401-403.

Ozkul, A., Ayhan, M., Yenisey, C., Akyol, A., Guney, E. &Ergin, F. A. (2010). The role of oxidative stress and endothelial injury in diabetic neuropathy and neuropathic pain. *NeuroEndocrinolLett*, *31*, 261-264.

Pirart, J. (1978). Diabetes mellitus and its degenerative complications: a prospective study of 4,400 patients observed between 1947 and 1973. *Diabetes Care,1*, 252–263.

Quattrini, C., Harris, N. D., Malik, R. A. &Tesfaye, S. (2007). Impaired skin microvascular reactivity in painful diabetic neuropathy. *Diabetes Care*, *30*, 655-659.

Rajbhandari, S. M., Jenkins, R. C., Davies, C. &Tesfaye, S. (2002). Charcot neuroarthropathy in diabetes mellitus. *Diabetologia*, *45*, 1085-1096.

Resnick, H. E., Stansberry, K. B., Harris, T. B., Tirivedi, M., Smith, K., Morgan, P. &Vinik, A. I. (2002). Diabetes, peripheral neuropathy, and old age disability. *Muscle Nerve*, *25*, 43–50.

Richardson, J. K., Thies, S. B., DeMott, T. K. & Ashton-Miller, J. A. (2004). A comparison of gait characteristics between older women with and without peripheral neuropathy in standard and challenging environments. *J Am GeriatrSoc*, *52*, 1532–1537.

Rochon, P. A. &Gurwitz, J. H. (1997). Optimising drug treatment for elderly people: the prescribing cascade. *BMJ*,*315*, 1096-1099.

Rogers, L. C., Frykberg, R. G., Armstrong, G., Boulton, A. J. M., Edmonds, M. & Ha Van, G. (2011). The Charcot Foot in Diabetes. *Diabetes Care*, *34*(9), 2123–2129.

Rosenstock, J., Tuchman, M., LaMoreaux, L. & Sharma, U. (2004). Pregabalin for the treatment of painful diabetic peripheral neuropathy: a double-blind, placebo-controlled trial. *Pain*, *110*, 628–638.

Rowe, J. W. & Kahn, R. L. (1987). Human aging: usual and successful. *Science*, *237*, 143-149.

Roy, M. L. & Narahashi, T. (1992). Differential properties of tetrodotoxinsensitive and tetrodotoxin-resistant sodium channels in rat dorsal root ganglion neurons. *J Neurosci*, *12*, 2104-2111.

Ruessmann, H. J. (2009). Switching from pathogenetic treatment with alpha-lipoic acid to gabapentin and other analgesics in painful diabetic neuropathy: a real-world study in outpatients. *J Diabetes Complications*, *23*, 174-177.

Ruhnau, K. J., Meissner, H. P., Finn, R., Reljanovic, M., Lobisch, M., Schutte, K., Nehrdich, D., Tritschler, H., Mehnert, H. & Ziegler, D. (1999). Effects of 3-week oral treatment with the antioxidant thioctic acid (alphalipoic acid) in symptomatic diabetic polyneuropathy. *DiabetMed*,*16*(12), 1040–1043.

Said, G., Slama, G. &Selva, J. (1983). Progressive centripetal degeneration of axons in small fibre diabetic polyneuropathy. *Brain*, *106*, (Pt 4), 791-807.

Salini, D., Harish, K., Minnie, P., Sundram, K. R., Arun, B. & Sandya, C. J. (2018). Prevalence of Charcot Arthropathy in Type 2 Diabetes Patients Aged over 50 Years with Severe Peripheral Neuropathy: A Retrospective Study in a Tertiary Care South Indian Hospital. *Indian J Endocrinol Metab.*, *22*, 107–111.

Sharma, K., Cross, J., Farronay, O., Ayyar, D., Sheber, R. & Bradley, W. (2002). Demyelinating neuropathy in diabetes mellitus. *Arch Neurol*, *59*, 758–765.

Sheetz, M. J. & King, G. L. (2002). Molecular understanding of hyperglycemia's adverse effects for diabetic complications. *JAMA*, *288*, 2579-2588.

Shun, C. T., Chang, Y. C., Wu, H. P., Hsieh, S. C., Lin, W. M., Lin, Y. H., Tai, T. Y. & Hsieh, S. T. (2004). Skin denervation in type 2 diabetes: correlations with diabetic duration and functional impairments. *Brain.*, *127*, 1593-1605.

Sofaer-Bennett, B., Walker, J., Moore, A., Lamberty, J., Thorp, T. & O'Dwyer, J. (2007). The social consequences for older people of neuropathic pain: a qualitative study. *Pain Med*,*8*(3), 263-270.

Stacher, G., Schernthaner, G. & Francesconi, M. l. (1999). Cisapride versus placebo for 8 weeks on glycemic control and gastric emptying in insulin-dependent diabetes: a double blind cross-over trial. *J ClinEndocrinol Metab.*,*84*, 2357-2362.

Steck, A. J. &Kappos, L. (1994). Gangliosides and autoimmune neuropathies: classification and clinical aspects of autoimmune neuropathies. *J Neuro lNeurosurg Psychiatry*,*57*, 26–28.

Stein, P. K., Barzilay, J. I., Domitrovich, P. P., Chaves, P. M., Gottdiener, J. S., Heckbert, S. R. & Kronmal, R. A. (2007). The relationship of heart rate and heart rate variability to non-diabetic fasting glucose levels and the metabolic syndrome: the Cardiovascular Health Study. *Diabet Med*, *24*, 855–863.

Stewart, J. D., Low, P. A. &Fealey, R. D. (1992). Distal small fiber neuropathy: results of tests of sweating and autonomic cardiovascular reflexes. *Muscle Nerve*, *15*, 661-665.

Strotmeyer, E. S., Cauley, J. A., Schwartz, A. V., de, R. N., Resnick, H. E., Zmuda, J. M., Shorr, R. I., Tylavsky, F. A., Vinik, A. I., Harris, T. B. & Newman, A. B. (2006). Reduced peripheral nerve function is related to lower hip BMD and calcaneal QUS in older white and black adults: the Health, Aging, and Body Composition Study. *J Bone Miner Res*, *21*, 1803–1810.

Summer, C. J., Seth, S., Griffin, G. W., Cornbalth, D. R. & Polydefkis, M. (2003). The spectrum of neuropathy in diabetes and impaired glucose intolerance. *Neurology*, *60*, 108-111.

Tang, J., Wingerchuk, D. M., Crum, B. A., Rubin, D. I. & Demaerschalk, B. M. (2007). Alpha-lipoic acid may improve symptomatic diabetic polyneuropathy. *Neurologist*, *13*, 164-167.

Tarride, J. E., Collet, J. P., Choiniere, M., et al. (2006). The economic burden of neuropathic pain in Canada. *J Med Econ*, *9*, 55–68.

Toth, C. C., Jedrzejewski, N. M., Ellis, C. L., Frey, W. H. (2010). Cannabinoidmediated modulation of neuropathic pain and microglial accumulation in a model of murine type I diabetic peripheral neuropathic pain. *Mol Pain*, *6*, 16.

Tuck, R. R., Schmelzer, J. D. & Low, P. A. (1984). Endoneurial blood flow and oxygen tension in the sciatic nerves of rats with experimental diabetic neuropathy. *Brain*, *107*, (Pt 3), 935-950.

Valensi, P., Le, D. C., Richard, J. L., Farez, C., Khodabandehlou, T., Rosenbloom, R. A. & LeFante, C. (2005). A multicenter, double-blind, safety study of QR-333 for the treatment of symptomatic diabetic peripheral neuropathy. A preliminary report. *J Diabetes Complications*, *19*, 247–253.

Valensi, P. (1998). Diabetic autonomic neuropathy: what are the risks? *DiabetsMetab*, *24*, 66-72.

Vareniuk, I., Pavlov, I. A., Drel, V. R., Lyzogubov, V. V., Ilnytska, O., Bell, S. R., Tibrewala, J., Groves, J. T. & Obrosova, I. G. (2007). Nitrosative stress and peripheral diabetic neuropathy in leptin-deficient (ob/ob) mice. *ExpNeurol*, *205*, 425-436.

Vinik, A., Mehrabyan, A., Colen, L. &Boulton, A. (2004). Focal entrapment neuropathies in diabetes. *Diabetes Care*, *27*, 1783–1788.

Vinik, A. I., Holland, M. T., LeBeau, J. M., Liuzzi, F. J., Stansberry, K. B. &Colen, L. B. (1992). Diabetic neuropathies. *Diabetes Care*,*15*, 1926–1975.

Vinik, A. I. & Richardson, D. (1998). Erectile dysfunction in diabetes.*Diabetes Rev*,*6*, 16-33.

Vinik, A. I., Suwanwalaikorn, S., Stansberry, K. B., Holland, M. T., McNitt, P. M. &Colen, L. E. (1995). Quantitative measurement of cutaneous perception in diabetic neuropathy. *Muscle Nerve,18*, 574–584.

Vinik, A. I. & Suwanwalaikorn, S. (1997). Autonomic neuropathy. In: DeFronzo RA, ed. Current Therapy of Diabetes Mellitus. St. Louis, MO: Mosby, 165-176.

Vinik, A. I., Pittenger, G. L., Milicevic, Z. & Cuca, J. (1998). Autoimmune Mechanisms in the Pathogenesis of Diabetic Neuropathy. In: Eisenbarth, RG., editor. *Molecular Mechanisms of Endocrine and Organ Specific Autoimmunity*. Vol. 1st ed. Georgetown: Landes Company., p. 217-251.

Vinik, E. J., Hayes, R. P., Oglesby, A., Bastyr, E., Barlow, P., Ford-Molvik, S. L. &Vinik, A. I. (2005). The development and validation of the Norfolk QOL-DN, a new measure of patients' perception of the effects of diabetes and diabetic neuropathy. *Diabetes TechnolTher*, *7*, 497–508.

Vydyanathan, A., Wu, Z. Z., Chen, S. R. & Pan, H. L. (2005). A-type voltagegated K+ currents influence firing properties of isolectin B4-positive but not isolectin B4-negative primary sensory neurons. *J Neurophysiol*, *93*, 3401-3409.

Wang, X. L., Zhang, H. M., Chen, S. R. & Pan, H. L. (2007). Altered synaptic input and GABAB receptor function in spinal superficial dorsal horn neurons in rats with diabetic neuropathy. *J Physiol*, *579*, 849-861.

Wilbourn, A. J. (1999). Diabetic entrapment and compression neuropathies. In: Dyck, P. J.; Thomas, PK., editors. *Diabetic Neuropathy*. Philadelphia: Saunders, p. 481-508.

Young, M. J., Boulton, A. J. M., MacLeod, A. F., Williams, D. R. R. &Sonksen, P. H. (1993). A multicenter study of the prevalence of diabetic peripheral neuropathy in the United Kingdom hospital clinic population. *Diabetologia,36*, 1–5.

Yu, R. K., Ariga, T., Kohriyama, T., Kusonoki, S., Maeda, Y. &Myatani, N. (1990). Autoimmune mechanisms in peripheral neuropathies. *Ann Neurol,27*, S30–S35.

Zhuang, H. X., Snyder, C. K., Pu, S. F. & Ishii, D. N. (1996). Insulin-like growth factors reverse or arrest diabetic neuropathy: effects on hyperalgesia and impaired nerve regeneration in rats. *ExpNeurol,140*, 198–205.

Ziegler, D., Low, P. A., Litchy, W. J., Boulton, A. J., Vinik, A. I., Freeman, R., Samigullin, R., Tritschler, H., Munzel, U., Maus, J., Schütte, K. &Dyck, P. J. (2011). Efficacy and safety of antioxidant treatment with α-lipoic acid over 4 years in diabetic polyneuropathy: the NATHAN 1 trial. *Diabetes Care*, *34*, 2054-2060.

Ziegler, D., Rathmann, W. & Dickhaus, T. (2008). Prevalence of polyneuropathy in pre-diabetes and diabetes is associated with abdominal obesity and macroangiopathy: the MONICA/KORA Augsburg Surveys S2 and S3. *Diabetes Care*, *31*, 464-469.

Ziegler, D., Schatz, H., Conrad, F., Gries, F. A., Ulrich, H. &Reichel, G. (1997). Effects of treatment with the antioxidant alpha-lipoic acid on cardiac autonomic neuropathy in NIDDM patients. A 4-month randomized controlled multicenter trial (DEKAN Study). Deutsche KardialeAutonomeNeuropathie. *Diabetes Care*, *20*, 369–373.

Zola, B. E. &Vinik, A. I. (1992). Effects of autonomic neuropathy associated with diabetes mellitus on cardiovascular function. *Coron Artery Dis.*, *3*, 33-41.

In: Current Challenges and Management … ISBN: 978-1-53617-304-8
Editor: Abhai Kumar

Chapter 4

Bone Diseases in Elderly Population: Challenges and Management

Yoganchal Mishra[1], Pradeep K. Shukla[2], PhD and Neelam Yadav[1,*], PhD

[1]Department of Biochemistry,
Dr. Rammanohar Lohia Avadh University, Faizabad, India
[2]Department of Physiology, College of Medicine,
University of Tennessee Health Science Centre, Memphis, TN, US

Abstract

Bone diseases are very common in the elderly. As we grow older our bone density decreases. This can lead to bone fracture and other bone diseases. The most common bone disease is osteoporosis, which is caused by thinning of the bone. Osteoporosis is also known as silent disease, because it remains undetected until people fracture their bone.

The second most common bone disease of the elderly is Paget's disease that affects the formation of bones in our body. Osteoarthritis is other common bone disease found in elder population. A significant amount of calcium, phosphorous and vitamin is required for the healthy

[*]Correspondence Author's Email: neelam2k4@gmail.com.

bone formation. Vitamin D plays a crucial role in the absorption of calcium in to the bone. Deficiency of calcium and vitamin D, hormone, lifestyle, and other genetic factors are responsible for defective bone formation and abnormal structure in older adults. This chapter intends to compile all information about bone diseases including osteoporosis, Paget's disease, osteoarthritis and osteomalacia and their challenges and management in the elderly population.

Keywords: osteoporosis, Paget's disease, calcium, osteoarthritis, vitamin D

INTRODUCTION

Aging in human is an inexorable and irreversible process characterized by morphological, functional and biochemical changes in the human body (Pinto et al., 2016). The musculoskeletal system of human body gradually changes and acquires specific structural and morphological characteristics, which mainly include loss of bone, muscle mass and strength (Araújoet al., 2014). In older age, untreated loss of bone mass (osteopenia or osteoporosis), loss of muscle mass and function (sarcopenia) are major health problem for the elderly population. Age related bone diseases osteopenia/osteoporosis and sarcopenia increase the risk of falls and fractures in older people and making them disable and more susceptible for the development of mobility limitations that ultimately affect their capacity for living independent life (Järvinen et al., 2008).

A variety of anatomical and physiological changes occur in advance age of human life (Table 1). These changes allow for the understanding of the pathophysiological differences between the elderly and the rest of the adult population. Muscle mass loss (sarcopenia) is one of the multiple age-related physical changes (Beaudartet al., 2014), which have been associated to the loss of physical activity (Morley et al., 2014). Due to the aging process, muscle mass loss is thought to be related to motor neuron loss in old age people (Dreyet al., 2014). Osteopenia (bone mass loss) is another age related problem, which can further lead to osteoporosis

(Sirolaand Kröger, 2011). The extent of loss in both conditions can be measured by dual energy x-ray absorptiometry (DXA) technique.

Table 1. Physiological and anatomical changes responsible for the bone diseases in elderly population

	Changes	Effects
Bones	Decreased bone mineral content	Osteoporosis Increased fractures and falls
Muscles	Loss of muscle mass Fat infiltration Less type II fibers	Fragility Falls Decreased strength and power
Body	Increased Body Mass Index(BMI) Increased body fat	Increased risk of disease

There are multiple treatment options for bone diseases in elderly population including the use of calcium, vitamin D, hormones and a balanced nutrition; however, physical activity and exercise are most recommended therapeutic approach for bone related disorders (Sirola and Kröger, 2011). The most common bone diseases in elder population are osteoporosis, Paget's disease, osteoarthritis, rheumatoid arthritis and osteomalacia. In this chapter, we discuss the causes, symptoms, pathophysiology, diagnosis and treatment of these major bone diseases of elderly.

TYPES OF BONE DISEASES

Osteoporosis

Osteoporosis is the most common bone disease in elderly (Cosmanet al., 2014), which is caused by the thinning of the bone. Osteoporosis (means- porous bone) is also known as silent disease, because it remains undetected until people factures a bone. The symptom associated with osteoporotic fracture is pain and it depends on the location of the fracture of bone (Kim and Vaccaro, 2006). The incidence of osteoporosis fracture increases with age (Cosmanet al., 2014). Due to advancement in socioeconomic conditions and many health related factors, the number of elder patients living with osteoporosis and the incidence of osteoporotic fractures will increase (Vandenbrouckeet al., 2017). This condition carries significant implications for individuals and society (Burge et al., 2007).

Table 2. Risk factors and complications of Osteoporosis

Risk factors	**Complications**
– Family history of osteoporotic fracture – Increasing age – Gonadal hormone deficiency – Obesity – Excessive alcohol intake (>4 drinks per day for men; >2 drinks per day for women), caffeine intake and tobacco use and smoking – Low calcium or vitamin D intake – Personal history of fracture – Low level of physical activity Information from U.S. Department of Health and Human Services (2004)*	a) Pain and disability- – 10 million Americans 50 years and older have osteoporosis of the hip – 1.5 million Americans have osteoporotic fracture (40% of women and 10% of men will have a fracture of the hip, spine, or wrist) b) Mortality – 10% to 20% increased mortality at one year after a fracture c) Long-term nursing home care – 20% of patients with a fracture Information from National Osteoporosis Foundation (2014)#

*U.S. Department of Health and Human Services. *Bone Health and Osteoporosis: A Report of the Surgeon General.* Rockville, Md.: U.S. Department of Health and Human Services, Office of the Surgeon General; 2004.

#National Osteoporosis Foundation. *Clinician's Guide to Prevention and Treatment of Osteoporosis*. Washington, DC: National Osteoporosis Foundation; 2014.

The main cause of osteoporosis is deficiency of hormones, as estrogen in women and androgen in men. Menopause is a foremost factor in older women, lower estrogen level increases risk for the osteoporosis. The common risk factors for osteoporosis include genetic factor, family history, deficiency of calcium and vitamin D, lack of physical activity, malabsorption, alcohol intake, smoking, low body mass, high-dose oral corticosteroids, and rheumatoid arthritis (Table 2) (Malay et al., 2015). Osteoporosis can be diagnosed by X-ray and bone density measurements; however, early diagnosis involves detection of calcium and vitamin D levels in patients (Guglielmi and Scalzo, 2010). Osteoporosis develops by three mechanism; less bone mass, excessive bone resorption and insufficient new bone formation. Hormones play an important role in control of bone resorption, therefore, lack of estrogen increases bone resorption, also decreasing the deposition of new bones in osteoporosis (Maria and Pedro, 2016). In addition, deficiency of calcium and vitamin D also leads to decreased bone deposition in older age osteoporosis patients. It may be prevented by regular intake of calcium and vitamin D (Moyer, 2013) and bone strengthening drugs alendronate, risedronate and calcitonin, to stop bone loss. Other bone formation drugs such as teriparatide are also helpful in prevention of osteoporosis (Adler et al., 2016).

Paget's Disease

The second most common bone disease of the elderly population is Paget's disease. It affects the formation of bones in the body. Paget disease is a skeletal disorder of bone remodeling that typically begins with excessive bone resorption followed by an increase in bone formation (Bouchette and Baktor, 2019). Subsequently, over a period of time, osteoblastic activity can result in sclerosis and deformation of bone. These new bones may be soft or deformed, which can result in pain and fracture (Ralston et al., 2019). Paget's disease of bone (osteitisdeformans) is generally diagnosed in human older than 50 years and usually manifests in one or several bones (Corral-Gudinoet al., 2013).

In this disease, affected bone is characterized by disorganization of architecture and lamellar pattern of collagen distribution. An increase in the rate of bone resorption at the areas of increased bone remodeling is initial abnormality in Paget's disease. Due to increase in resorption activity, large numbers of osteoblasts are recruited to the remodeling sites, which result in an increase in the amount of new bone formation (Meunieret al., 1980). These osteoblasts form new osteoid tissue very rapidly and it is deposited in a disorganized woven pattern replacing the lamellar pattern found in normal bone remodeling. This new rapidly formed bone is structurally weaker than normal bone and can bow or fracture more easily. In addition, bone marrow becomes infiltrated with an excess of fibrous connective tissue and blood vessels, leading to hyper vascularity in Paget's disease (Lyles et al., 2001).

The most commonly involved bones include skull, vertebrae, pelvis, tibia and femur. Skeletal deformity is hallmark of the Paget's disease, which may manifest as an increase in size and abnormal shape of a bone. Due to rise in skin temperature over the affected bone, the increased vascularity of the surrounding soft tissues and the bones is the characteristic of Paget's disease. Other bones of skull, clavicles, and jaws are also prominent for deformity. Another, important sign of Paget's disease is bone pain, which often develops in later stage of the disease (Singer, 2015).

A variety of symptoms may result from Paget's disease of bone (Table 3). Musculoskeletal and neurological complications (hearing loss) are most common in older age patients with Paget's disease.Complications associated with spinal stenosis are less common; however, cardiac output increases in advance stage of the disease (Haworth, 1953). One report has shown that atherosclerosis, aortic stenosis and intracardiac calcification are more common in older patients (Hultgren, 1998).

Table 3. Impact of Paget's disease of bone

Medical conditions	Impact
Musculoskeletal disorders	Bone deformity, Acetabular protrusion, Bone pain, Fractures, Osteoarthritis
Cardiovascular disorders	Increased cardiac output, Angina and heart failure, Endocardial calcification Aortic stenosis, Atherosclerosis
Neurological disorders	Increased CSF pressure, Hearing Loss, Spinal stenosis, Cranial nerve deficits, Vascular steal syndrome
Metabolic disorders	Hypercalcemia,Nephrolithiasis, Hypercalciuria Hyperuricemia
Neoplastic disorders	Giant cell tumor, osteosarcoma, fibrosarcomachrondrosarcoma

Osteosarcoma and Giant cell tumors of bone occur in less than 1% of patients with Paget's disease (Haibachet al., 1985; Singer and Mills, 1993). These types of bone tumors develop only in the affected pagetic bone. Hypercalcemia and nephrolithiasis are unusual complications; however, hyperuricemia is sometimes, seen in Paget's disease patients (Kanis, 1991).

Osteoarthritis and Rheumatoid Arthritis

Two other common diseases found in elderly population are osteoarthritis (OA) and rheumatoid arthritis. The majority of seniors over the age of 75 have osteoarthritis in at least one joint. It occurs when cartilage at the ends of the bones wears down and restricts the bones movement. On the other hand, rheumatoid arthritis is caused by inflammation of the joints and similar to osteoarthritis, can be very painful.

Osteoarthritis (OA) is the most common joint disease and major cause of disability in people aged >65 years. OA is a chronic arthropathy, affects joints including cartilage, ligaments, joint lining and underline bones. In this disease, osteophyte formation (bone spurs); cartilage loss subchondral bone sclerosis leads to pain, disability and reduction in quality of life (Glyn-Jones et al., 2015). The common risk factors for OA are genetics, obesity, joint injury and anatomical abnormalities in the elderly population. Structural changes in OA patients include narrowing of the joint space, osteophyte formation, and bone remodeling around the joints can be visualized by radiography. This disease is most common in the knees, hips, hands and spine, but it can arise in any synovial joint of the body in elder people (Glyn-Jones et al., 2015).

Osteomalacia

Osteomalacia is a common metabolic disease, characterized by a deficient mineralization of bone without a loss in bone matrix. It is a condition associated with increased bone fragility, bone pain, and fractures (Ralston and McInnes, 2014). The word osteomalacia means soft bones (osteo - bone, malacia- soft). It is a failure to mineralize the newly formed organic matrix (osteoid) of bone. The softening of the bones occurs due to deficiency of vitamin D (Cardinal and Gregory, 2009). Common reasons of deficiencyinclude limitedexposure to sunlight, abnormalities in vitamin D metabolism, malnutrition, low levels of phosphate (hypophosphataemia) and drug-induced inhibition of bone mineralization (Ralston and McInnes, 2014). Due to the reduced ability of the skin to synthesize vitamin D and reduced synthesis in the kidney, older age people are at the higher risk (Kinyamuet al., 1997).

Second cause of osteomalacia is direct inhibition of mineralization of bone. This may be due to use of bisphosphonates to treat osteoporosis and Paget's disease of the bone, excessive use of fluoride or aluminum intoxication often associated with patients who have chronic renal failure and are undergoing dialysis and taking phosphate binding drugs (Ralston and McInnes, 2014).

Vitamin D deficiency is a common problem in the older population having darker skin pigmentation (Cardinal and Gregory, 2009). It is also more prevalent in obese people (Cardinal and Gregory, 2009). Due to deficiency of calcium and vitamin D, muscle cramps, numbness and tingling in legs may occur in osteomalacia. Early symptoms of osteomalacia may be non-specific such as bone and joint pain, especially in lower back, hips, and legs at night, persistent fatigue and tenderness, however, at the later stage muscles may become weak and stiff, which can make many activities difficult in elderly population.

Aging and Bone Loss

Bone mass loss (osteopenia) often progresses to osteoporosis, a condition characterized by the reduced bone mineral density and increased rate of bone loss (Sirola and Kröger, 2011). Bone mineral density decreases with age. Therefore, the probability of suffering from osteopenia or osteoporosis and related skeletal fragility increases (Sirola and Kröger, 2011).

Treatment and Management of Bone Diseases

Bone loss and natural aging are associated with each other, but neither was defined in the pathological term. Human population with aging is significantly affected by bone loss (Vanden brouckeet al., 2017). There is an urgent need to understand the systemic management of bone loss with increasing age. Here, we are focusing on three main known bone diseases - osteoporosis, Paget's disease and rheumatoid arthritis, in which aging is considered as an augmenting factor.

Osteoporosis

The National Osteoporosis Foundation (NOF) recommends treatment of men and postmenopausal women with a personal history of hip or vertebral fracture, in which T-score of −2.5 or less, or a combination of low bone mass with a T-score between −1 and −2.5 range. Moreover, a 10-year probability of hip fracture of at least 3%, or any major fracture of at least 20%, is calculated by the FRAX, a Fracture Risk Assessment Tool (Cosmanet al., 2014). The World Health Organization's (WHO) recommendations are less specific (Jeremiah et al., 2015), stating that people with osteoporosis or at its risk should be considered for treatment. Randomized controlled trials of treatment have shown reduction of fractures for only two groups: those with a T-score of less than –2.5 and those who have already experienced a hip or vertebral fracture (Unnanuntanaet al., 2010). Fragility fracture is a known symptom of osteoporosis, but low bone mass density (BMD) can also be used as a marker before and for the fragility fracture (Kling et al., 2014; Report, 2014). Dual-energy X-ray Absorptiometry (DXA) is a known standard test, which is frequently used for diagnosis in people without an osteoporotic fracture.

Various pharmacological agents including bisphosphonates (alendronate, risedronate, ibandronate, zoledronic acid), peptide hormones (teriparatide [the 1,3,4 amino acid fragment of parathyroid hormone] and calcitonin), estrogen (in the form of menopausal hormone therapy), and selective estrogen receptor modulators (raloxifene for postmenopausal women) have been used for the treatment of osteoporosis (Amizukaet al., 2009; Tuet al., 2018; Wang et al., 2019). Main aim of using these pharmacological agents is to prevent bone resorption. New biologic agent (Denosumab), dietary calcium and vitamin D supplements are also commonly used for the osteoporosis treatment (Saito et al., 2019; Souberbielleet al., 2019). Recently, U.S. Food and Drug Administration (FDA) approved a selective estrogen receptor modulator (Bazedoxifene) with conjugated estrogen for the prevention of osteoporosis (Yavropoulouet al., 2019).

Paget's Disease

Paget's disease is a second most common bone disease after osteoporosis that is mostly seen in old population. Studies report that 2-5% people aged 50 years and older, and 10% of those aged 80 years and older are affected. Usually, it is diagnosed at the age of 58. It involves a dysfunction of osteoclasts that causes rapid bone remodeling, resulting in disorganization, expansion, and distortion of the architectural structure of bones. It is usually diagnosed by the X-rays or by the elevated alkaline phosphatase level. Paget's disease is often asymptomatic (in 80-90% of cases), but when symptoms appear, localized pain is noticed. With increasing age, there is an increase in prevalence of Paget's disease, which shows male predominance and affects femur, pelvis, spine, and skull. Bone deformities and fractures can complicate the disease's condition. Pharmacological agents are used to 1) reduce pain and inflammation, 2) reduce the amount of bone turnover. NSAIDs and Bisphosphonates, which inhibit excessive bone loss, are frequently used for Paget's disease management based on history, symptoms and severity. A potent bisphosphonate zoledronic acid (intravenously) and alendronate and risendronate (orally) are also being used to treat disease symptoms. Intranasal calcitonin is an alternative option for Paget's disease patients, who want to avoid oral or intravenous injection of bisphosphonates. Surgery is another option to clear bone deformity, fractures, neurologic dysfunction (abnormal narrowing in the spinal canal) and degenerative joint disease or malignant transformation to sarcoma. Physical therapy, exercise, and muscle strengthening program provide beneficial effects along with medications (Kravetset al., 2018; Winter et al., 2016).

Rheumatoid Arthritis

Rheumatoid arthritis (RA) is a chronic progressive inflammatory disease of the synovial joints and has strong association with age. The prevalence of RA is more in old age population. Chronic RA affects 2-3% of general population. Almost one-third of RA patients are more than 60 years of age, and also, elderly patients with RA are at particular risk for other diseases including cardiovascular, neoplastic and infectious complications (Cauduroet al., 2006). Additionally, RA in the elderly may have different clinical and biological features, with different responses to the treatment. There is no cure for RA, but clinical studies showed that the pharmacological agents are able to provide benefits by modifying disease symptoms (disease modifying therapy). Medication is recommended based on the symptoms and duration of the disease (Englbrechtet al., 2019; Cioffiet al., 2016).

Nonsteroidal anti-inflammatory drugs (NSAIDs) can reduce pain and decrease inflammation. Over-the-counter NSAIDs include ibuprofen and naproxen sodium. Major side effects associated with NSAIDs are stomach irritation, heart problems and kidney damage. Majority of old population suffering from RA has secondary disease complications, which limit the use of NSAIDs. Steroids such as prednisone are also frequently used for RA management by reducing inflammation, pain and joint damage. Clinicians often prescribe a corticosteroid to reduce acute clinical symptoms with the goal of gradually narrowing off the medication. Number of side effects including thinning of bones, weight gain and diabetes are associated with steroid treatment in RA patients. Disease-modifying anti-rheumatic drugs (DMARDs) are also being used for RA treatment. These drugs can slow the progression of rheumatoid arthritis, and save the joints and other tissues from permanent damage. Common DMARDs include methotrexate, leflunomide, hydroxychloroquine, and sulfasalazine. DMARDs also have different side effects including liver damage, bone marrow suppression and severe lung infections, which limit the beneficial effects in RA patients (Kilcheret al., 2018; Gualtierottiet al., 2018; Abbasiet al., 2019; Bazzichiet al., 2019).

Recent studies showed that number of biological agents, also known as biologic response modifiers have beneficial effects. These new DMARDs include abatacept, adalimumab, anakinra, baricitinib, certolizumab, etanercept, golimumab, infliximab, rituximab, sarilumab, tocilizumab and tofacitinib. These drugs can target parts of the immune system that illicit inflammation and causes joint and tissue damage. These types of drugs also increase the risk of infections. In people with rheumatoid arthritis, higher doses of tofacitinib can increase the risk of blood clots in the lungs. Biologic DMARDs are usually most effective when paired with a nonbiologic DMARD, such as methotrexate (Smolenet al., 2014; Drugs, 2018).

Adequate calcium and vitamin D supplementation have long been identified as essential nutrients to maintain bone health and calcium homeostasis as well. Studies show that calcium and vitamin D therapy along with pharmacological treatments of bone diseases like osteoporosis; Paget's disease; RA; and osteoarthritis plays a potential role in the management of these and similar bone diseases (Hwang, 2019; Suzuki et al., 2019; Polyzoset al., 2011).

CONCLUSION AND FUTURE PERSPECTIVE

Bone diseases are very common in the elderly population. Vitamin D is imperative for strong bones, produced by the body when it is exposed to sunlight. This sunshine vitamin supports the body to use calcium from the food. Typically, its deficiency causes rickets, a skeletal disorder that affects children and adults both. But, any aged person who does not have frequent exposure to sunlight, or suffering from milk allergies or follows vegan diet strictly, is at risk of vitamin D deficiency too. Also, it is common among the people over age 50 and risk increases with the increasing age. Inadequacy of vitamin D promotes low bone density, increased risk of developing osteoporosis, risk of fracture and secondary hyperparathyroidism. By rectification of vitamin D deficiency, skeletal health can be maintained and risk of osteoporosis and other bone diseases can be reduced. Although, the vital role of vitamin D in bone health and calcium homeostasis has been shown, a complete mechanism of occurrence of skeletal diseases, contributed by vitamin deficiency is not known yet. Next-generation sequencing (NGS), next next-generation sequencing and other biomedical technologies are achieving their new heights. With the advancement in these technologies, the genomic insights, about the factors involved in vitamin D regulating genes and age-related changes in epigenetic regulation of vitamin D receptor (VDR) functioning and co-activator proteins, would be able to elucidate significant understanding about dysfunctions of calcium homeostasis with increasing age. These genomic studies will discover vitamin D target genes as biomarkers for the potential pharmacological interventions to maintain calcium homeostasis with increasing age.

REFERENCES

Abbasi, M. Mousavi, M. J., Jamalzehi, S., Alimohammadi, R., Bezvan, M. H., et al., (2019). Strategies toward rheumatoid arthritis therapy; the old and the new. *J Cell Physiol* 234: 10018-10031.

Adler, A., El-Hajj F. and Ghada B. (2016). Managing osteoporosis inpatients on long-term bisphosphonate treatment: Report of atask force of the American Society for Bone and Mineral *Research. J Bone Miner Res* 31: 16-35.

Amizuka, N., Li, M., Tamura, M. and Oda, K. (2009). Hormones and osteoporosis update. Histological aspects on the action of parathyroid hormone (PTH) and PTH-related peptide (PTHrP) on bone and cartilage. *Clin Calcium* 19: 935-943.

Araújo, A. P., Bertolini, S. M. M. G. and Junior J. M. (2014). Morpho-physiologial alterations resulted from the process of musculoskeletal system aging and its consequences for the human body. *Perspectivas: biológicas e saúde.* 4:22–34.

Bazzichi, L., Nacci, F., Sinigaglia, L., Bianchino, L. and Caporali R. (2019). Subcutaneous tocilizumab alone or with a csDMARD in rheumatoid arthritis patients: subanalysis of Italian data from a multicenter phase IIIb/IV trial. *Clin Rheumatol* 38: 841-849.

Beaudart, C., Reginster, J. Y., Slomian, J., Buckinx, F., Locquet, M. and Bruyère, O. (2014). Prevalence of sarcopenia: the impact of different diagnostic cut-off limits. *J Musculoskelet Neuronal Interact.* 14(4): 425–31.

Bouchette, P.and Baktor, S. W. (2019). Paget Disease.*StatPearls (Internet),*25(2): e34-e39.

Burge, R., Dawson-Hughes, B., Solomon, D. H., Wong, J. B., King A. and Tosteson A. (2007). Incidence and economic burden of osteoporosis-related fractures in the United States, 2005-2025.*J Bone Miner Res* 22(3): 465-475.

Cardinal, R. and Gregory C. (2009). Osteomalacia and vitamin D deficiency in a psychiatric rehabilitation unit: case report and survey. *BMC Research Notes* 2: 82.

Cauduro, S. A., Moder, K. G., Luthra, H. S. and Seward, J. B. (2006). Echocardiographically guided pericardiocentesis for treatment of clinically significant pericardial effusion in rheumatoid arthritis. *J Rheumatol* 33: 2173-2177.

Cioffi, G. Viapiana, O., Ognibeni, F., Dalbeni, A., Orsolini, G., Adami, S., et al., (2016). Clinical profile and outcome of patients with rheumatoid arthritis and abnormally high aortic stiffness. *Eur J PrevCardiol,* 23: 1848-1859.

Corral-Gudino, L., Borao-Cengotita-Bengoa, M., Del Pino-Montes, J. and Ralston, S. (2013). Epidemiology of Paget's disease of bone: a systematic review and meta-analysis of secular changes. *Bone* 55: 347–352.

Cosman, F., deBeur, S. J., LeBoff, M.S., Lewiecki, E.M., Tanner, B., Randall, S. et al., (2014). Clinician's Guide to Prevention and Treatment of Osteoporosis. *Osteoporos Int* 25: 2359-2381.

Drey, M., Krieger, B., Sieber, C. C. et al., (2014). Motoneuron loss is associated with sarcopenia. J *Am Med Dir Assoc.* 15(6):435–39.

Drugs for rheumatoid arthritis. (2018). *Med Lett Drugs Ther* 60 (1552): 123-128.

Englbrecht, M. Alten, R., Aringer, M., Baewald, C. G., Burlhardt, H., Eby, N. et al., (2019). New insights into the prevalence of depressive symptoms and depression in rheumatoid arthritis - Implications from the prospective multicenter VADERA II study. *PLoS One,* 14: e0217 412.

Glyn-Jones, S., Palmer, A. J., Agricola, R., Price, A. J. Vincent, T. L. et al., (2015). Osteoarthritis. *Lancet* 386 (9991): 376-87.

Gualtierotti, R., Parisi, M. and Ingegnoli F. (2018). Perioperative Management of Patients with Inflammatory Rheumatic Diseases Undergoing Major Orthopaedic Surgery: A Practical Overview. *AdvTher* 35: 439-456.

Guglielmi, G. and Scalzo, G. (2010) Imaging tools transform diagnosisof osteoporosis. *DiagnosImagEur* 26: 7-11.

Haibach, H., Farrell, C. and Dittrich, F. J. (1985) Neoplasms arising in Paget's disease of bone: A study of 82 cases. *Am J ClinPathol* 83:594–600.

Haworth, S. (1953). Cardiac output in osteitisdeformans. *Clin Sci.* 12:271–275.

Hultgren, H. N. (1998). Osteitisdeformans (Paget's disease) and calcific disease of the heart valves. *Am J Cardiol* 81:1461–1464.

Hwang, S. W. (2019). Can vitamin D supplementation help control inflammation in inflammatory bowel disease beyond its classical role in bone health? *Intest Res* 17: 157-159.

In Bone Health and Osteoporosis: A Report of the Surgeon General Reports of the Surgeon General (2004).

Järvinen, T. L., Sievänen, H. and Khan, K. M., Heinonen, A. and Kannus, P. (2008). Shifting the focus in fracture prevention from osteoporosis to falls. *BMJ* 336 (7636):124–126.

Jeremiah, M. P., Unwin, B. K., Greenawald, M. H. and Casiano V. E. (2015). Diagnosis and Management of Osteoporosis. *Am Fam Physician* 92: 261-268.

Kanis, J. A. (1991). Radiological features. In: Kanis JA (ed.) Pathophysiologyand Treatment of Paget's Disease of Bone. MartinDunitz, London, UK, pp. 41–88.

Kilcher, G. Hummel, N., Didden, E. M., Egger, M. and Reichenbach, S. (2018). Rheumatoid arthritis patients treated in trial and real world settings: comparison of randomized trials with registries. *Rheumatology (Oxford)* 57: 354-369.

Kim, D. and Vaccaro, A. (2006). Osteoporotic compression fractures of the spine; current options and considerations fortreatment. *Spine J* 6: 479-487.

Kinyamu, H., Gallagher, J., Balhorn, K. et al., (1997). Serum vitamin D metabolites and calcium absorption in normal young and elderly free-living women and in women living in nursing homes. *American Journal of Clinical Nutrition* 65 (3): 790-797.

Kling, J. M., Clarke, B. L. andSandhu, N. P. (2014). Osteoporosis prevention, screening, and treatment: a review. *J Womens Health (Larchmt)* 23: 563-572.

Kravets, I. (2018). Paget's disease of Bone: Diagnosis and Treatment. *Am J Med* 131: 1298-1303.

Lyles, K.W., Siris, E. S., Singer, F. R. and Meunier P. J. (2001). A Clinical Approach to Diagnosis and Management of Paget's Disease of Bone. *J of bone and Mineral Res.* 16 (8): 1379-1387.

Malay, S., Rajeev, B. and Irappa, M. (2015). Osteoporosis in chronicobstructive pulmonary disease. *Clin Med Insights Circ Respir Pulm Med* 9: 5-21.

Maria, H. and Pedro, G. (2016) Bone cells dynamics during periimplantitis: A theoretical analysis. *J Oral Maxillofac Res* 7: e6.

Meunier, P. J, Coindre J., Edouard C. M. and Arlot M.E. (1980). Bonehistomorphometry in Paget's disease: Quantitative and dynamic-analysis of pagetic and non-pagetic bone tissue. *Arthritis Rheum* 23**:** 1095–1103.

Miljkovic, N., Lim, J.Y., Miljkovic, I. and Frontera, W. R. (2015). Aging of skeletal muscle fibers. *Ann Rehabil Med.* 39(2):155–62.

Morley, J. E., Anker, S. D. and Von haehling S. (2014). Prevalence, incidence, and clinical impact of sarcopenia: facts, numbers, and epidemiology-update. *J Cachexia Sarcopenia Muscle*. 5(4):253–59.

Moyer, V. (2013). Vitamin D and calcium supplementation to prevent fractures in adults: U.S. preventive services task force recommendation statement. *Ann Intern Med* 158: 691-696.

National Osteoporosis Foundation. (2014). *Clinician's Guide to Prevention and Treatment of Osteoporosis*. Washington, DC: National Osteoporosis Foundation.

Pinto, C. L., Botelho, P. B., Carneiro, J. A. and Mota, J. F. (2016). Impact of creatine supplementation in combination with resistance training on lean mass in the elderly. *J Cachexia Sarcopenia Muscle*. 7(4):413– 21.

Polyzos, S. A., Anastasilakis, A. D., Makras, P. and Terpos, E. (2011). Paget's disease of bone and calcium homeostasis: focus on bisphosphonate treatment. *Exp Clin Endocrinol Diabetes* 119: 519-524.

Ralston, S. H., Corral-Gudino, L., Cooper, C., Francis, R. M., Fraser, W. D., Gennari L. et al., (2019). Diagnosis and Management of Paget's Disease of Bone in Adults: A Clinical Guideline. *J. Bone Miner. Res.*Feb 25: e3657.

Ralston, S., McInnes, I. (2014). Rheumatology and bone disease. In Walker B., Colledge, N., Ralston S. et al., *(Eds)* Davidson's Principles and Practice of Medicine. 22nd edition. Churchill Livingstone Elsevier, Edinburgh.

Saito, S. Sugo, Y., Tsuburai, T., Kurasawa, K., Nakamura, T., Yoshikata, H. et al., (2019). Activated vitamin D3 formulations can be safely used as concomitant medication for prevention of denosumab-induced hypocalcemia in women with postmenopausal osteoporosis. *J Obstet Gynaecol Res* 45: 908-914.

Singer, F. R. (2015). Paget's disease of bone-genetic and environmental factors. *Nat Rev Endocrinol* 11: 662-671.

Singer, F. R. and Mills, B. G. (1993). Giant cell tumor arising in Paget's disease of bone. Recurrences after 36 years. *ClinOrthop*293: 293–301.

Sirola, J. and Kröger, H. (2011). Similarities in acquired factors related to postmenopausal osteoporosis and sarcopenia. *J Osteoporos*. 536735: 1-14.

Smolen, J. S., van der Heijde, D., Machold, K. P., Aletaha, D. and Landewe, R. (2014). Proposal for a new nomenclature of disease-modifying antirheumatic drugs. *Ann Rheum Dis* 73: 3-5.

Souberbielle, J. C., Cormier, C., Cavalier, E., Breuil, V, Debiais, F, Fardellone, P. et al., (2019). Vitamin D Supplementation in France in patients with or at risk for osteoporosis: Recent data and new practices. *Joint Bone Spine,* S1297-319X (19): 30067-3.

Suzuki, T., Nakamura, Y. and Kato H. (2019). Calcium and vitamin D supplementation with 3-year denosumab treatment is beneficial to enhance bone mineral density in postmenopausal patients with osteoporosis and rheumatoid arthritis. *TherClin Risk Manag* 15: 15-22.

Tu, K. N., Lie, J. D. Victoria Wan, C. K. Cameron M., Austel, A. G. et al., (2018). Osteoporosis: A Review of Treatment Options. *P & T* 43: 92-104.

U.S. Department of Health and Human Services. (2004). *Bone Health and Osteoporosis: A Report of the Surgeon General.* Rockville, Md.: U.S. Department of Health and Human Services, Office of the Surgeon General.

Unnanuntana, A., Gladnick, B. P., Donnelly, E. and Lane, J. M. (2010). The assessment of fracture risk. *J Bone Joint Surg Am* 92: 743-753.

Vandenbroucke, A., Luyten, F. P., Flamaing, J. and Gielen E. (2017). Pharmacological treatment of osteoporosis in the oldest old. *ClinInterv Aging* 12: 1065-1077.

Wang, Q. Yao, L., Xu, K., Jin, H., Chen, K., Wang, Z. et al., (2019). Madecassoside inhibits estrogen deficiency-induced osteoporosis by suppressing RANKL-induced osteoclastogenesis. *J Cell Mol Med* 23: 380-394.

Winter, E. M., Hamdy, N. A., deJonge, R. T., Eekhoff, E. M., Zillikens, M. C. and Appelman-Dijkstra, N. M. (2016). Paget's disease of bone: diagnosis and treatment. *Ned TijdschrGeneeskd* 160: D254.

Yavropoulou, M. P., Makras, P. and Anastasilakis, A. D. (2019). Bazedoxifene for the treatment of osteoporosis. *Expert Opin Pharmacother,* 20: 1201-1210.

In: Current Challenges and Management … ISBN: 978-1-53617-304-8
Editor: Abhai Kumar

Chapter 5

Osteoporosis in Female: Strategies for Prevention, Promotion, and Restoration of Bone Health

Vivek Dixit PhD[1,*], James Pegrum[2,†], Bhavuk Garg[1,‡], Nishank Mehta[1], Vijay Kumar[3§], Dinesh K Dhanwal[4] and Rajesh Malhotra[1]

[1]Department of Orthopaedics, All India Institute of Medical Sciences, New Delhi, India

[2]Nuffield Orthopaedics Centre, NHS Trust, Oxford University Hospitals, Oxford, UK

[3]Department of Geriatric Medicine, All India Institute of Medical Sciences, New Delhi,

[4]NMC Specialty Hospital, Abu Dhabi, UAE

---

* Corresponding Author's Email: vivek_sgpgi@yahoo.com.

Dr. Vivek Dixit Research Scientist-III, Department of Orthopaedics, All India Institute of Medical Sciences, New Delhi, India.

† James Pergum MBBS

‡ Bhavuk Garg MS

§ Nishank Mehta MS

ABSTRACT

Preservation of bone health is necessary for women. Due to increase in life expectancy in India, the age related metabolic bone diseases such as osteoporosis are increasing rapidly too. Osteoporosis is a skeletal disorder in which the bone becomes fragile and susceptible to fractures and is manifested as a myriad of signs and symptoms consecutively. Although, osteoporosis is common in both men and women but in women, it is conceptually linked to menopause and therefore it is imperative that monitoring and treatment should be performed timely in order to maintain bone health of almost 50% of the population. Postmenopausal women are at increased risk of cardiovascular disease (CVD), cancer and diabetes due to declining levels of intracellular oestrogen and its receptors, which results in postmenopausal syndrome and vitamin D deficiency. Over last two decades, vitamin D deficiency (VDD) is being increasingly recognized as a major health issue, particularly for women. Postmenopausal women are more susceptible to vitamin D deficiency due to the dependency of the vitamin D receptor (VDR) on oestrogen. Vitamin D deficiency may be further exacerbated by lifestyle changes resulting in limited sunlight exposure. The influence of Vitamin D insufficiency in osteoporosis will be discussed later in this review. Several studies show that vitamin D renders an important role on both physical and mental wellbeing. Vitamin D deficiency was found to be associated with muscle weakness, handgrip strength, falls, depressed mood, CVD, cancer, cognitive impairment and dementia. There is encouraging evidence that treatment of vitamin D insufficiency may provide a simple, cost-effective modality for management and prevention of these post-menopausal health conditions. Therefore, Vitamin D supplementation is one of the most important and cost effective modalities that can be implemented to prevent osteoporosis. In recent years, literature from the west has also addressed the poor bone health status amongst females with a special emphasis to the Asian population.

Keywords: vitamin D deficiency (VDD), parathyroid hormone (PTH), bone mineral density (BMD)

1. INTRODUCTION

Preservation of bone health is important for women as bone health is linked to physiological changes. Besides other risk factors, several hormones play a major role in maintenance of bone health and any alteration in hormones leads to osteopenia and consequently osteoporosis. Worldwide, osteoporosis is a significant health problem (WHO, 2003). World Health Organisation (WHO) describes osteoporosis by comparing bone mineral density (BMD) with the average BMD of a young person i.e., T-score <–2.5. It is estimated that more than 75 million people are affected by osteoporosis in USA, Europe and Japan. Additionally, the economic burden for osteoporotic fractures constitutes 2.8 million disability-adjusted life years (DALYs) annually in the USA and Europe alone (Kanis JA, 2000). Osteoporosis prevalence varies from 5% to 50% among women aged between 50-85 years of age and the comparable figures among men and women are 2.4% and 20% respectively (Kanis JA, 2000). The prevalence of osteoporosis among Indian women ranges from 8 to 62% (Anuradha V K, 2015).

One of the key concerns with managing osteoporosis is to reduce fracture burden. Osteoporotic fractures can result in serious complications with chronic pain, loss of independence and particularly in the geriatric age group, is potentially life threatening. Worldwide, around 9 million osteoporotic fractures occur every year with more than 4.5 million occurring in the USA and Europe alone whereas in developing countries, the estimated risk for a hip, wrist and vertebral fracture are seen in the order of 30-40% over lifetime (Cooper C, 1992).

Osteoporosis is a silent disease because it progresses without symptoms. It involves the gradual loss of bone tissue or bone density and results in bones so fragile that they break under the slightest strain and thus often may be under diagnosed and under treated due to unavailability of an expert especially in community-based primary healthcare setups. People are often unaware of the frequent link between a broken bone and osteoporosis. The commonest osteoporotic fracture sites are proximal femur, vertebral, and distal forearm. Therefore, it is important for all women aged above 65 to be carefully screened for osteoporosis (WHO, 2003). However, young postmenopausal women are also at risk and thus, screening in the younger age groups may also be advocated. The diagnosis following an osteoporotic fracture results in increased morbidity and mortality and is considered too late (Johnell, O, 2004). The 10 year and lifetime risk of sustaining an osteoporotic fracture alongside potential risk factors are summarized in Table 1.

Table 1. Lifetime risk of Osteoporotic fracture (WHO, 2003)

Risk of fractures in Women & Men	Current age (years)			
	50	60	70	80
Lifetime risk				
Men	20.7	14.7	11.4	9.6
Women	53.2	45.5	36.9	28.6
10-year risk				
Men	7.1	5.7	6.2	8.0
Women	9.8	13.3	17.0	21.7

2. Classification of Osteoporosis

There are basically two types of osteoporosis i.e., Type I and type II. Type I refer as postmenopausal osteoporosis and generally develops in women after menopause due to decrease or no production of estrogen in the body. Since estrogen works as protector of bone health and thus its deficiency leads to an increase in the resorption of bone (the bones loses substance). The type II osteoporosis generally occurs in 7th decade of life and affects both trabacular and cortical bones. The other type is disease and drug related osteoporosis where certain disease & drugs such as Drugs for the cancer therapy, epilepsy, blood pressure medication, mood altering drugs and excessive hormonal therapy (Table 2). Apart from all these factors, the occurrence of osteoporosis or low BMD is broadly depends genetically. Genes play a major role in bone metabolism. Certain mutations in candidate genes which are responsible for the regulation for bone mineral homeostasis may alter the bone metabolism further creates an imbalance between bone formation and bone resorption.

3. Bone Metabolism

Bone mineral homeostasis plays an important phenomenon under bone metabolism where bone resorption and bone formation takes place. In elderly female the resorption exceeds the formation. The amount of bone loss is referred as bone turnover (Seeman E., 2003).

Among all the major factors which lead to bone loss in elderly the most important one appears to be gonadal sex hormone deficiency. Genetic and biochemical factors play major role in sex hormone deficiency. Vitamin D deficiency (VDD)/hyperparathyroidism which triggers bone loss (Labrie F, 2010). These conditions inversely affect and mitigate peak bone mass and further result in bone loss. It is an established fact that the trabecular bone loss starts around 30 years of age, before gonadal sex steroid deficiency develops, whereas cortical bone loss typically follows menopause which begins around 60 years of age. (Seeman E., 2003), (Labrie F, 2010).

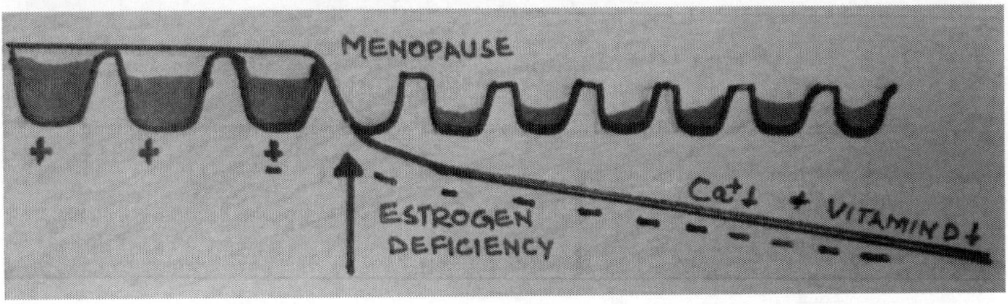

Figure 1. Pathophysiology of bone loss in women.

Oestrogen deficiency after menopause results in accelerated bone resorption and negatively affects bone density which contrasts with the gradual decline in BMD seen in men (Figure 1), (Matsushita H, 2015). Anti-resorptive agents work as catabolic agents for the treatment of osteoporosis primarily by mitigating osteoclast cells whereas teriparatide which is an osteoanabolic agent stimulates osteoblast cells in order to form a new bone (Labrie F, 2010), (Matsushita H, 2015). The current research & development is focused on such new compounds which can stimulate bone formation than resorption for the treatment of osteoporosis (Table 3).

Table 2. Types of Osteoporosis

Types of Osteoporosis	Description
Type 1	Occurs between 55-75 yrs & affects trabecular bone
Type II	(Senile or age related osteoporosis) Occurs after 70 yrs of age and affects both cortical & trabecular bone
Secondary Osteoporosis	Disease or drug related
Genetic factors	up to 85% of the variance in BMD are determined genetically

Table 3. Treatment currently available for osteoporosis

Anti-resorptive therapies	Anabolic therapies
Bisphosphonates	Teriparatide (1-34 fragment of PTH) Daily subcutaneous injections)
Alendronate	Strontium renelate (mechanism Unclear)
Residronate	
Ibandronate	
Zoledronic acid (Annual intravenous Injection)	
Reloxifene	
Calcitonin (daily nasel spray or subcutaneous injection)	
Estrogen replacement therapy (women)	
Ipriflavone	
Denosumab (6 monthly subcutaneous Injection)	

3.1. Modeling and Remodeling of Bone

Bone growth occurs as a result of modeling in which renewal of bone substance and change in size and shape of bone takes place whereas bone health is maintained by remodeling in which replacement of old bone with new bone (stress damage, microfractures, etc.), maintenance of mechanical strength (replacement of fatigued bone, prevention of excessive aging, supply of bone marrow with growth factors and mineral homeostasis (calcium release) takes place (Garg B, 2018). (Figure 2)

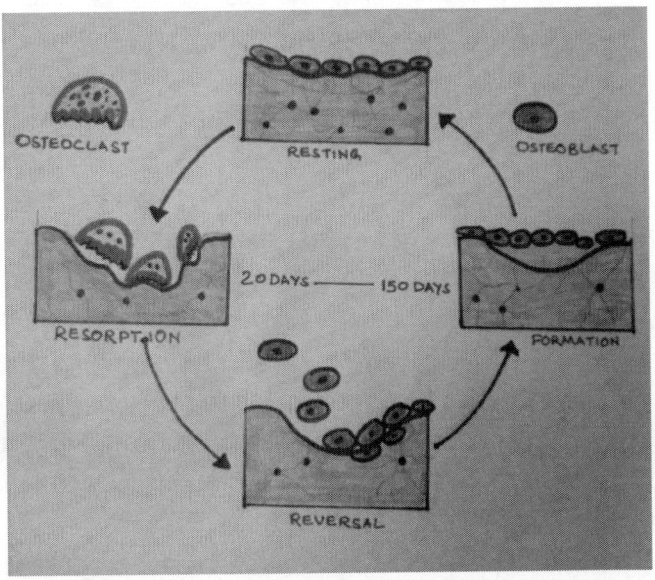

Figure 2. Bone remodeling cycle.

4. Genetic Factors

Genetic factors constitute a major role in the occurrence of osteoporosis. Genes play an important role as reflected by heritability of many components of bone strength. This hypothesis has also been strongly supported by the findings of the scientific group conducted a genome-wide association studies (GWAS) where small effects (Single nucleotide polymorphism-SNP) from dozens of common variants in or closely associated genes were observed (Ralston, 2010). With regard to genetic association of osteoporosis, studies have noted SNPs difference in the genetic code (unlike mutation) that is not always a basis of disease but it determines the heterogeneity of physical phenotypes among individuals and may have a role to play in the development of a disease (Vupputuri MR, Goswami R, 2006). The commonest (idiopathic) osteoporosis carries a strong heritable component however it is not communicated according to Mendelian law of inheritance as a single gene disorder. Therefore, SNPs contribute only a few percentages to the genetic risk of osteoporosis in populations and can be better understood by gene-environment interactions (Ferrari S., 2008). Genome wide association studies (GWAS) analysed thousands of SNPs in each individual and identified genes associated with osteoporosis (VDR, SOST, ESRI, COL1A1, COL1A2, LRP5, TFGb, TNFRSF11b, TNSF11, MHC and 1p36). However, GWAS analysis further suggests that many other genes are implicated which still require replication (Garnero P, 2005).

Cohort studies shown that up to 85% of the variance in BMD are determined genetically (et al., 2009). However; molecular studies have identified several candidate genes responsible for this problem. The vitamin D receptor gene (VDR) is extensively studied among candidate genes but the association between VDR polymorphisms and bone density is inconclusive and inconsistent in different populations. The association between VDR genotypes and the chance of fracture in postmenopausal women independently of BMD bone turnover has been shown. But the whole mechanisms by which VDR genotypes influence bone strength is yet to be determined (Ferrari S., 2008, Garnero P, 2005).

5. Major Osteoporotic Fractures

Osteoporosis is a silent disease but brings noisy outcomes. There is always a risk of fracture with osteoporosis. Fractures are the costliest outcome of the disease and may result into morbidity and even mortality.

Fractures limits the routine activity of person and the chances of second fracture remains a fear since the occurrence of first fracture. In osteoporosis, fractures of hip, spine and wrist are common fractures.

5.1. Hip Fracture

Needless to say, hip fractures are painful and restrict mobility. Hip fractures causes 20-30% mortality within the first year. Additionally, only One third (30%) of patients with hip fracture able to regain function (Elffors I, et al. 1994, Johnell O, 1992, Ferencz V, 2015, NICE, 2011). Therefore, co-morbidities with hip fractures lead to an even worse outcome (Johnell, O, 2004). The incidence of hip fractures gradually increases with age with rates of 2 per 1 lakh person-years in women aged <35 years and exponentially rises to 3032 per 1 lakh person-years in women aged ≥85 years. In men, the incidence rates are 4 and 1909 per 1 lakh person-years respectively in the west (WHO Bulletin, 2003). In the year 1990, more than 1.66 million people were affected by hip fractures worldwide. Around 1.19 million and 463 000 in women and men respectively had hip fractures (Cooper, C., et al., 2011). However; the fracture rate varies in different countries. In Europe and North America particularly Scandinavian region of Europe, the highest rates are seen. Projections suggest that the prevalence of osteoporotic hip fractures in Asia and Africa will increase rapidly in near future (Cooper C, 1992). Bone density is the key factor and has a potent relationship to fracture, however fractures may arise in women even without osteoporosis, as a result of falls (Table 6). Therefore additional risk factors are useful to forecast 10-year probability of fracture (Table 1) (Gogate Y, 2012).

Demographics of world are changing rapidly with majority of elderly people living in developing nations only. A study revealed that by 2050, out of all hip fractures, 50% will be occur in Asian region only (Dhanwal DK, 2013) and soon South Asia (India) may face a great burden of such fractures in coming decades. Keeping in view the increased life expectancy and rapid growth in population, these alarming findings should be taken into account now by policy makers to strengthen strategies for the optimization of hip fractures.

5.2. Spinal Fractures

Worldwide, back pain is also a common presentation. Osteoporotic vertebral fractures (VCF's) result in pain, disability and spinal deformity and cause deterioration in quality of life (Mithal A,2012) and are often characterised by immobility and physical frailty. It is estimated that there is a 5% mortality rate with such fractures over the following 5 years (Garg B et. al, 2017). Osteoporotic vertebral fractures have recurrent course, further ranging in patients between 20–44% within one year (Cooper C, 1992). The lifetime recurrence of vertebral fracture exceeds up to 85% (Johnell, O., 2004). The highest numbers of VCFs were recorded in the last decade worldwide. In clinical settings, VCFs are difficult to manage if presented with co-morbid factors that may limit aggressive interventions.

5.3. Fractures of Wrist

There is a paucity of data available with regards to the epidemiology of the fractures of wrist in osteoporotic patients except few epidemiological studies from Asia (Sandeep J., 2012). The studies show that fracture rates varies among population, although the overall gender rates are similar both in men and women from non-Asian regions (vanStaa TP, 2001). Studies reveals that fractures in men tend to occur in young age whereas there is a preponderance of females in the elderly group due to osteoporosis. The other reasons of such fractures are due to poor balance and physical inactivity (Sandeep J., 2012).

6. FRAX IN FRACTURE PREDICTION

FRAX® is a computer-based algorithm which is an important web based tool to assess fragility fracture risk (hip, spine and wrist) in osteoporosis. It is an important tool to be used for primary care which can predict fracture probability easily albeit, with certain limitations. Thus, a fair and close clinical judgement is needed to interpret the results of FRAX (Figure 3) (Gogate Y, 2012).

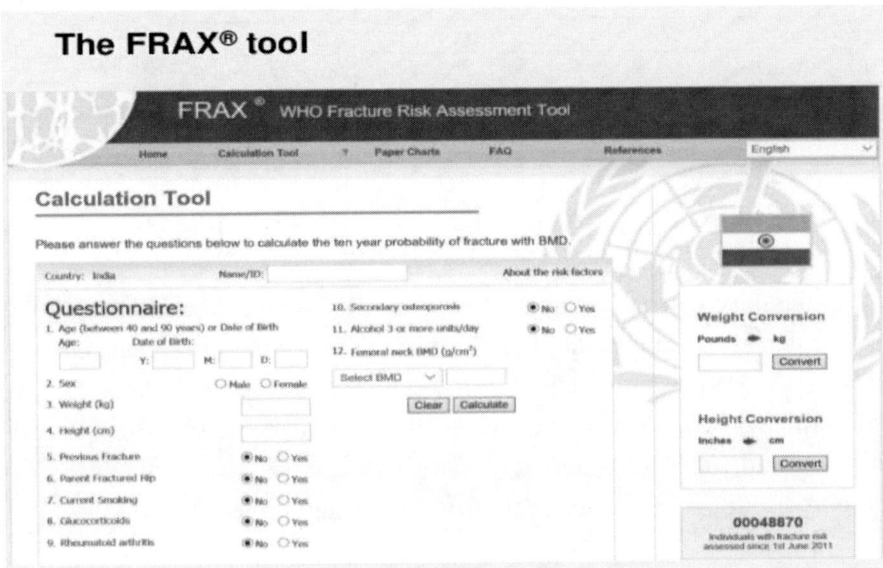

Figure 3. FRAX calculation tool for 10 year probability of fracture.

Department of Orthopaedics at All India Institute of Medical Sciences, New Delhi (author's department) runs a special outpatient clinic (OPD) as 'fragility fracture clinic' weekly. Elderly patients with metabolic bone diseases such as osteoporosis and osteopenia, patients with osteoporotic fractures are being treated.

Table 4. Risk factors for bone loss, development of osteoporosis and fracture

Non Modifiable	Other associated disorders	Behavioural
Ageing	Rheumatoid arthritis	Physical inactivity
Female	Liver disorders/ malabsorption/ Inflammatory bowel disease (IBD)	Low calcium intake
Previous history of fracture	Disorders of parathyroid gland	Smoking/Alcohol/tobacco
Deformity/ kyphosis	Prolonged immobilization	No sun seeking
Height loss	-	Clothing pattern
Low body mass	-	Low calcium diet (<500 mg/day)

7. Osteoporosis: Diagnosis and Tests

To diagnose osteoporosis and assess the risk of fracture determination of Bone density is important. This exam is used to measure bone mineral density (BMD). It is most commonly performed using dual-energy x-ray absorptiometry (DXA or DEXA) or bone densitometry. However a complete medical history and physical exam are needed in diagnosis of osteoporosis along with other tests (from blood and urine) (Table 5)

8. Life Style and Bone Health

Diet & exercise plays a critical role in overall health. Therefore, prevention strategies at the time of menopause should begin with screening and careful assessment for risk factors (Table 4). Once timely screening of certain risk factors is identified, this will help women to undergo standard care. Other evidence-based prevention strategies which are important under overall lifestyle management include a healthy diet, moderate exercise, cessation of smoking, curtailing alcohol consumption and meditational activities (Park DI, 2015). Lack of exercise and physical activity are major contributory factors for low BMD (Aggarwal N1, et al., 2011). Physical activity positively affects peak bone mass and also mitigates the bone loss with aging and thus reduces the chance of osteoporosis. Results from the EPIC-Potsdam study on peri and postmenopausal women also showed that physical activity is helpful in prevention of obesity (Menzel J, 2015).

Table 5. Diagnostic tools for the treatment and management of Osteoporosis

Diagnostic Tools/Parameters	Application/function
Bone densitometry (DEXA).	To determine bone mineral density (BMD)
X-ray	To identify fractures
Radionuclide bone scan	• Helpful in early prediction of osteoporosis • Fracture assessment and also for regional bone changes after anti-osteoporotic treatment
Bone mineral homeostasis	Bone mineral homeostasis parameters such as Vitamin D (25 (OH) D, parathyroid hormone (Intact iPTH), calcium (Total calcium, Urinary calcium and 24hours dietary calcium), Phosphorous (Po4), Alkaline phosphatise (ALP)
Bone turn over markers (BTM's) • (BALP & P1NP as Bone formation markers) • BCrb & Urinary NTX as Bone resorption markers)	To analyse and monitor the treatment response in osteoporosis

Fall rates are high and brings costly outcome particularly in elderly. Vitamin D and exercise both have been advocated to minimize the fall risk among elderly. Exercise can be helpful in reducing fall-related injuries among community-dwelling elderly however exercise alone does not appear help in bone formation (Notelovitz, M., et al., 1991). Breer et al. found that 83.8% of elderly had Vitamin D deficiency out of which only 75% were participating in physical activity more than once a week (Breer, S. et al., 2012).

Exercises	Functions
Endurance, or aerobic, activities	Breathing and heart rate
Strength exercises	Muscles
Balance exercises/GAIT	Prevent falls
Flexibility exercises	Cycling, swimming, etc.

Like muscle, the impact of exercise on bone is positive. Exercise regulates bone mineral homeostasis which regulates osteoblastogenesis resulting in stronger bones. The habit of exercise in younger age can help prevent bone loss. Exercising can also help us maintain muscle strength, coordination, and balance, which in turn helps to prevent falls and related fractures. Following common exercise are found useful in studies (Gómez-Bruton A, 2017).

8.1. Exercises and Bone Health

Improved quality of life, it is never too late to start exercising. Exercise modalities require a controlled environment. Muscle power exercises are superior to balance exercises Balance & Muscle strengthening (Not brisk walk) for older adults. Regular physical activity can:

- Increases the muscle strength
- Improve in maintaining balance and posture (Prevention of falls to reduce disability & Fracture
- Decrease the risk of bone fracture
- Relieve or decrease pain
- Positive mood and sense of overall wellbeing

8.2. Benefits of Exercises in Bone Health!

Although lifting weights makes bones stronger. Regular resistance exercises, Even without any additional weights positively influences bone density. Running, cycling, jumping and swimming are also effective including Low-impact strength training. Exercise triggers the gene regulation in bone metabolism by promoting osteoblast cells (osteobalstogenesis).

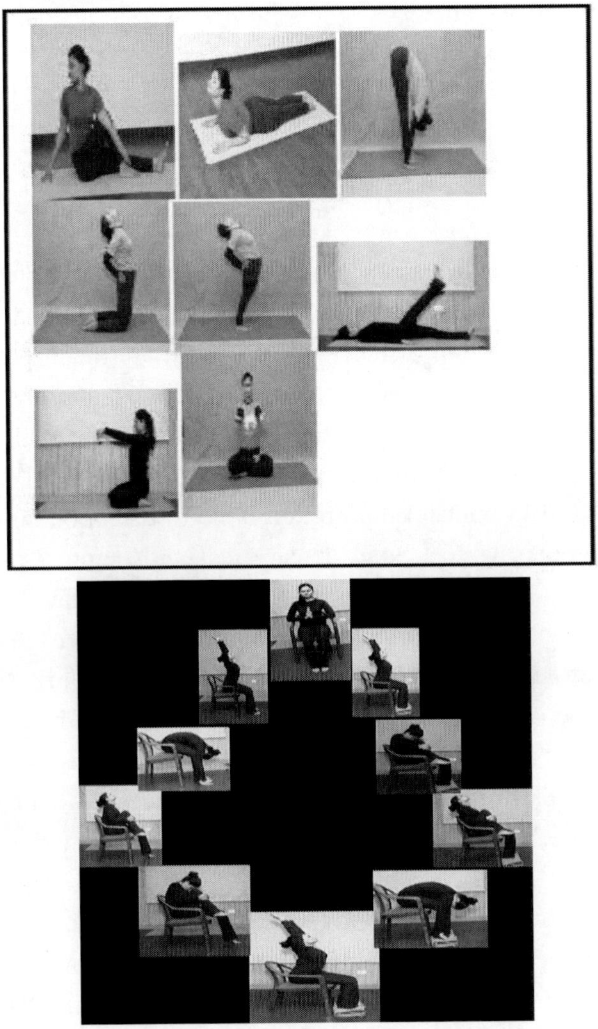

Photo 1. Exercises for muscles and bone health.

Exercise benefits by

- Stimulate bone formation (new bone tissue)
- Retain calcium in the bones
- Increase bone density
- Reduces the risk of fractures

9. Fall Prevention

Although, fall events can be critical at any stage of life but among elderly, the chances of fall events are much higher than young people as in frail elderly the reflexes are usually poor. People are much prone for falls due to variety of risk factors (Table 6). There is a close association between weaker bone, osteoporosis and fall. Falls are especially dangerous for people who are unaware that they have low bone density. If the patient and the doctor fail to connect the broken bone to osteoporosis, the chance to make a diagnosis with a bone density test and begin a prevention or treatment program is lost. From the author's institute (AIIMS, New Delhi) fall prevention education is an important component under the umbrella of fragility fracture network Indian fragility fracture network (IFFN). The authors department has a facility of GAIT laboratory where motion and balance training is also given. The department of Orthopaedics has a facility of 'SAATHI' instrument helpful in training of balance and fall prevention in elderly. The fall related risk factors among elderly are given in following table.

The introduction of oestrogen substitution therapy alone is found potent against bone mineral loss, but combination of therapy with exercise together may increase total BMD (Prince, 1991). Therefore in elderly women, exercise may stimulate calcium absorption, while the oestrogenic effects on calcium facilitate in regulation of bone mineralisation process (Figure 2).

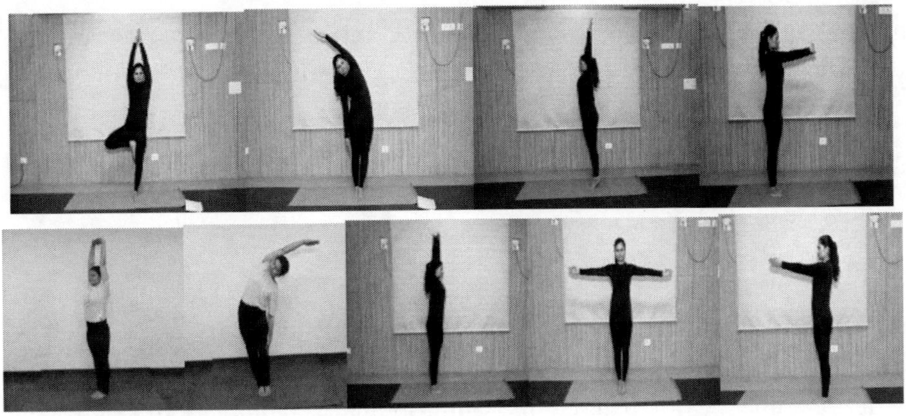

Photo 2. Fall prevention excercises.

Table 6. Risk factors for falling among the elderly

Intrinsic factors	Extrinsic factors	Environmental factors
General deterioration associated with ageing	Personal hazards	Indoor/home hazards
Balance, gait, or mobility problems	Multiple drug therapy	Outdoor hazards
• Visual impairment • Impaired cognition or depression "Blackout"		

Sonneville et al., 2012 and colleagues found that vitamin D mitigates the possibility of stress fractures with its protective effect. The authors also noticed a 50% reduction in the incidence of fractures in women who performed high impact activity. Thus, the importance of vitamin D over calcium is relatively greater (Sonneville et al., 2012).

Vitamin D deficiency in women wearing veiled clothing is also supported by (Allali F, et al., 2009). Lack of sun exposure and wearing veiled were contributory factors for vitamin D deficiency. The resulting insufficiency resulted in higher bone turnover (Allali F, et al., 2009). Studies have also shown higher level of bone loss with vitamin D deficiency in Muslim women (Diamond H T, 2002).

Ishii et al. have shown that higher body mass index (BMI) is associated with higher BMD but with lower composite strength indicators in the cohort of peri and postmenopausal women. The finding suggests that increase in BMD is insufficient alone to compensate the increase impact forces during event of fall (Table 6, Figure 5) (Ishii S, 2014).

10. Nutrition and Bone Health

It is well known that food habits and health behaviours are significantly associated with bone health. Several studies have attempted to find out the link between nutrition and bone health. Park et al. revealed the dietary habits, health behaviours, anthropometric calculation and BMD showed significant deficiencies in vitamin D and calcium with excessive cholesterol and sodium consumption (Park DI, 2015). Other unhealthy dietary and health practices include excessive coffee intake, low milk consumption, night time snacking, etc. (Park DI, 2015).

Although cross-sectional and retrospective studies come up with mixed opinions a study in a cohort of peri-menopausal women shows that low fat dairy products along with major nutrient such as protein calcium and vitamin D were significantly associated with greater bone health gain with low fracture rate (Aggarwal N1, et al., 2011). These findings were further supported by Tenforde et al., demonstrated that women's who consumed greater than 1500 mg of calcium daily had much less likely to get a stress fracture (Tenforde AS, 2010). The sufficient calcium consumption during childhood days also appears to be important. Wentz et al. showed that milk consumption during mid-school years are positively correlated with BMD at hip region (Wentz, L, et al., 2012). Lower levels of calcium intake (500-1000 mg/ day) have been shown to be unsuccessful in post-menopausal women (Hirani, V, 2005). A population-based trial recommends the dose of vitamin D should be 2000 IU/day according to recommended dietary allowance (RDA) for vitamin D to escort 97.5% of the population to levels of 80 nmol/L or higher (Hyppönen E, 2007). Good sources of calcium include: milk, cheese and other dairy foods. Calcium can be obtained both from dairy and non-dairy products. This highlights the importance role of vitamin D dietary supplementation.

10.1. List of Calcium Rich Eatables

Green leafy vegetables, such as broccoli, cabbage and okra, but not spinach
Soya beans/ Soya drinks (with added calcium)
Cheese
Milk
Yogurt
Tofu
Nuts/seeds/beans/ Lentils
Dry fruits especially Almonds
Bread and anything made with fortified flour
Whey Protein
Fish (Sardines and Canned Salmon)

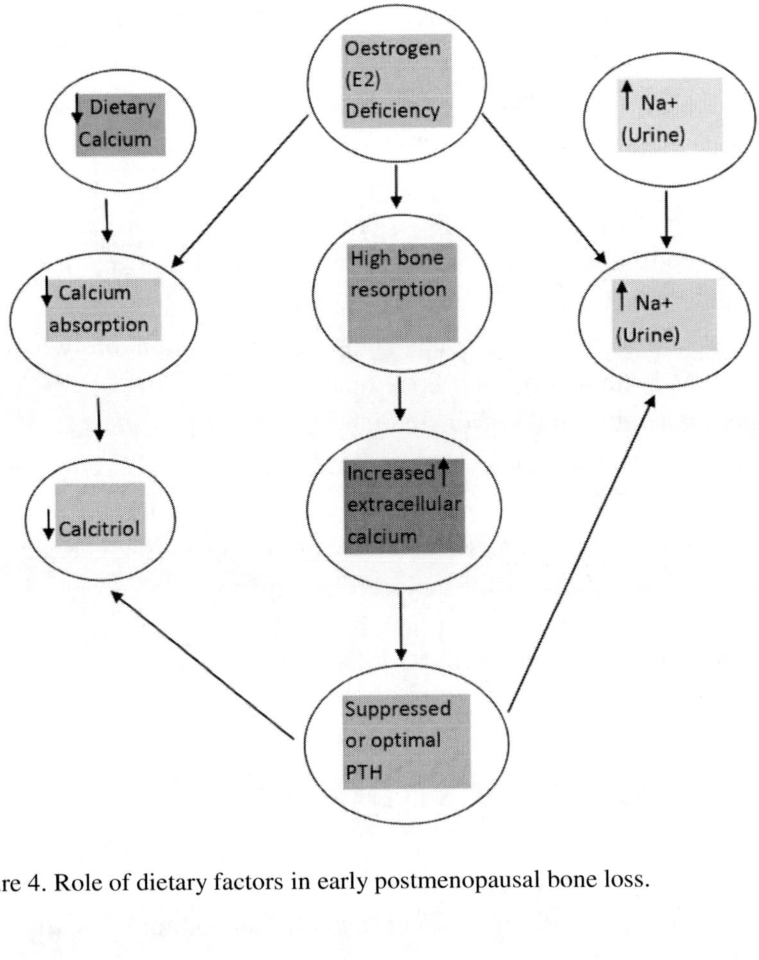

Figure 4. Role of dietary factors in early postmenopausal bone loss.

11. Postmenopausal Osteoporosis

In women, the onset of menopause is a crucial phase to get prepared for prevention and restoration of bone health. Impaired metabolism with other co-morbid diseases such as obesity, diabetes, CVD, cognitive decline, dementia, depression, cancer and osteoporosis constitutes as postmenopausal syndrome in women (Kuchuk NO, 2009). However, hormonal therapy after menopause as a prevention strategy is not appreciated by recent studies as these interventions may not be fully valid for women at this juncture (Figure 4). According to world bank report, the incidence of Postmenopausal osteoporosis PMO which was 470 million in 1990 is expected to reach 1.3 billion by 2030 (76% women from developing countries) In India, it is projected that by the year 2030 the population of women with PMO will be the 2nd highest in the world, second to China only. The average prevalence of osteoporosis is 25%-30% in women above 50 years (Milenković S, 2010). Postmenopausal women are more susceptible for the risk of osteoporosis because of the decline in oestrogen and vitamin D levels resulting into weaker bones. Bone strength in women after menopause depends upon the integration of two main features such as bone density and bone quality (LaFleur J et al., 2016). A recent study on healthy Indian women older than 50 years showed a 17.1% incidence of vertebral fractures and the prevalence of osteoporosis based on BMD was 35.7%. Based on such results the number of women requiring therapy for osteoporosis is nearly 50% (Anuradha V K, 2015). VDD seems to be higher especially in postmenopausal women with osteoporosis and with history of fracture (Neuprez A, 2017). However, VDD is preventable in community.

12. Vitamin D Deficiency

Several studies have uniformly discussed about the wide range of vitamin D deficiency (VDD) in Indian population including from children to elderly from urban to rural and from planes to hills with a prevalence rate between 70 to 100% despite the generous sun exposure in India (Dixit V, 2018). Deficiency of vitamin D not only affects musculoskeletal health but is also associated with a wide range of acute and chronic diseases too including risk factors for the development of osteopenia and osteoporosis as well (Table 4) (Goswami R, 2000). The common risk factors for VDD including low exposure to sun, atmospheric pollution, darker skin pigmentation, low physical activity or impaired intestinal absorption, indoor confinement of children during the day, high rise buildings and sedentary life style (Holick MF., 2007, Harsh Arora, 2016, Ritu G, 2014). The major cause of VDD is the lack of sun exposure in moderation (Goswami R, 2008). Studies have shown that even low-lying vitamin D levels are associated with muscle weakness, low BMD and hip fractures (Matthias Wacker, 2013, Lips, P. 2011, Yoshida, T. 2012). Vitamin D deficient premenopausal women have also found increased risk of breast and colon cancers (Manar Atoum, 2017).

In postmenopausal women, deficiency is exacerbated by the loss of oestrogen and age-related alteration in the vitamin D receptor VDR and vitamin D synthesis (Garnero P, 2005). Oestrogen and vitamin D deficiency can further enhance the risk of malignancy, bone loss, diabetes, hypertension, depression, falls and osteoporotic fractures (Ferrari S., 2008). Evidence shows that vitamin D deficiency may affect the vascular system and the brain, resulting in cognitive impairment and dementia (Holick MF., 2007).

In Indian climate vitamin D deficiency is common and found at varying latitudes resulting in urban north and South Indian women having lower BMD (Goswami R, 2008). Additional risk for deficiency includes female gender, advance age, reduce sunlight exposure, darker skin pigmentation, dietary habits, winter season, and lack of fortified dairy products (Harinarayan CV, 2009). Although, sunlight is the most cost-effective and easiest way to optimise vitamin D deficiency but a recent study reveals that ultra violet B rays (UVB) between 290-310 nm are at their peak between 11:00 AM to 01:00 PM (Marwaha RK, et al., 2016) but it appears difficult for working professionals to go out for 'sun break' in this time frame. A study was done among university level students shows poor level of knowledge, awareness and attitude for vitamin D and sunshine (Arora H, Dixit V, 2016).

Prevalence of vitamin D deficiency by regions varies from 53.4% to 81.8% (Ritu G, 2014, Harinarayan CV, 2009). Among osteoporotic populations, the frequency of vitamin D congregation varies from 12.5% to 76% (Kuchuk NO, 2009). In elderly female, the prevalence of 25-hydroxyvitamin D concentrations ≤20 ng/ml ranged from 1.6% (community-living) to 86% (institutionalized women) in population and confirms by various studies (Gaugris S, 2005). A high prevalence of hypovitaminosis D (66.67%) has been also seen in healthy asymptomatic postmenopausal women in northern part of India (Kalra S, 2011) and these figures are in concordance with neighbouring states as well (Goswami R, 2008). Results from a study conducted in 29 countries studied a large group of postmenopausal women showed the average concentration of 25-hydroxyvitamin D within the serum was 61.2nmol/l (Spiro A, 2014). The OFELY study also showed 73% of postmenopausal had the average concentration of 25(OH) D lower than 75nmol/l (Sornay-Rendu E, 2005).

12.1. Vitamin D Deficiency and Secondary Hyperparathyroidism

A concomitant rise in parathyroid hormone typically occurs with vitamin D deficiency (Kuchuk NO, 2009). The correlation between vitamin D and PTH is often very strong and therefore it is not uncommon to find vitamin D inadequacy among elderly subjects with elevated levels of PTH. Inadequacy of vitamin D leads to secondary hyperparathyroidism (SHPT) followed by rapid bone turnover and bone loss (Milenković S, 2010). The desirable 25-hydroxyvitamin D levels attained from examining the 25-hydroxyvitamin D–PTH relationship should be carefully taken into consideration. A recent study shows that around 83% of postmenopausal women had secondary hyperparathyroidism but interestingly there were sizable number of subjects (27%) who had normal PTH levels despite vitamin D deficiency (Dixit V, 2018). This study also shows the cut-off point of vitamin D which was 25ng/ml from where PTH begins to rise. So far the 25-hydroxyvitamin D is higher than 30 ng/ml and calcium intakes greater than 17.5 mmol/day, are needed to arrest promotion in PTH levels (Maggio D, et al. 2005).

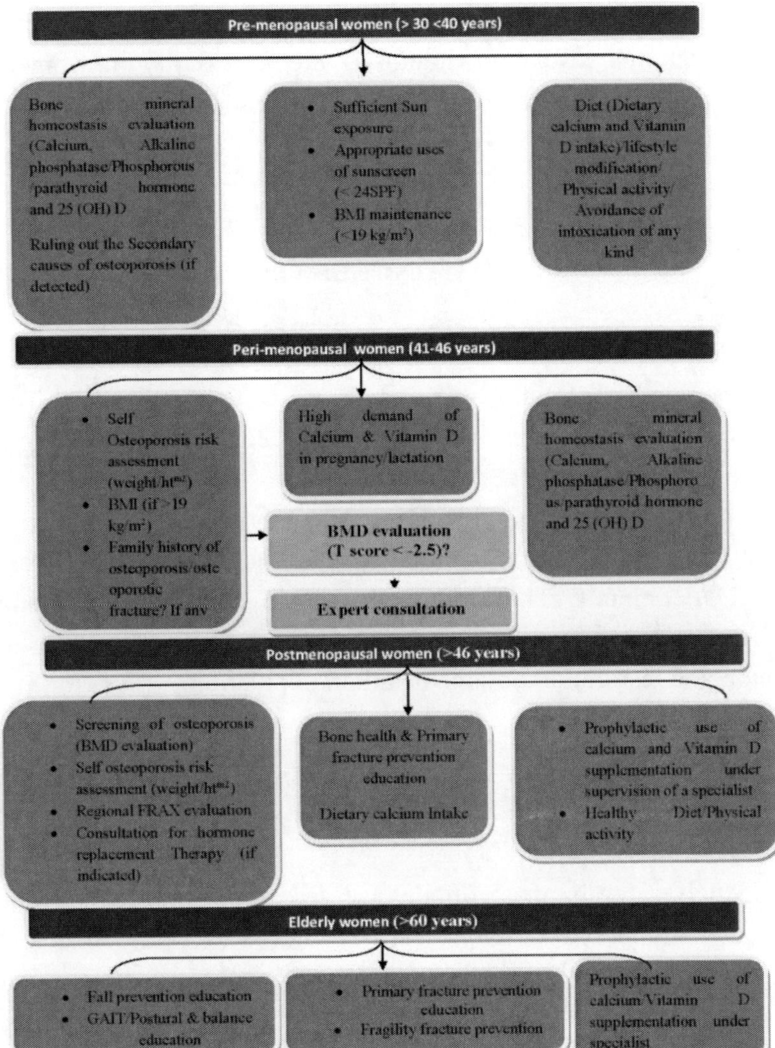

Figure 5. Flow diagram of Prevention, promotion and Restoration of bone health in women.

Gender-specific impact of aging affects the vitamin D serum levels and also the age-specific association of parathyroid hormone (PTH). Study of the same ethnic group revealed a negative relationship between vitamin D and PTH which is regulated by age factor rather sex specific (Arabi A, 2010). Data also show that decline of vitamin D starts after 50 years of age in women whereas in men vitamin D decline begins after 70 years. Therefore, optimal levels of vitamin D are necessarily in women at a younger age to avoid the age-associated compensatory hyperparathyroidism (Heaney RP. 2005).

13. Conclusion

Poor bone health status in females is a big concern. With increasing age and population growth, osteoporosis is set to rise in Asia. Tailored strategies including awareness, bone health education and community screening programmes are required to close the gap between health behavioural understanding and practice. The exposure to sunlight and food fortification with vitamin D alone appears inadequate to address the vitamin D deficiency. Thus more widespread advocacy of Vitamin D supplementation programme is needed to be done for the prevention, promotion and restoration of bone health in population.

14. Key Message

- Much of the burden of bone disease can potentially be avoided if at-risk individuals are identified and appropriate interventions (both preventive and therapeutic) are made in a timely manner. The evidence suggests that health care providers frequently fail to identify and treat individuals at high risk for future osteoporosis or other disorders of bone, even those who have already had a fracture.

- It is important to evaluate the risks for poor bone health at all ages. Therefore, assessment of calcium and vitamin D intake, physical activity, and adverse behaviors such as smoking/alcohol should be a routine part of health care for all individuals.
- Those in greatest need should receive a full assessment of bone health. Diagnostic methods (DEXA Scan) are available that can help to identify those in the population who are at highest risk of fracture.
- Both the public and health care professionals need to be aware of a number of known (Prevalence and Incidence), easy-to-identify risk factors for osteoporosis and other bone diseases.
- Providers should be aware of a number of red flags that might signal potential problems with an individual's bone health at different ages. One of the most important flags is a previous fragility-related fracture.
- While osteoporosis is clearly the most common bone disease, health care providers must also actively look for other bone diseases. Diseases such as hyper-parathyroidism, rickets, osteomalacia, and Paget's disease can often be identified by being aware of the warning signs and/or through simple biochemical measurements. Early identification of such diseases is critical, since treatment at an early stage can often be highly effective.
- Bone mineral density or BMD testing should be performed on any patient for whom risk factor analysis indicates a strong potential for osteoporosis. Formal guidelines have been developed recommending BMD testing in certain populations, including postmenopausal women over age 65, younger women with multiple risk factors, and men and women with fragility fractures or who have other diseases or take medications that can greatly increase the risk of fracture.
- Individuals who are diagnosed with osteoporosis should be further assessed for secondary, treatable causes of the disease, particularly men and premenopausal women who suffer a fragility fracture.

- All elderly individuals should be given education about primary fracture prevention and fall prevention programs by health care providers
- Metabolic bone disease particularly, Osteoporosis should be kept under national health schemes/programs
- Nationwide, registry programs are required such as Fracture Liaison Services (FLS), under the umbrella of fragility fracture network of India (IFFN).

Acknowledgments

The authors acknowledge Centre for Integrative Medicine (CIMR), for providing guidance on role of Yoga in bone health. The authors are also grateful to Mrs. Mohini Sinde, Senior Research Fellow & Certified Yoga Therapist at CIMR, AIIMS, New Delhi for providing photographs related to Yoga & Pranayama. The authors are also thankful to Ms. Khyati Bhadula, Medical Social Worker for her assistance in drawing figures for this chapter.

References

Aggarwal, N1; Raveendran, A; Khandelwal, N; Sen, RK; Thakur, JS; Dhaliwal, LK; Singla, V; Manoharan, SR. Prevalence and related risk factors of osteoporosis in peri- and postmenopausal Indian women. *J Midlife Health.*, 2011 Jul, 2(2), 81-5.

Allali, F; El Aichaoui, S; Khazani, H; Benyahia, B; Saoud, B; El Kabbaj, S; Bahiri, R; Abouqa, lR; Hajjaj, Hassouni. High prevalence of hypovitaminosis D in Morocco: relationship to lifestyle, physical performance, bone markers, and bone mineral density. *Semin Arthritis Rheum*, 2009, 38, 444-51.

Anuradha, V. Khadilkar; Rubina, M Mandlik. Epidemiology and treatment of osteoporosis in women: an Indian perspective. *International Journal of Women's Health*, 2015, 7, 841-849.

Arabi, A; Baddoura, R; El-Rassi, R; El-Hajj Fuleihan, G. Age but not gender modulates the relationship between PTH and vitamin D. *Bone*, 2010, 47, 408–412.

Breer, S; et al., Stress fractures in elderly patients. *Int Orthop*, 2012. 36, 2581-7.

Bulletin of the World Health Organization, 2003, 81 (9).

Cooper, C; Melton, LJ. III. Epidemiology of osteoporosis. *Trends in Endocrinology and Metabolism*, 1992, 314, 224-9.

Cooper, C; et al., Secular trends in the incidence of hip and other osteoporotic fractures. *Osteoporosis Int*, 2011, 22, 1277-88.

Dhanwal, DK; Siwach, R; Dixit, V; Mithal, A; Jameson, K; Cooper, C. Incidence of hip fracture in Rohtak district, North India. *Arch Osteoporosis*, 2013, 8, 135.

Diamond, HT; Levy, S; Smith, A; Day, P. High bone turnover in Muslim women with vitamin D deficiency. *MJA*, 2002, 177, 139-141.

Dixit, V; Pegrum, J; Batra, S; Dhanwal, D; Garg, B. Is there a need of Vitamin D supplementation programme in India (VDSPI)? A letter to the Editor. *J Clin Orthop Trauma.*, 2018 Mar, 9 (Suppl 1), S56-S57.

Dixit, V; Tripathi, R. L; Dhanwal, D. K. All 25-hydroxyvitamin D-deficient Indian postmenopausal women do not have secondary hyper-parathyroidism. *Arch Osteoporos.*, 2018 May 27, 13(1), 62.

Elffors, I; Allander, E.; Kanis, JA; Gullberg, B; Johnell, O; Dequeker, J; et al. The variable incidence of hip fracture in southern Europe: the MEDOS Study. *Osteoporosis International*, 1994, 4, 253-63.

Ferencz, V; Horváth, C; Huszár, S; Bors, K. Assessment of risk factors for fractures in postmenopausal women with osteoporosis. *ORV Hetil*, 2015, 156, 146-53.

Ferrari, S. Human genetics in osteoporosis. *Best Pract Res Clin Endocrinol Metab*, 2008b, 22, 723-35

Ferrari, S. Human genetics in osteoporosis. *Best Pract Res Clin Endocrinol Metab*, 2008b, 22, 723-35

Garg, B; et al. Non-surgical management of acute osteoporotic vertebral compression fracture: *A review Journal of Clinical Orthopaedics and Trauma*, 8 (2017) 131–138

Garg, B; Batra, S; Dixit, V. An unexpected healing of an established non union of the radial neck through teriparatide: A case report and review of literature. *J Clin Orthop Trauma.*, 2018 Mar, 9(Suppl 1), S103-S105.

Garnero, P; Munoz, F; Borel, O; Sornay-Rendu, E; and Delmas, PD. Vitamin D Receptor Gene Polymorphisms Are Associated with the Risk of Fractures in Postmenopausal Women, Independently of Bone Mineral Density. *J Clin Endocrinol Metab*, 2005, 90, 4829–4835.

Gaugris, S; Heaney, RP; Boonen, S; Kurth, H; Bentkover, JD; Sen, SS. Vitamin D inadequacy among post-menopausal women: a systematic review, *QJM*, 2005, 98, 667-76.

Gogate, Y; Bhadada, SK. FRAX: Facts and Fantasy. *Indian J Endocr Metab*, 2012, 16, Suppl S2, 224-6

Gómez-Bruton, A; Matute-Llorente, Á; González-Agüero, A; Casajús, JA; Vicente-Rodríguez, G. Plyometric exercise and bone health in children and adolescents: a systematic review. *World J Pediatr.*, 2017 Apr, 13(2), 112-121.

Goswami, R; Gupta, N; Goswami, D; Marwaha, RK; Tandon, N; Kochupillai, N. Prevalence and significance of low 25-hydroxyvitamin D concentrations in healthy subjects in Delhi. *Am J Clin Nutr.*, 2000 Aug, 72(2), 472-5.

Goswami, R; Kochupillai, N; Gupta, N; Goswami, D; Singh, N; Dudha, A. Presence of 25(OH)D deficiency in rural north Indian village despite abundant sunshine. *J Assoc Physicians India*, 2008, 56, 755-57.

Harinarayan, CV; Joshi, SR. Vitamin D status in India--its implications and remedial measures. *J Assoc Physicians India.*, 2009 Jan, 57, 40-8.

Harsh, Arora; Vivek, Dixit; Nidhi, Srivastava. Evaluation of knowledge, practices of vitamin d and attitude towards sunlight among indian students. *Asian J Pharm Clin Res*, Vol 9, Issue 1, 2016, 308-313

Harsh, Arora; Vivek, Dixit; Nidhi, Srivastava. Evaluation of knowledge, practices of vitamin d and attitude towards sunlight among indian students. *Asian J Pharm Clin Res*, Vol 9, Issue 1, 2016, 308-313

Heaney, RP. The Vitamin D requirement in health and disease. *Steroid Biochem Mol Biol.*, 2005, 97, 13–9.

Hirani, V; Primatesta, P. Vitamin D concentrations among people aged 65 years and over living in private households and institutions in England: population survey. *Age Ageing*, 2005, 34, 485-91.

Holick, MF. Vitamin D deficiency. *N Engl J Med*, 2007, 357, 266–81.

Hyppönen, E; Power, C. Hypovitaminosis D in British adults at age 45 y: Nationwide cohort study of dietary and lifestyle predictors. *Am J Clin Nutr*, 2007, 85, 860–8.

Ishii, S; Cauley, JA; Greendale, GA; Nielsen, C; Karvonen-Gutierrez, C; Ruppert, K; Karlamangla, AS. Pleiotropic effects of obesity on fracture risk: the Study of Women's Health across the Nation. *J Bone Miner Res*, 2014, 29, 2561-70.

Johnell, O; Gullberg, B, Allander, E; Kanis, JA. The apparent incidence of hip fracture in Europe: a study of national register sources. MEDOS Study Group. *Osteoporosis International*, 1992, 2, 298-302.

Johnell, O; and, JA. Kanis, An estimate of the worldwide prevalence, mortality and disability associated with hip fracture. *Osteoporos Int*, 2004, 15, 897-902.

Kalra, S; Kalra, B; Khandelwal, Sk. Vitamin D deficiency in Healthy Postmenopausal Women in Haryana. *World J Life Sci. and Medical Research*, 2011, 1, 11-14.

Kanis, JA; Johnell, O; Oden, A; Jonsson, B; De Laet, C; Dawson, A. Risk of hip fracture according to the World Health Organization criteria for osteopenia and osteoporosis. *Bone*, 2000, 27, 585-90.

Kuchuk, NO; van Schoor, NM; Pluijm, SM; Chines, A; Lips, P. Vitamin D status, parathyroid function, bone turnover, and BMD in postmenopausal women with osteoporosis: global perspective. *J Bone Miner Res*, 2009, 24, 693-701.

Labrie, F. DHEA, important source of sex steroids in men and even more in women. *Prog Brain Res*, 2010, 182, 97-148.

LaFleur, J; et al. Fracture Rates and Bone Density among Postmenopausal Veteran and Non-Veteran Women from the Women's Health Initiative. *Gerontologist*, 2016, 56 Suppl 1, S78-90.

Lips, P; van Schoor, NM. The effect of vitamin D on bone and osteoporosis. *Best Pract. Res. Clin. Endocrinol. Metab.*, 2011, 25, 585–591.

Maggio, D; Cherubini, A; Lauretani, F; Russo, CR; Bartali, B; Pierandrei, M; Ruggiero, C; Macchiarulo, MC; Giorgino, R; Minisola, S; Ferrucci, L. 25(OH)D Serum Levels Decline With Age Earlier in Women Than in Men and Less Efficiently Prevent Compensatory Hyperparathyroidism in Older Adults. *Journal of Gerontology: Medical Sciences*, 2005, 60A, 11, 1414–1419.

Manar, Atoum; Foad, Alzoughool. Vitamin D and Breast Cancer: Latest Evidence and Future Steps. *Breast Cancer (Auckl).*, 2017 11, 1–8.

Marwaha, RK; Yenamandra, VK; Sreenivas, V; Sahay, R; Baruah, MP; Desai, A; Kurvilla, S; Joseph, S; Unnikrishnan, AG; Lakshmy, R; Apoorva, C; Sharma, VK; Sethuraman, G. Regional and seasonal variations in ultraviolet B irradiation and vitamin D synthesis in India. *Osteoporos Int.*, 2016 Apr, 27(4), 1611-1617.

Matsushita, H; Wakatsuki, A. Osteoporosis: a gender specific disease. *Nihon Rinsho.*, 2015, 73, 639-43.

Matthias, Wacker; Michael, F. Holick. Vitamin D—Effects on Skeletal and Extraskeletal Health and the Need for Supplementation. *Nutrients.* 2013 Jan, 5(1), 111–148.

Menzel, J; di Giuseppe, R; Wientzek, A; Kroke, A; Boeing, H; Weikert, C. Physical Activity, Bone Health, and Obesity in Peri-/Pre- and Postmenopausal Women: Results from the EPIC-Potsdam Study. *Calcif Tissue Int*, 2015, 97, 376-84.

Milenković, S; Dimić, A; Stanković, A; Aleksić, I; Petrović, D. Vitamin D status in women with postmenopausal osteoporosis. *Acta Medica Medianae*, 2010, 49.

Mithal, A; Kaur, P. Osteoporosis in Asia: a call to action. *Curr Osteoporos Rep.*, 2012 Dec, 10(4), 245-7.

Neuprez, A; Bruyère, O; Collette, J; Reginster, JY. Vitamin D inadequacy in Belgian postmenopausal osteoporotic women. *BMC Public Health*, 2007, 7, 64.

NICE, The Management of Hip Fracture in Adults. National Clinical Guideline Centre (NICE) London: National Clinical Guideline Centre, 2011, CG124.

Notelovitz, M; et al., Estrogen therapy and variable-resistance weight training increase bone mineral in surgically menopausal women. *J Bone Miner Res*., 1991, 6, 583-90.

Park, DI; Choi-Kwon, S; Han, K. Health behaviors of Korean female nursing students in relation to obesity and osteoporosis. *Nurs Outlook*, 2015, 63, 504-11.

Park, DI; Choi-Kwon, S; Han K. Health behaviors of Korean female nursing students in relation to obesity and osteoporosis. *Nurs Outlook*, 2015, 63, 504-11.

Prince, RL; et al., Prevention of postmenopausal osteoporosis. A comparative study of exercise, calcium supplementation, and hormone-replacement therapy. *N Engl J Med*, 1991, 325, 1189-95.

Ritu, G; Ajay, Gupta. Vitamin D Deficiency in India: Prevalence, Causalities and Interventions. *Nutrients*., 2014 Feb, 6(2), 729–775.

Sandeep, J. Sebastin, Kevin, C. Chung. An Asian Perspective on the Management of Distal Radius Fractures. *Hand Clin*., 2012 May, 28(2), 151–156.

Seeman, E. Invited Review: Pathogenesis of osteoporosis. *J Appl Physiol*, (1985). 2003 Nov, 95(5), 2142-51.

Seremak-Mrozikiewicz, A; Drews, K; Mrozikiewicz, PM; Bartkowiak-Wieczorek, J; Marcinkowska, M; Wawrzyniak, A; Slomski, R; KalakR; Czerny, B; Horst-Sikorska, W. Correlation of vitamin D receptor gene (VDR) polymorphism with osteoporotic changes in Polish postmenopausal women. *Neuro Endocrinol Lett*, 2009, 30, 540-6.

Sonneville, KR; GC; Kocher, MS; Pierce, LM; Ramappa, A; Field, AE. Vitamin d, calcium, and dairy intakes and stress fractures among female adolescents. *Archives of Pediatric and Adolescent Medicine*, 2012, 166, 595-600.

Sornay-Rendu, E; Munoz, F; Garnero, P; Duboeuf, F; Delmas, PD. Identification of osteopenic women at high risk of fracture: the OFELY study. *J Bone Miner Res*, 2005, 20, 1813-9.

Spiro, A; Buttriss, JL. Vitamin D: An overview of vitamin D status and intake in Europe. *Nutr Bull*, 2014, 39, 322-350.

Stuart, H; Ralston, André G. Uitterlinden. Genetics of Osteoporosis., *Endocrine Reviews*, Volume 31, Issue 5, 1 October 2010, Pages 629–662.

Tenforde, AS; Sayres, LC; Sainani, KL; Fredericson, M. Evaluating the relationship of calcium and vitamin D in the prevention of stress fracture injuries in the young athlete: a review of the literature. *PMR*. 2010 Oct, 2(10), 945-9.

Van Staa, TP; Dennison, EM; Leufkens, HG; Cooper, C. Epidemiology of fractures in England and Wales. *Bone*., 2001, 29, 517, 29, 517–522.

Vupputuri, MR; Goswami, R; Gupta, N; Ray, D; Tandon, N; Kumar, N. Prevalence and functional significance of 25-hydroxyvitamin D deficiency and vitamin D receptor gene polymorphisms in Asian Indians. *Am J Clin Nutr*., 2006 Jun, 83(6), 1411-9.

Wentz, L; et al., Dietary and training predictors of stress fractures in female runners. *Int J Sport Nutr Exerc Metab*, 2012, 22, 374-82.

WHO scientific group on the assessment of osteoporosis at primary health care level, Summary meeting report. Brussels, Belgium, 5-7 may 2004.

Yoshida, T; Stern, PH. How vitamin D works on bone. *Endocrinol. Metab. Clin. North Am*., 2012, 41, 557–569.

In: Current Challenges and Management … ISBN: 978-1-53617-304-8
Editor: Abhai Kumar

Chapter 6

AGING EYE: AN INSIGHT TO COMMON VISION PROBLEMS AND ASSOCIATED CHALLENGES

Sanjay Kumar Ojha[1,2], PhD, Vijay Kumar Singh[1], PhD, K. M. Ashwin[1], MSc, Mukesh Damala[1], MSc, K. Shiva Vaishnavi[1,2], BOpt, Om Prakash Narayan[1], PhD and Vivek Singh[1,*], PhD

[1]Brien Holden Eye Research Center and Center for Ocular Regeneration (CORE), LV Prasad Eye Institute, Hyderabad, Telangana, India
[2]Pandorum Technologies Pvt. Ltd., Bangalore, India

ABSTRACT

As the global older population escalates due to increased life span, increase in the prevalence of age-related eye problems resulting with age progression will pose devastating personal and socio-economic consequences. Among several age-related eye diseases, few common

* Corresponding Author's Emails: singhvivekbhu@gmail.com, viveksingh@lvpei.org.

diseases such as presbyopia and cataract can be easily identified and treated. Few age-related eye changes including Dry eyes and Vitreous detachment condition can be managed with medications. Other major age-related eye diseases such as Glaucoma, age-related Macular Degeneration and Diabetic Retinopathy may lead to irreversible visual impairment or blindness requiring immediate medical intervention. Education, awareness program, comprehensive dilated eye exam, proper diet and a healthy lifestyle are very useful for prevention, detection and treatment of such diseases.

Keywords: age-related eye diseases, cataracts, glaucoma, macular degeneration, diabetic retinopathy, diet, health

1. INTRODUCTION

An age-related ocular disease which risks the elder population to lead an independent life, have expensive treatments. The world's population is ageing globally and expected to reach 2.1 billion by 2050 and 3.1 billion in 2100 (Steverson, 2017). World Population Prospects: The 2017 Revision, Key Findings and Advance Tables). As the world ages, there will be more complications in eye conditions with high risk in treatment even using modern-day expensive technologies. The situation demands immediate intervention to prevent partial or complete vision loss which can begin with a rehabilitation program such as education and public awareness regarding the problem. A routine eye examination is needed even if there are no symptoms to avoid further vision loss (Maylahn et al., 2005).

Ocular trauma remains the primary reason of unavoidable monocular blindness across the world, although epidemiology of such events is not well documented. It occurs mostly in working-age population leading to a considerable impact on socio-economic, personal and occupational life. Medical costs, worker's compensation and loss of productivity together produce huge short and long term expenses (Nowak & Smigielski, 2015).

A study based on the vast number of participants has offered new evidence regarding the incidence of visual loss as well as major age-related ocular disorders. Particularly, the epidemiology of refractive errors and glaucoma have been well studied providing insights into the public health implications as well as into age-related changes in the eye (Nowak & Smigielski, 2015).

Certain parts of the eye become less elastic making an impact on the capacity to focus at close range. Cells clumping causing floaters and several other changes in the eye are a natural part of ageing (Nowak & Smigielski, 2015). These changes occur as the age increases and they stop the elders to enjoy an active lifestyle or leading an independent lifestyle. Although there are a lot of scientific advancements like stem cell technology for the treatment of corneal diseases, they are still not adequate for the management of age-related eye diseases (Funderburgh et al., 2018; Shanbhag et al., 2019). In the current chapter, we have tried to gather information regarding age-related eye disorders and their management.

2. Ageing-Related Eye Problems

Several eye-related problems are generally more common in elders and they can occur at any age. These diseases of considerable public health markedly affect the patient's independence, physical, emotional, and social health (Tisdale et al., 2018; Rovner et al., 2014). As people age, they are at greater risk to develop some age-related ocular disorders such as cataract, diabetic retinopathy, age-related macular degeneration, glaucoma and dry eye (Table 1). Preventive measures such as multivitamins and management of health situation may prevent these diseases.

Table 1. Detailed information on age-related eye disorders

Disease	Age of onset	Risk factor	Symptoms	Diagnosis	Treatment
Age-related Macular degeneration	>50	Age sex Smoking Genetic susceptibility Cardiovascular	Blurred vision Decreased visual acuity Distorted near vision Visual distortion,	Amsler grid Fundus Fluorescein Angiography Optical Coherence	Antioxidant and mineral supplement Anti-VEGF Photodynamic Radiation Surgery

Table 1. (Continued)

Disease	Age of onset	Risk factor	Symptoms	Diagnosis	Treatment
		Hypertension Obesity hyperopia	metamorphopsia, micropsia Vague visual complaints	Tomography (OCT)	
Cataract	>40	Diabetes Steroid use, UV exposure, Smoking, Retinitis, Uveitis, Prior ocular surgery, Genetic	Blurred vision Glare poor night vision second sight Decreased contrast and the decreased ability to discern colors	comprehensive dilated eye exam	Controlled smoking, extracapsular cataract extraction, phacoemulsification, and small incision cataract surgery
Glaucoma	>40	Age Family history Sex Thin cornea	Severe eye pain. Nausea and vomiting (accompanying the severe eye pain) Sudden onset of visual disturbance, Blurred vision. Reddening of the eye	Tonometry, Ophthalmoscopy Perimetry Gonioscopy Pachymetry	prostaglandin analogues Carbonic anhydrase inhibitors Mitotics ρ kinase inhibitors laser trabeculoplasty Trabeculectomy deep sclerectomy, viscocanal ostomy, and canaloplasty
Diabetic retinopathy	Variable (depends on the onset of diabetes)	Diabetes hypertension, hyperlipidemia, nephropathy	Blurred vision. Fluctuating vision. Impaired color vision. Vision loss.	Slit-lamp examination dilated fundus examination Fluorescein angiography Ocular coherence tomography Hemoglobin A1c	anti-VEGF drugs Surgery
Dry eye disease	>50	Age, asthma, eczema, allergy, cataract surgery, arthritis, migraine and Hypertension	Burning, Itching, Tearing, foreign body sensation Redness, Blurry vision Light sensitivity Eye pain headache Heavy eyelids Eye fatigue	Corneal sensation Tear breakup time Fluorescein staining Schirmer test MMP-9 Tear film interferometry	Artificial tears, artificial tear gel and ointments and lacrisert punctal plugs, Warm compresses, Eyelash scrubs Tear enhancing Drug, Topical steroids. Omega-3 fatty acids supplement

2.1. Age-Related Macular Degeneration

In the developed world, age-related macular degeneration (AMD) is the major cause of severe vision loss in adults. In the USA alone, AMD was reported to affect over 1.7 million people in 2004 which is likely to increase to 3 million in 2020 due to rapid ageing of the population (Werdich et al., 2010). In developed economies, age-related macular degeneration is a major cause of irreversible vision loss in people with 65 years of age and older. Although the etiology of AMD is still not clear, vascular abnormality and defective circulatory system have been assumed to be a major factor in the pathogenesis. It is classified into two types i.e., non-exudative AMD and neovascular AMD. Neovascular AMD is characterized by the presence of choroid neovascular membrane (CNVM) due to abnormal blood vessels, which grow from the choroid pathologically into or under the retina (Figure 1A). Although CNVM is present in only 10% of patients with AMD, it is responsible for more than 90% of cases where severe vision loss is seen due to hemorrhage and fibrosis.

Moreover, vascular endothelial growth factor-A (VEGF-A) through its role in angiogenesis and vascular permeability has been implicated in the pathogenesis of neovascular AMD. Patients with AMD have shown an increase in VEGF-A level in excised CNV membranes, as well as VEGF-A level, is also increased in macular pigment epithelial cells during the preliminary stages of AMD (Kaiser et al., 2007). Although there have been astounding advances in the management of neovascular AMD since the last decade, the major effective treatment to date is Ranibizumab (Mitchell et al., 2010). Further studies for the search of new therapeutics and improved treatment are underway. Currently, photodynamic therapy (PDT) along with verteporfin (photosensitizer) has been approved for management of neovascular AMD. PDT along with verteporfin is an angio-occlusive treatment targeting and specifically destructing CNV through an activated photochemical reaction but does not address the reason for CNV development. Whereas, pegaptanib and ranibizumab specifically target and inhibits VEGF-A preventing angiogenesis (Kaiser et al., 2007).

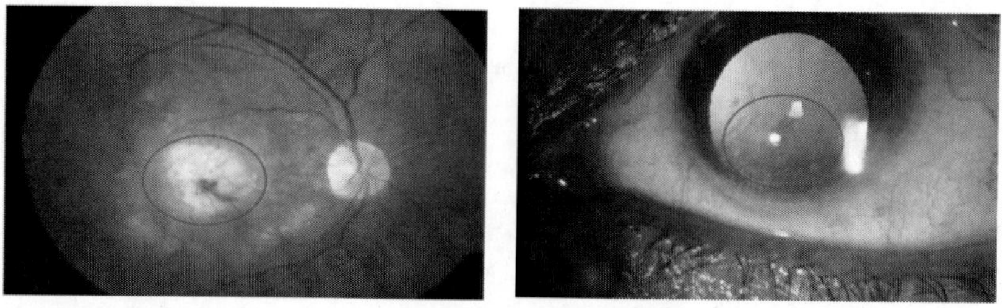

(A) (B)

Figure 1. A. This fundus image represents the signs of ARMD having Drusens, hard exudates, hemorrhages. B. This slit lamp image represents the retro illumination in a cataract patient having grade 2 nuclear sclerosis and cortical cataract.

Moreover, patients with AMD population, the continuously escalating social and budgetary burden of frequent visits, injection fees and large pharmaceutical costs, necessitate the development of new treatment requiring minimal cost.

2.2. Cataract

Cataract is a major health care problem in all parts of the world. Untreated, Cataract may form into a blinding condition and it remains the most predominant reason for visual deficiency comprehensively in spite of viable treatment. Increase in population of old residents and their tendency to have diseases along with age-related eye disease requiring medical procedure will drastically increase the medical expense (Lee et al., 2017). A recent report on cataract epidemiology shows that cataract is responsible for 47.8% of the world's 37 million blind, with 82% of cataract blindness occurring in those 50 years and older (Beaver et al., 2019).

Cataract is an obsessive condition in which the lens becomes opaque, in this manner diminishing the measure of light achieving the retina (Figure 1B). The reasons for cataract development are various, including quality changes and protein post-translational modification.

The recent studies have shown that the major protein in a lens is crystallin. It is a highly concentrated protein in the lens and accounts for lens transparency and refractive properties. Lanosterol is an ampipathic molecule which is synthesized by lanosterol synthase, encoded by LSS gene. Zhao et al., (Zhao et al., 2015) have recently revealed mutations in the LSS gene in cataract and postulated that due to mutation in the LSS gene there was protein aggregation. The study further suggests treatment with lanosterol prevents protein aggregation in the lens and prevents cataract.

Sex and socioeconomic levels play a role in disparities in cataract treatment. The majority of studies found that women have a higher rate of cataracts than men (Zhu et al., 2016). The age-standardized prevalence of cataract blindness in 2010 was 0.19% for women and 0.13% for men (Zhu et al., 2016). Numerous reasons for this have been theorized, including the fact that women live longer than men and have more time for cataracts to develop. Another theory proposes that women are less vocal than men about their need for sight and 'suffer in silence' (Stevens et al., 2013).

Cataract surgery is the most commonly performed ophthalmic procedure and has become one of the most common and successful procedures in ophthalmology (Zhu et al., 2016, Stevens et al., 2013). Phacoemulsification and manual small-incision cataract surgery (SICS) are two different kinds of surgery done for cataract. A study to compare the safety and efficacy of phacoemulsification and SICS to treat white cataracts in southern India showed that both techniques achieved excellent visual outcomes with minimal complications (Venkatesh et al., 2010). However, compared to phacoemulsification, SICS is relatively quick, less expensive and less technology-dependent and therefore it may be a more suited procedure in the developing world. Further to maximize the outcome of cataract surgery, three topical pharmaceutical agents: an antimicrobial, a potent corticosteroid and a non-steroidal anti-inflammatory drug (NSAID) are recommended post-operatively (Duong et al., 2011).

2.3. Glaucoma

Glaucoma is a neurodegenerative disorder due to impairment to the internal layers of the retina and distortion of the optic nerve head. With ageing, degeneration of retinal ganglion cells (RGCs) and their axons results in an irreversible loss of vision. Extracellular matrix (ECM) changes identified with regular maturing create a stiffer extracellular condition all through the body. These age-related changes leading to visual tissue solidification assumes a noteworthy role in a critical number of ophthalmic pathologies (Liu et al., 2018).

Glaucoma is the foremost source of irreversible visual field imperfections and visual impairment with a projection to influence more than 80 million individuals worldwide by 2020 (Quigley & Broman, 2006). Currently, it is reported to affect 2-3% of the world's population over the age of 40, making it the second major cause of blindness following cataracts (Chae et al., 2013).

Like other neurodegenerative disease, glaucoma predominance connects with growing age. As there is increase in human population life expectancy, there is also chance for emerging a bigger financial burden because of rising cases of visual loss.

It is realized that raised intraocular pressure (IOP) is the essential hazard factor for glaucoma. As of late, an ever-increasing number of confirmations demonstrate that vascular shortage likewise assumes a significant role in the pathogenesis of glaucoma. The vascular study of glaucoma speculates that altered blood supply to the optic nerve head adds to optic nerve head injury (Figure 2A). Color Doppler imaging (CDI) has been acquainted as of late with ophthalmology as a non-intrusive imaging technique to monitor bloodstream speeds of retrobulbar vessels (Mokbel & Ghanem, 2011). The normal IOP of the human eye is recommended to be 10-21mmHg (Wamg et al., 2018).

Recently, corticosteroids have been known to raise intraocular pressure (IOP) and this rise has been correlated with the length of treatment, corticosteroid type and individual weakness. Moreover, steroid seems to deliver an IOP rise over a time of weeks in both typical and glaucomatous eyes. Most patients with raised IOP after corticosteroid utilization can be effectively cured with topical glaucoma treatment (Mokbel & Ghanem, 2011).

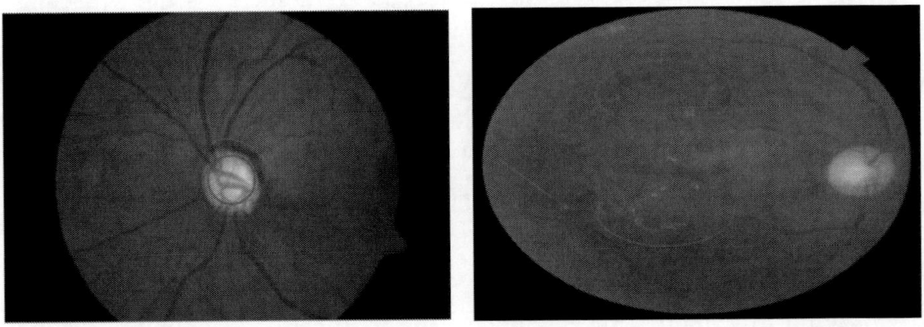

(A) (B)

Figure 2. A. This optic disc represents the features of glaucoma like Infero-TEMPORAL localized notch, supero-temporal excavation, Superior and Inferior wedge RNFL defect, Inf > Sup, 0.9 CDR. B. This fundus image represents the signs of PDR having hard exudates, dot and blot hemorrhages, neovascularization, macular edema.

Since many years the only conventional and common method used globally to reduce IOP in ocular hypertension or in open-angle glaucoma patient is selective laser trabeculoplasty (SLT).To make more noteworthy progress in glaucoma care, it is necessary to minimize the weight of interminable joined therapeutic treatment and expand care by utilizing optional treatment choices, SLT, or minimally invasive glaucoma surgery (MIGS) (Francis et al., 2016). This also suggests we ought to think about laser and explicitly SLT not if all else fails, when restorative treatment has flopped, however as a second or third step in our administration calculation and rehash it if important. In reality, SLT may help with postponing or notwithstanding keeping away from filtration medical procedure, which could be significant for certain patients (Katsanos et al., 2018).

2.4. Diabetic Retinopathy

Diabetic retinopathy (DR) is one of the main reasons for vision impairment in developed countries and the complexity of diabetes is what actually influences the eyes. Diabetic retinopathy is an illness because of diabetic endless hyperglycemia described by small scale vascular inconveniences in the retina, where neuronal components responsible for vision are found (Figure 2B). There are many reasons responsible for DR, primary being the age and puberty due to hormone level changes. Other than these factors, there are several other factors like anaemia, obesity, smoking and hyperlipidemia which are the main reasons leading to DR (Gudla et al., 2018).

Diabetes influenced an estimated 415 million individuals globally in 2015, with this increasing incidence the number of populations with diabetes living longer and there is a rise in the number of individuals with DR and visual impairment caused due to it (Sabanayagam et al., 2019). Diabetic macular edema (DME) is the utmost reason for vision impairment in patients with DR. Recently, DR screening projects have been executed worldwide. While most screening projects uses traditional fundus photography with skilled operators, newly developed technologies have shown more current imaging modalities and picture examination programming that can possibly improve screening meticulousness and lessen the monetary weight of these inescapably costly projects (Fenner et al., 2018)

In the last decade, intravitreal anti-vascular endothelial growth factor (VEGF) agents are the primary treatment for DME. Still, due to many restrictions such as regular injections, economical challenges and less support from patients during clinical practice, the use of anti-VEGF drugs is limited. Intravitreal corticosteroids have exhibited clinical advantages in the treatment of DR case when it rejects the anti-VEGF therapy. Actually, as far as DR treatment is concerned, laser photocoagulation plays a significant role. However, it is tough for patients with serious visual impairment to accomplish reading or driving with presently accessible therapeutics (Wang, & Lo, 2018).

2.5. Dry Eyes

A suitable and constant layer of liquid, tears is constantly needed on the upper surface of the eye to keep it moist and function well. Dry eye syndrome is affected by a chronic absence of enough lubrication and wetness on the surface of the eye (Seen & Tong, 2018). Magnitudes of dry eye problem start with eye irritation and may range up to scarring of the anterior segment to inflammation (Figure 3). The main reason for dry eyes is nonfunction of meibomian gland which consequences to lipid tear scarcity. Dry eye is likely to affect 7.4% to 33.7% of the global population (Yeo & Tong, 2018). There are several factors which are responsible for dry eyes mainly smoking, autoimmune disease, post-menopausal hormonal changes etc. Along with this, there are environmental risk factors like dust, wind and excess use of computers and television (Yeo & Tong, 2018).

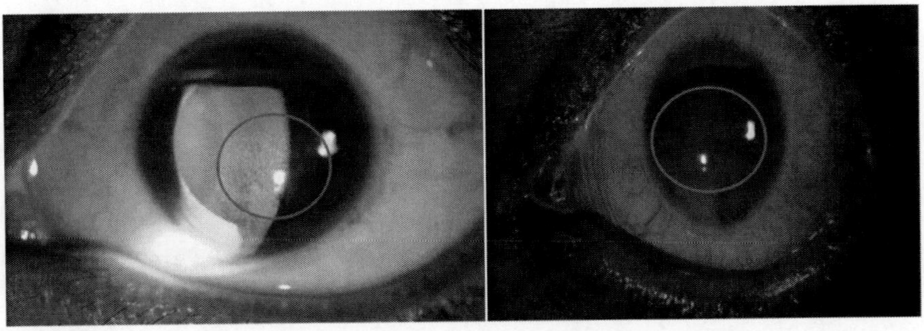

A B

Figure 3. This slit lamp photograph represents the cornea image of the dry eye condition having superficial punctate keratitis (A), and the other image is the fluorescein dye stained (B).

The details regarding types, symptoms and available treatment have been represented in Figure 4. Aqueous deficient dry eye affecting the lacrimal gland and it is further sub-classified into the Sjögren's syndrome (SS) and non-Sjögren's syndrome (NSS). Sjögren's syndrome is due to inflammation of the lacrimal gland, it is mainly found in the older adult or middle-aged person. Non-Sjögren's syndrome is due to the lack of lacrimal gland, lacrimal duct obstruction, use of systemic drugs etc. Evaporative dry eye syndrome is either intrinsic or extrinsic. The intrinsic syndrome is caused due to meibomian gland deficiency, defective blinking and lid aperture disorder. The extrinsic syndrome is caused due to Vit-A deficiency, use of topical drugs and contact lenses. The third mucous deficient dry eye is mainly due to very few numbers of goblet cell or declined function of goblet cells. At the age of 50years or older than this are more prone to conjunctiva apoptosis. Therefore, at the age of 50 years or more, mucous deficient dry eye syndrome is predominant. Presentaly tears substitute, topical cyclosporine (CsA), Vit-A, a nanomicellar farmulation of topical cyclosporine CsA 0.09% approved to incresae tear production in DED (Sun Pharmaceuticals India), surgical intervention etc. are available.. Currently, the use of tear substitutes, emulsions, gels, ointments is recommended. Whereas, eyelid hygiene as well as warm compression encourages the production of tears and therefore reduces the discomfort due to dry eyes.

3. Preventive Measures

Ageing is frequently connected with a phase of life combined with ailment and weakness, and also the collection of physiological, mental and economic status which may unfavourably influence health conditions. Aged individuals could have a greater commonness of perpetual health disorders, various risk factors may instigate more aged individuals to an unfortunate wholesome status creating over or undernourishment. Deprived and poor nourishment are common and occur in considcrable numbers in older individuals. However, the indications of ailing health (weight reduction, perplexity, discombobulation and poor hunger) may lead to wrong diagnosis (Turconi, 2010).However, attributable to various stabilization methods, it has been able to determine a variety of health-advancing products by improving well being in adults and elderly people with low physical capability. There is a huge gap in people's awareness and comprehension of eye ailment that should be understood for eye health advancement exercises (Livingston et al., 1998).

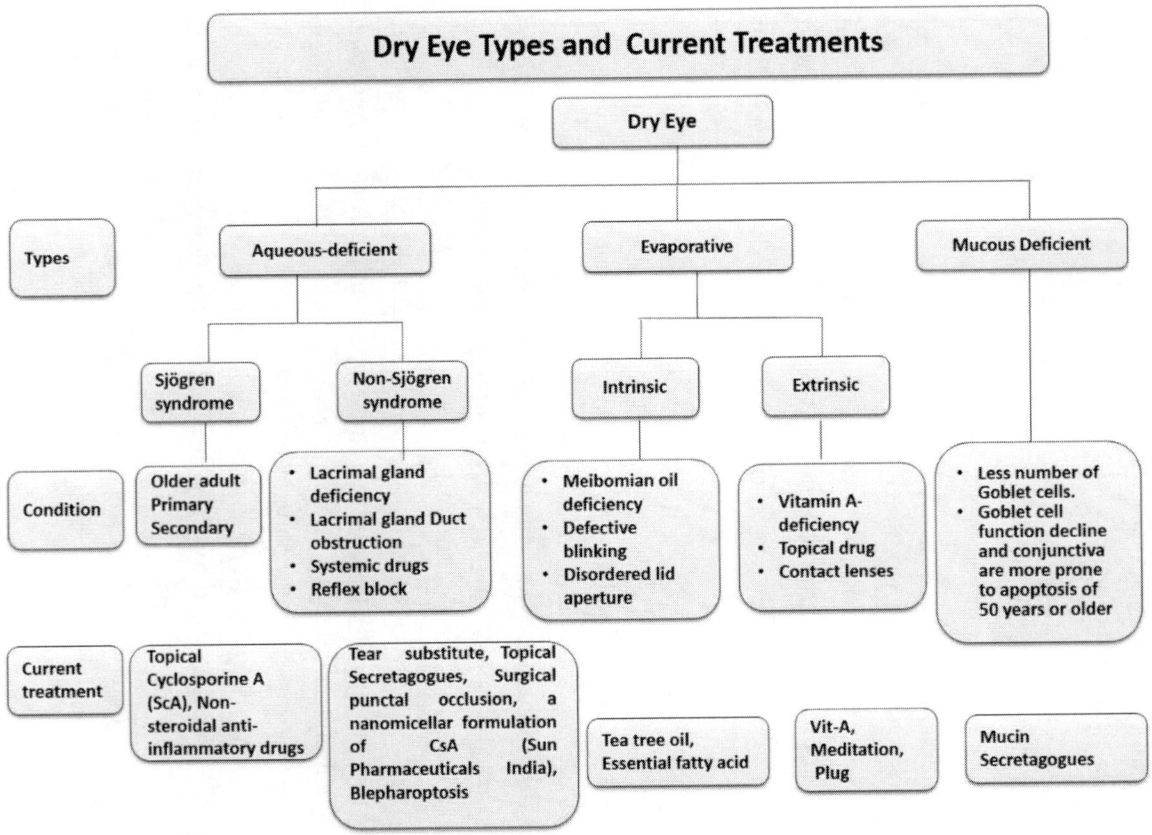

Figure 4. Schematic representation of dry eye disease (DED) classification, symptoms and the currently available treatment.

Intraocular pressure (IOP) assessment plays a major role in glaucoma diagnosis and management. The earlier findings suggest that the quantity of glaucoma drugs isn't meeting the quality of patient satisfaction and further clinical facility required to confirm and examine glaucoma cases. (Rossi et al., 2010). Specialists and the whole ophthalmic care group ought to know about this occurrence and try to limit the damage by doing more work in a ophthalmic area (Raqqad & Liu, 2010; Rosen et al., 2011).

As of now, completely robotized PC projects are accessible to the electronic record. The doctor or ophthalmologist can pursue the patient from the workplace through the web (Mostafa et al., 2010). Most cataract medical procedure patients want not to just appreciate brilliant non-spectacle adjusted far vision, yet additionally non-corrected near vision without glasses.

In the developing world, the lack of protein in the diet is an important and very common medical issue. Natural products including fruits and vegetables are good sources of micro and macronutrients, minerals, and are rich in fibres that provide fundamental supplements to the human wellbeing. Phytochemicals being a strong antioxidant obtained from plants, have gained a lot of consideration as of late. Polyunsaturated fatty acids especially long-chained are the major constituents of the construction and function of the retina, any disability in their supply either through maternal or dietary supply may lead to imperfect retinal development, morphology and capacity. Long-chained polyunsaturated fatty acids, an antecedent could be provided simply through meat and seafood diets to the people who depend primarily on eating regimen for their antecedents. Recently, the use of limbal stem cells is trending for treatment of various kinds of limbal stem cell deficiency (Basu et al., 2016; Kethiri et al., 2017) corneal ulcers and other ocular diseases (Singh et al., 2015).

ACKNOWLEDGMENTS

This work was supported by the Hyderabad Eye Research Foundation, Hyderabad, India. Support in part was provided by Champalimaud

Translational Centre for Eye Research, L V Prasad Eye Institute, Hyderabad, India; Science and Engineering Research Board - Core Research Grant (SERB-CRG) (Vivek Singh: CRG/2018/003514) and DBT grant (Vivek Singh: BY/PR28299/MED/32/632/2018), Government of India. Thanks to Photography and EMR department of LV Prasad Eye Institute for providing the relevant images of a diseased eye. All consents were taken for the use of these images as per the Institutional guidelines.

REFERENCES

Basu, S., Sureka, S. P., Shanbhag, S. S., Kethiri, A. R., Singh, V., & Sangwan, V. S. (2016). Simple limbal epithelial transplantation: long-term clinical outcomes in 125 cases of unilateral chronic ocular surface burns. *Ophthalmology*, *123*(5), 1000-1010.

Beaver, Hilary A. "Cataracts and cataract surgery." In *Geriatric Ophthalmology*, pp. 15-26. Springer, Cham, 2019.

Chae, B., Cakiner-Egilmez, T., & Desai, M. (2013). Glaucoma medications. *Insight (American Society of Ophthalmic Registered Nurses)*, *38*(1), 5-9.

Duong, H. Q., Westfield, K. C., & Singleton, I. C. (2011). Comparing Three Post-Op Regiments for Management of Inflammation Post Uncomplicated Cataract Surgery. *Are Steroids Really Necessary*, 2.

Fenner, B. J., Wong, R. L., Lam, W. C., Tan, G. S., & Cheung, G. C. (2018). Advances in retinal imaging and applications in diabetic retinopathy screening: A review. *Ophthalmology and therapy*, *7*(2), 333-346.

Francis, B. A., Loewen, N., Hong, B., Dustin, L., Kaplowitz, K., Kinast, R. & Ichhpujani, P. (2016). Repeatability of selective laser trabeculoplasty for open-angle glaucoma. *BMC ophthalmology*, *16*(1), 128.

Fu, J., Mou, D. P., Li, S. N., Wang, X. Z., & Hao, L. (2011). Mid-Term Results of Filtering Surgery in Corticosteroid-Induced Glaucoma Patients. *J Clinic Experiment Ophthalmol*, *2*, 142.

Funderburgh, J., Basu, S., Damala, M., Tavakkoli, F., Sangwan, V., & Singh, V. (2018). Limbal stromal stem cell therapy for acute and chronic superficial corneal pathologies: one-year outcomes. *Investigative Ophthalmology & Visual Science*, *59*(9), 3455-3455.

Gudla, S., Tenneti, D., Pande, M., & Tipparaju, S. M. (2018). *Diabetic retinopathy: pathogenesis, treatment, and complications in Drug delivery for the retina and posterior segment disease* (pp. 83-94). Springer, Cham.

Kaiser, P. K., & Do, D. V. (2007). Ranibizumab for the treatment of neovascular AMD. *International journal of clinical practice*, *61*(3), 501-509.

Katsanos, A., Konstas, A. G., Mikropoulos, D. G., Quaranta, L., Voudouragkaki, I. C., Athanasopoulos, G. P., & Teus, M. A. (2018). A review of the clinical usefulness of selective laser trabeculoplasty in exfoliative glaucoma. *Advances in therapy*, *35*(5), 619-630.

Kethiri, A. R., Basu, S., Shukla, S., Sangwan, V. S., & Singh, V. (2017). Optimizing the role of limbal explant size and source in determining the outcomes of limbal transplantation: An in vitro study. *PloS one*, *12*(9), e0185623.

Lee, C. M., & Afshari, N. A. (2017). The global state of cataract blindness. *Current opinion in ophthalmology*, *28*(1), 98-103.

Liu, B., McNally, S., Kilpatrick, J. I., Jarvis, S. P., & O'Brien, C. J. (2018). Ageing and ocular tissue stiffness in glaucoma. *Survey of ophthalmology*, *63*(1), 56-74.

Livingston, P. M., McCarty, C. A., & Taylor, H. R. (1998). Knowledge, attitudes, and self-care practices associated with age-related eye disease in Australia. *British journal of ophthalmology*, *82*(7), 780-785.

Maylahn, C., Gohdes, D. M., Balamurugan, A., & Larsen, B. A. (2005). *Peer-reviewed:* Age-related Eye Diseases: An Emerging Challenge for Public Health Professionals. *Preventing chronic disease*, 2(3).

Mitchell, P., Korobelnik, J. F., Lanzetta, P., Holz, F. G., Pruente, C., Schmidt-Erfurth, U. & Wolf, S. (2010). Ranibizumab (Lucentis) in neovascular age-related macular degeneration: evidence from clinical trials. *British Journal of Ophthalmology*, *94*(1), 2-13.

Mokbel, T. H., & Ghanem, A. A. (2011). Diagnostic value of color Doppler imaging and pattern visual evoked potential in primary open-angle glaucoma. *J Clinic Experiment Ophthalmol*, *2*(1), 127.

Mostafa, A. M., Kassem, R. R., & Abdel-Meguid, A. A. E. (2010). Factors Affecting Compliance to Two-Hour Versus Six-Hour Occlusion Therapy Regimens for Treatment of Strabismic Amblyopia. J Clinic Experiment Ophthalmol 1: 110. doi:10.4172/2 155-9570.1000110.

Nowak, M. S., & Smigielski, J. (2015). The prevalence and causes of visual impairment and blindness among older adults in the city of Lodz, Poland. *Medicine*, *94*(5).

Quigley, H. A., & Broman, A. T. (2006). The number of people with glaucoma worldwide in 2010 and 2020. *British journal of ophthalmology*, *90*(3), 262-267.

Raqqad, N. A., & Liu, C. (2010). Mascara: a cause of thermal burn after cautery for eyelid lesion excision; a case report. *J Clinic Experiment Ophthalmol*, *1*, 105.

Rosen, J. E., Yoffe, S., Meerasa, A., Verma, M., & Gu, F. X. (2011). Nanotechnology and diagnostic imaging: new advances in contrast agent technology. *J Nanomed Nanotechnol*, *2*(5), 115-126.

Rossi, G. C. M., Pasinetti, G. M., Briola, A., & Bianchi, P. E. (2010). Effect of Glaucoma Medications on Quality of Life Examined by Generic and Vision Specific Instruments. J Clinic Experiment Ophthalmol 1: 106. doi: 10.4172/2155-9570.1000106.

Rovner, B. W., Casten, R. J., Hegel, M. T., Massof, R. W., Leiby, B. E., Ho, A. C., & Tasman, W. S. (2014). Low vision depression prevention trial in age-related macular degeneration: a randomized clinical trial. *Ophthalmology*, *121*(11), 2204-2211.

Sabanayagam, C., Banu, R., Chee, M. L., Lee, R., Wang, Y. X., Tan, G. & Mitchell, P. (2019). Incidence and progression of diabetic retinopathy: a systematic review. *The Lancet Diabetes & Endocrinology*, *7*(2), 140-149.

Salvi, S. M., Akhtar, S., & Currie, Z. (2006). Ageing changes in the eye. *Postgraduate medical journal*, *82*(971), 581-587.

Seen, S., & Tong, L. (2018). Dry eye disease and oxidative stress. *Acta ophthalmologica*, *96*(4), e412-e420.

Shanbhag, S. S., Nikpoor, N., Donthineni, P. R., Singh, V., Chodosh, J., & Basu, S. (2019). Autologous limbal stem cell transplantation: a systematic review of clinical outcomes with different surgical techniques. *British Journal of Ophthalmology*, bjophthalmol-2019.

Singh, V., Shukla, S., Ramachandran, C., Mishra, D. K., Katikireddy, K. R., Lal, I. & Sangwan, V. S. (2015). Science and art of cell-based ocular surface regeneration. In *International review of cell and molecular biology* (Vol. 319, pp. 45-106). Academic Press.

Stevens, G. A., White, R. A., Flaxman, S. R., Price, H., Jonas, J. B., Keeffe, J., ... & Taylor, H. (2013). Global prevalence of vision impairment and blindness: magnitude and temporal trends, 1990–2010. *Ophthalmology*, *120*(12), 2377-2384.

Steverson, United Nations, Department of Economic and Social Affairs, Population Division (2017). World Population Prospects: The 2017 Revision, Key Findings and Advance Tables.

Tisdale, A. K., Agrón, E., Sunshine, S. B., Clemons, T. E., Ferris, F. L., & Chew, E. Y. (2019). Association of dietary and supplementary calcium intake with age-related macular degeneration: Age-Related Eye Disease Study report 39. *JAMA ophthalmology*, *137*(5), 543-550.

Turconi, G. (2010). Healthy Aging: Nutritional Intervention to Improve and Extend Quality of Life among Older People. *Nutrition & Food Sciences*.

Venkatesh, R., Tan, C. S., Sengupta, S., Ravindran, R. D., Krishnan, K. T., & Chang, D. F. (2010). Phacoemulsification versus manual small-incision cataract surgery for white cataract. *Journal of Cataract & Refractive Surgery*, *36*(11), 1849-1854.

Wang, W., & Lo, A. (2018). Diabetic retinopathy: pathophysiology and treatments. *International journal of molecular sciences*, *19*(6), 1816.

Wang, Y. X., Xu, L., Wei, W. B., & Jonas, J. B. (2018). Intraocular pressure and its normal range adjusted for ocular and systemic parameters. The Beijing Eye Study 2011. *PloS one*, *13*(5), e0196926.

Werdich, X. Q., Ruez, T., & Singh, R. P. (2010). Prevalence and severity of blepharitis symptoms and signs amongst patients with age-related macular degeneration. *Investigative Ophthalmology & Visual Science*, *51*(13), 5122-5122.

Yeo, S., & Tong, L. (2018). Coping with dry eyes: a qualitative approach. *BMC ophthalmology*, *18*(1), 8.

Zhao, L., Chen, X. J., Zhu, J., Xi, Y. B., Yang, X., Hu, L. D., ... & Wu, F. (2015). Lanosterol reverses protein aggregation in cataracts. *Nature*, *523*(7562), 607.

Zhu, R. R., Shi, J., Yang, M., & Guan, H. J. (2016). Prevalences and causes of vision impairment in elderly Chinese: a socioeconomic perspective of a comparative report nested in Jiangsu Eye Study. *International journal of ophthalmology*, *9*(7), 1051.

In: Current Challenges and Management … ISBN: 978-1-53617-304-8
Editor: Abhai Kumar

Chapter 7

METABOLOMICS: TOWARDS HEALTH CARE CHALLENGES AND MANAGEMENT IN ELDERLY POPULATION

Sonia Gandhi**, PhD and Isha Gupta, JRF
Institute of Nuclear Medicine and Allied Sciences (INMAS), DRDO, India

ABSTRACT

Ageing is a complex biological process which varies from one individual to another. There has been an exponential increase in ageing in India due to increased life expectancy which in turn is raising the demand for more holistic care. With the increase in older population, risk factor also increase which in turn needs more research focus towards ageing process, age related diseases and longevity. Studies have shown that various genetic and metabolic pathways gets affected due to ageing process but there is still a need to predict biomarkers and understand the correlation between various pathways which influence the ageing process. Metabolomics can be one potential technique which can help in bridging the gap between genotype and downstream ageing phenotypes.

---

* Corresponding Author's Email: sonia@inmas.drdo.in.

Metabolomics is paving its way as a diagnostic tool in clinical research and can be a solution to many ageing maladies in elderly population which are presently unanswered. In this chapter we present metabolomics as a potential tool for developing biomarkers of age and age-related diseases, to metabolic pathway and network analysis. Future of ageing research in elderly population lies in integration of various 'omics' platforms which will help in identifying the causes of ageing and developing interventions to prevent the consequences thereby improving the lifespan.

1. INTRODUCTION

The world population has reached from 3.3 billion in 1965 to 7.5 billion in 2017 due to rapid development in the field of science and technology. Around 11.5% of 7.5 billion world population is above 60. The people of 60 or above come under the category of elderly population according to National Policy on Older Persons, January 1999. The number of people falling under elderly category will exceed the number of children below the age of 15 years. While in Asia, the elderly population will increase from 10.5% to 22.4% by 2050. India is going to contribute 158.1 million populations of elderly people. India is also going to be labelled as "*an aging nation*" in the coming future but the pace of drift is slower as compared to the other countries [1, 2, 3].

The major reason behind this drift is demographic transition. Demographic transition is stage where birth rate falls below the death rate due to decline in fertility and mortality rate while escalation in survival rate [4]. This is the "older-older age wave" that has been going around the globe [5]. Developing nations such as India are affected worst by this wave because this segment of population is aging with each passing day [6]. Aging is a complex and irreversible process which involves gradual decline in the age-specific fitness components of an organism due to internal physiological deterioration [7] and is a component of the genetic routine of an organism. Aging process leads to decline in ability to tackle stress and physical alertness [8]. Therefore, the health of this section of society is a major concern for the Government of India because they suffer from high mortality and morbidity. Population health continuum of elderly is divided into four categories for better understanding: Healthy and active, at risk but healthy, coping with disease and severely ill. Maximum population lie in the middle two categories of the continuum. At risk but healthy and coping with disease require higher health care expenditure while severely ill population require constant medical support for survival. This continuum model can help to understand and implement the progress in the field of health. In other words, old age is one of the major reasons behind chronic diseases. According to report of National council Aging, 2014, 92% of elderly suffer from at least one chronic disease while 77% from at least two chronic diseases [9]. Most of the elderly suffer from the sensory changes such as hearing loss, visual acuity, vestibular function, immunosenescence, urologic changes, somatic and multiple chronic diseases (cardiovascular, hypertension, cancer, osteoarthritis, diabetes milletus, osteoporosis), and psychological changes (cognitive aging, dementia, depression) which is presented in the Figure 1. Morbidity of elderly people is higher in urban areas as compared to rural areas. Hypertension is the most common ailment followed by arthritis. The diseases leading to the death among elderly population are cardiovascular diseases followed by respiratory ailments [10]. Elderly population needs medical support and care to tackle the demographic transition which can be a hindrance to the development of our nation. Due to this trend, the human ageing is being debated and researched worldwide. Future of ageing research requires expertise from vast areas to (i) identify the socio-cultural, psychological, economic and public health implications of human ageing; (ii) understand the molecular, biological and physiological factors of human ageing and (iii) identify factors that promote health in later life and/or protect against ageing-related disease and dysfunction.

High rates of morbidity and mortality are associated with elderly population due to various infectious diseases. The success of the medical science is accompanied by several social, economic and psychological problems in older persons, in addition to the medical problems and hence the care for elderly population is emerging as a point of public and private concern. The treatment for many of these problems requires lifelong drug therapy, physical therapy and long-term rehabilitation [11]. Proteomic and metabolomic profiling has a great potential in identifying the underlying causal mechanisms that link genotype to phenotype. Ageing and age related changes can be attributed to failure of coordination between biological network of RNAs, proteins and metabolites that are responsible for modulating longevity across various tissues and cellular organelles [12]. Potentially powerful hypothesis related to ageing and age-related diseases can be studied not only by up or down regulation of the levels of proteins or metabolites but also by inter correlation of these molecules in larger networks. Here, metabolomics can work as a disease diagnostic tool because some questions are not answered by other branch of science.

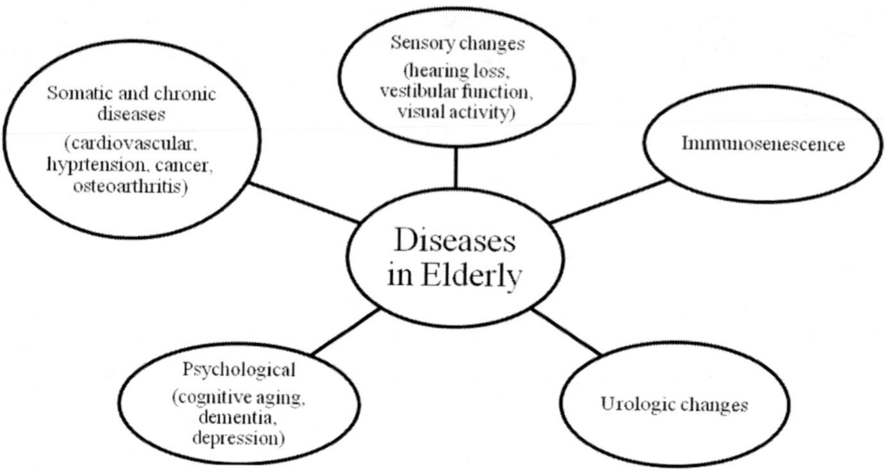

Figure 1. Various diseases in elderly population.

In this chapter, we deal with potential of metabolomics in ageing research which goes from individual biomarker of ageing and diseases to metabolic pathways and network analysis. Further, various 'omics' techniques can be integrated to give a complete insight of molecular causes and consequences of ageing.

2. What Is Metabolomics and Metabonomics?

The study of the dynamics of an organism comes under the branch of Omics which is an important part of biomedical sciences. Omics is that branch of science which characterizes and quantifies the biological molecules such as genes, transcriptomes, proteins and metabolites. Therefore, this branch is divided into four main layers: Genomics, Transcriptomics, Proteomics and Metabolomics [13]. This chapter focuses on the young branch of Omics i.e., Metabolomics which is a fast developing robust field. More than 3700 articles have been published in the two decades on various aspects of metabolomics [14]. This branch evaluates the metabolomes (amino acids, carbohydrates, fatty acids) present in the biological samples at a particular time point which provides less complex and more precise data than the other three omics. Other omics field provide information of what is happening inside the living organism while metabolomics provides an entire "snapshot" of the physiology of the living organism. Metabolome term was first defined by Oliver et al. in 1998 [15]. Metabolome is the set of metabolites which are end products or intermediates of processes involved in the metabolism. Metabolites are also obtained from the diet and other exogenous sources. Metabolomics and metabonomics are used interchangeably by the researchers wherein Metabolomics is ''the study of the measurement of metabolite concentrations, fluxes and secretion in cells and tissues where there is a direct connection between the genetic activity, protein activity and the metabolic activity itself'' while metabonomics is ''the study of the quantitative measurement of the multivariate metabolic responses of multicellular systems to pathophysiological stimuli or genetic modification''. This branch shortens the gap between genotype and phenotype. Metabolomics has wide applications in the field of therapeutics, disease biomarkers, toxicology, drug discovery etc. Still some challenges such as heterogeneity and chemical complexity of metabolites, development of extraction protocols, limitations of various techniques and high throughput measurement are needed to be resolved.

The two methodologies used for the analysis are untargeted and targeted metabolomics. Untargeted metabolomics is to analyse the broadest range of metabolites present in the samples without the prior knowledge of the metabolites while targeted metabolomics is to analyse the specific metabolites on the account of prior knowledge. Targeted metabolomics methodology is more sensitive and selective as compared to untargeted metabolomics. These methodologies are used to validate and to develop the workflow of metabolomics. Hence, the information obtained from it can be used to validate and to develop the workflow of metabolomics. Untargeted approach still remains a challenge for researchers to identify the complete set of metabolites.

Different biological samples such as urine, plasma, serum, saliva, cerebrospinal fluid, bile, seminal fluid, saliva, amniotic fluid, blister fluids, dialysis fluids and tissues can be examined. Fluids secreted or excreted from a living organism carry the biochemical information related to stress, disease, drug toxicity etc. Other variations or perturbation in the human system can also affect the composition of the fluids. Urine composition is complex; therefore, complete analysis is difficult. This complexity shows the problem of diagnostic variation and the influence of variation on diagnosis. Whole blood samples pose various limitations. Serum and plasma contains mainly water but serum is devoid of clotting agent and less viscous as compared to plasma. In tissue analysis, researcher can study the localized responses to stimuli, which provides the biochemical information of diseases. It requires extraction of all the metabolites from the tissues into a liquid form. More than 3,500 metabolites have been discovered and added to human metabolome project (HMP) by Wishart and his co-workers.

Different analytical tools are used to study the human metabolome such as Nuclear magnetic resonance (NMR) spectroscopy, Fourier transform- Infrared (FT-IR) spectroscopy, High- performance Liquid Chromatography (HPLC) and Gas Chromatography (GC) and Mass spectrometry (MS). The minimum criteria to be fulfilled by these approaches are sensitivity, selectivity and comprehensiveness. Hence, the major analytical techniques are NMR spectroscopy and MS combined with multivariate data analysis methods to identify the metabolites and metabolic pathways which are related to a specific phenotype. NMR spectroscopy is the technique which differentiates the sample on the basis of natural abundance of NMR-active nuclei. Spectral data of MS is represented as natural abundance vs. ratio of mass to charge (m/z). It provides the information of accurate mass of ion and distinguishing fragment. MS provides higher sensitivity while NMR spectroscopy provides higher reproducibility. MS helps in the identification of the masses of molecules. Samples can be directly injected to the MS, but production of thousands of ions suppresses signals. So, substances are first separated with the help of different chromatography techniques (usually High performance liquid chromatography and Gas chromatography) on the basis of their retention time which further increases the sensitivity of the MS. This type of coupling between two techniques is known as hyphenated technology. NMR is a reproducible, non-destructive, non-invasive, non-equilibrium and robust technique. It provides information through spin relaxation and molecular diffusion properties of molecular dynamics and mobility of metabolites. Amount of sample required for acquisition of spectra is quite low and the time required for acquisition is also less for NMR. Preferences of tools depend on the type of sample, availability of resources and objective of the study.

2.1. Various Analytical Techniques for Metabolomics

There has been rapid development of a range of analytical platforms in metabolomics field which can enable separation, detection, characterization and quantification of various metabolites and related metabolic pathways. Single analytical platform cannot be applied to detect all metabolites in a biological sample due to its complex nature and large metabolome. Various analytical platform being widely used in metabolomics research are:

2.1.1. Mass Spectroscopy

Mass spectrometry is one of the most widely applied techniques in metabolomics, as it is a combination of rapid, sensitive and selective qualitative and quantitative analyses with the ability to identify metabolites. The separation of metabolites is carried out using GC or LC before MS detection [16].

2.1.2. Gas Chromatography–mass Spectrometry (GC-MS)

GC-MS is a combination of high sensitivity and resolution with a reproducible fragmentation pattern of the separated molecules. GC-MS is the principal technique for separation and detection of metabolites that are naturally volatile at temperatures up to 250°C (e.g., fatty acids, aliphatic alcohols, and esters essential oils). It also applies to groups of non-volatile, polar (mainly primary) metabolites, such as amino acids, sugars, and organic acids, by converting these into volatile compounds through chemical derivatization. However, incomplete derivatization can cause the problem of more than one peak for the same compound [17] and complex plant secondary metabolites, such as phenolic glycosides, are difficult to be analyzed by GC.

2.1.3. Liquid Chromatography-mass Spectrometry (LC–MS)

One of the very versatile techniques in metabolomics, LC-MS is capable of facilitating the analysis of several large groups of secondary metabolites. Advances in chromatographic techniques together with advances in column chemistry have resulted in a significantly improved separation potential. The only restriction to the technique being those molecules which can be ionized, either as positively or as negatively charged ions, before moving through the MS. It can be used for wide range of analytes in terms of molecular weight and polarity along with quantitative precise molecular weight determination [18].

2.1.4. Capillary Electrophoresis–Mass Spectrometry (CE–MS)

CE is being used as an alternative separation technology, particularly for charged metabolites, and is combined with MS for extra selectivity and sensitivity [19]. High-resolution chromatographic separation and sensitive detection of water soluble extracts make a strong combination suitable for the analysis of a diverse range of polar and water-soluble primary and secondary metabolites. This technique has bioanalytical applications such as analysis of proteins, peptides, amino acids, and mixture of saccharides, has been reviewed by Klampfl [20].

2.1.5. Ion Mobility Mass Spectrometry

Ion mobility mass spectrometry (IMMS) is a gas phase process in which ions are separated by their different mobility in a buffer gas under the influence of an electric field. It is a high throughput technique which is suited for isomers separation. IMMS systems have been used for targeting specific small biomolecules, such as amino acids, carbohydrates, glucose, caffeine, neurometabolites, and drugs.

2.1.6. Fourier Transform–infrared Spectroscopy (FT-IR)

This technique is considered as the basic among the spectroscopic techniques with the features such as fast, high throughput, non-destructive, and non-selective [21]. It is a method of choice for initial screening owing to its low cost as compared to other spectrometric and spectroscopic techniques [22].

2.1.7. MALDI-ToFMS

Matrix-assisted laser desorption ionization time-of-flight mass spectrometry (MALDI-ToFMS) shows application in metabolomics technology in detection and quantitation of high molecular weight biomolecules from biofluids and intact tissue (plant and animal) [23]. MALDIToFMS can prove useful in studies where ESI-MS would present complex spectra due to multiple charging effects.

2.1.8. Nuclear Magnetic Resonance (NMR) Spectroscopy

In metabolomics studies, NMR spectroscopy provides a rapid, unbiased, reproducible, non-destructive, high throughput method with minimal sample preparation [24]. The technique, especially 1H NMR is used extensively in clinical and pharmaceutical applications since it provides detailed structural information of small organic molecules and biofluids. Typically, biofluids such as urine, bile, blood plasma and tissue extract have been investigated. NMR based metabolomics has been used in various areas such as toxicology [25], disease progression [26], drug efficacy monitoring [27] and biomarker discovery. NMR can also be used for the analysis of samples that are composed of diverse compound mixtures. NMR based metabolomics is being used in applied situations such as quality characteristics or identifying potential biochemical markers to detect product contamination and adulteration.

2.1.9. Hyphenated Techniques

Hyphenation between various separation and detection techniques are being explored to improve upon various aspects of metabolomics. Researchers are working on developing and providing instrumental platforms and methods for analyzing metabolites present in a sample using comprehensive analytical techniques. The various techniques such as UV, IR, FT-IR, and FT-MS spectroscopies, nuclear magnetic resonance (NMR), liquid chromatography (LC), capillary electrophoresis, and LC or gas chromatography (GC) combined with mass spectrometry (LC-MS and GCMS) are being explored. Comprehensive two-dimensional (2D) GC coupled to time-of-flight mass spectrometry (GC × GC–TOFMS) has emerged as a powerful chemical analysis tool to study complex samples in metabolomics studies. Metabolomic analysis has also been performed with linear ion traps or the QTRAP which provides resolution along with MS/MS capabilities. There has been considerable interest in laser desorption ionization (LDI) techniques such as MALDI (matrix-assisted laser desorption ionization), SELDI (surface-enhanced laser desorption ionization), or desorption/extractive electrospray ionization (EESI). Analytical method needs to be carefully chosen in order to have an excellent initial strategy for getting a metabolic profile that can ultimately be used to identify key biochemical leads to further or more focused studies.

2.2. Metabolomics Workflow

Metabolomics is highly interdisciplinary requiring a specialized workflow which is presented in Figure 2. The first step of workflow is to design the experiment because at this stage outline is defined which includes aims and the subjects which have to involve in this experiment. Thereafter ethical approval is obtained to conduct it, which is followed by sample preparation and data acquisition. After acquisition, data pre-processing and interrogation are done. Identification of metabolite which alters the particular pathway is identified and quantified. The result of this study can also be verified and justified by other orthogonal approach such as genomics and proteomics. In this way, different omics fields are integrated [13, 28, 29].

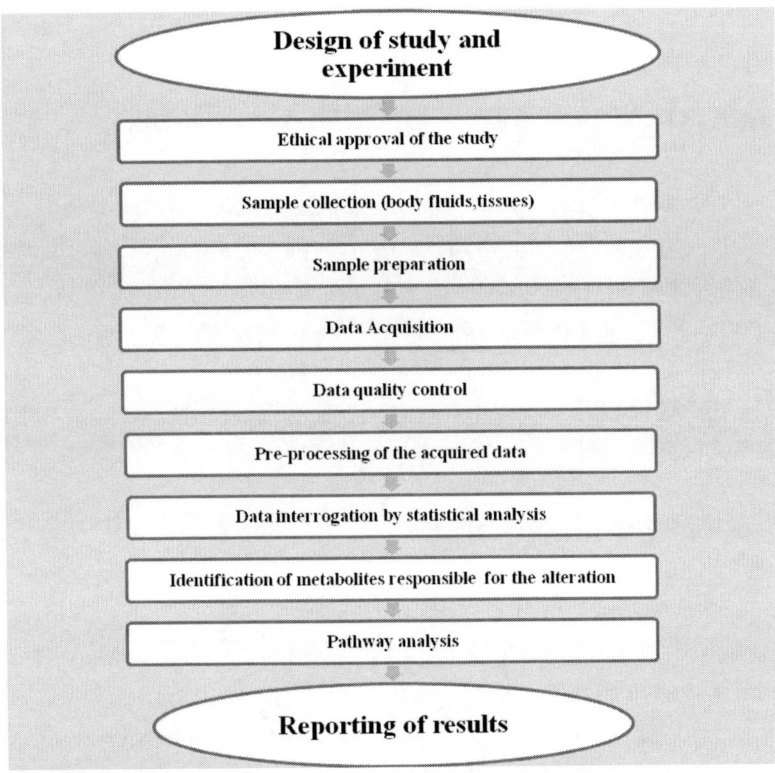

Figure 2. Flowchart depicting study design for Metabolomics.

Complex datasets are obtained from the above analytical techniques; therefore, chemometric and pattern recognition (PR) analysis methods are needed to interpret the results. There are tools such as XCMS Online, Metabo Analyst which can be used for statistical analysis. However, choosing correct test can be difficult. Researchers can take the help of developed databases of metabolites such as METLIN, HMDB, GMD and MassBank. These databases contain the information of concentration range of metabolites which can be matched with the data obtained from NMR spectroscopy and MS. Pathway mapping tools such as mummichog and metabolite set enrichment analysis (MSEA) can be used. Coordination of Standards in Metabolomics (COSMOS) is providing complete data sharing for standardization of metabolomics for helping new researchers in this flourishing field. Despite all of these developments, data processing becomes a tedious job.

3. Application of Metabonomics

Metabolomics is the future of the rapid developing and progressive science. This can predict the disease as well as the status of the disease by linking genotype with phenotype. It can also study the therapeutic response of the drug. This omics has application in many research areas such as disease diagnosis, therapeutics, etc. Figure 3 depicts few of the areas where metabolomics is paving its way.

3.1. Identification of Biomarkers

Biomarker is crucial for the prediction of the disease dynamics in the living organism. Biomarker is a biological molecule that is identified and quantified as an indicator of the disease progression or response to the treatment. This omics can help to identify the new pathways involved in disease. Novel biomarkers can be determined to detect, track and monitor any disease and the effectiveness of the treatment. In this way customized drug treatment can be provided by clinicians. Hence, this can be a breakthrough in the field of medical sciences [30].

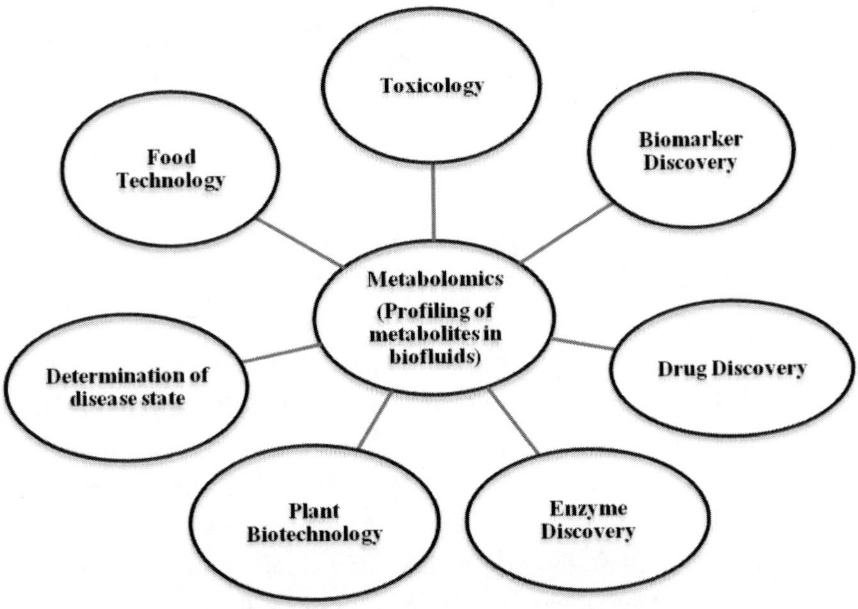

Figure 3. Application of Metabolomics in various research fields.

3.2. Herbal Medicine

Preference for herbal medicines over conventional drugs has gained popularity. Administration of herbal medicines raise many safety issues such as dosing regimen, identification of active ingredient, presence of any contaminants, preparation method. This issue has not been resolved. Metabolic fingerprint of *Euonymus alatus* (Thuhb) siebold administered for atherosclerosis was determined by LC-DAD/ESI-MS/MS. LC-MS metabolomics approach has been used to identify biomolecules such as flavonoids, monoterpene glycosides present in Chinese medicine, PHY906 and has great potential is herbal medicine [30].

3.3. Determination of Disease State

Pathogenesis of the diseases such as disease onset and progression can also be determined by metabolomics. Concentration level of branched amino acids, fatty acids, ornithine and acylcarnitines can predict the wellness of a person [31].

3.4. Drug Discovery and Disease Diagnostics

Drug discovery and disease diagnostics is one area which involves lot of complexity and expertise. It involves many disciplines such as biochemistry, pharmacology, clinicians etc. to integrate together. These areas involve two phases: preclinical and clinical phases which involve step by step approach to reach the next level (Figure 4). Metabolomics can contribute a lot to this science by discovering markers of its efficacy or toxicity which will help in drug discovery and personalization of medicine. 165 volunteers were recruited to identify the metabolic pathway affected by the dose of aspirin. It was found that aspirin affects the purine pathway. Metabolomics approach can be an alternative to angiography which is used for coronary artery disease [31-33].

4. Role of Metabonomics in Disease Diagnosis in Elderly Population

This topic is going to discuss about the diagnosis of diseases and how researchers are using metabolomics in disease diagnosis. Diagnosis is a basic model for treatment and prognosis of the disease. There are few common diseases which are found quite prevalent in elderly population and early diagnosis and better treatment can enhance the quality of life to large extent. Few of the common problems which elder population face are:

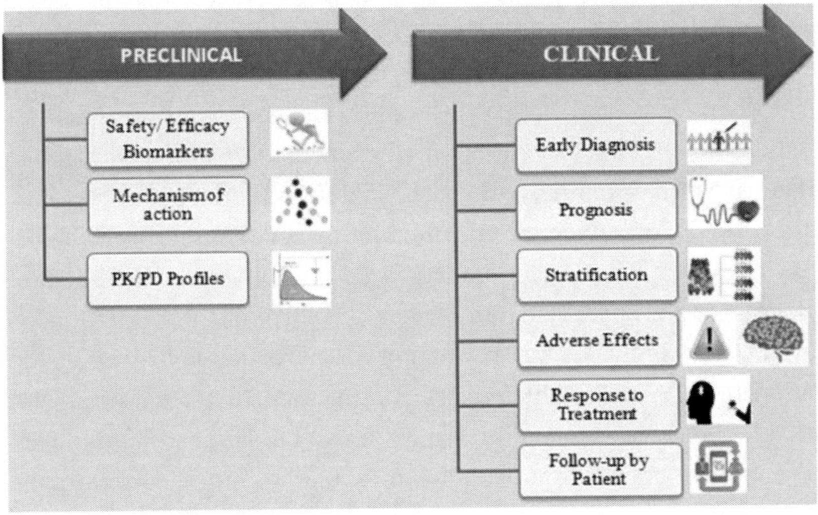

Figure 4. Application of metabolomics in preclinical & clinical domains of disease diagnosis and prognosis.

4.1. Dementia

Around 50 million people are suffering from dementia in 2017 and this number will double after every 20 years [34]. Alzheimer's disease (AD) starts in the hippocampus region of the brain by aggregation of amyloid β protein and hyper phosphorylated tau protein [35]. Liang et al. collected serum from 256 AD patients and 218 controls and with the help of ultra-HPLC with TOF-MS, 6 metabolites were identified. The levels of sphinganine-1-phosphate, phenyllactic acid and ornithine increased while that of inosine, hydroxanthine and 3-dehydrocarnitine decreased [36]. Valine, choline, arginine, dimethylarginine (DMA) values were found higher than the classical biomarkers of AD [34].

4.2. Parkinson's Disease (PD)

This is the second most prevalent neurodegenerative disorder in elderly population. Similar to AD, the number of cases will double up by 2030.

The main challenges associated with PD are its diagnosis and thereafter prognosis [34]. Ahmed et al. collected plasma samples from 43 drug resistant PD patients and 37 healthy people. He assessed 22 metabolites by targeted approach. The concentration of 17 metabolites including glutarate, glucolate, isocitrate, citrate, gluconate, malate, suberate, methylmalonate, galactitol, succinate, glycerol, ethanolamine, acetate, ascorbate, threonate, trimethylamine and methylamine decreased while 5 metabolites including propylene glycol, pyruvate, myoinositol, sorbitol and ethylmalonate increased. This indicates up regulation in pyruvate levels while down regulation in TCA metabolites in the plasma samples of patients. Citrate, acetate, glucitol, pyruvate and myoinositol can be the potential biomarkers for PD [38]. Tohgei et al. noticed down regulation in the concentration of δ-aminobutyric acid (GABA), asparate, and glutamate. In cerebrospinal fluid samples, the decrease in the concentration of glycine was noticeable [39]. Jiménez et al. studies only showed increased level of GABA in CSF samples of PD patients. The level of glutamine, glycine and asparagines increased while aspartate decreased in plasma samples [40]. The research conducted by Mally et al. found decrease in the level of glutamate similar to research of Toghi et al. They also observed decrease in the level of alanine, isoleucine and lysine in the CSF. The levels of valine increased while that of methionine and arginine decreased [41].

4.3. Inflammatory Bowel Disease (IBD)

IBD is a chronic inflammation disease of the intestinal tract. Ulcerative colitis (UC) and Crohn's disease (CD) are two different inflammatory bowel diseases (IBD) which can lead to chronic gastrointestinal disease. Hence, the cases with these diseases in elderly population are expected to increase in the coming future. Metabolic profiling technique can be used to explore the different stages involved in the development of IBD. In the advanced state of IBD, variation was noticed in the sphingomyelins, plasmalogens, triglycerides, cholesterol and phospholipids. Lipid dependent process gets affected in the inflammatory state of IBD. The UC and CD patients were differentiated by characterising the metabolites in serum, plasma and urine samples. The levels of aminoacids, methanol, formate, mannose and 3-methyl-2-oxovalerate increased while that of citrate and urea decreased in serum and plasma. Similarly, the level of xylose, mannitol, carnitine and allantoin increased while that of hippurate and betaine decreased in urine samples [42-44].

4.4. Arthritis

Synovial fluids samples were collected from patients suffering from different forms arthritis such as crystal arthropathy, septic arthritis etc. Synovial fluid is obtained from the filtrate of plasma synovial membrane. It is mainly composed of hyaluronic acid which provides lubrication of joint. Rheumatoid arthritis (RA) patient's synovial fluid contains proteins, metabolites and inflammatory cells. Lactate/alanine ratio is high in RA cases than osteoarthritis (OA). Drugs such as paracetamol, ibuprofen and 35 metabolites were characterised in the fluid. Osteoarthritis and inflammatory arthritis showed similar results. Aceylated glycoprotein, cholesterol, lipid and lactate can serve as potential biomarkers to identify the severity of the disease. Young et al. collected serum samples from early RA cases in which Lactate and lipid was found to be the potential biomarker [45-47].

4.5. Depression

According to 2017 report of World Health Organisation, 300 million people are affected by major depressive disorder (MDD). MDD cases are needed to be diagnosed because more than 10% cases can attempt suicide. Depression is found to be a major concern in elderly population [48]. 10-20% of old people struggle with this disease. Most of the times, Bipolar disorders (BD) cases are misdiagnosed as MDD cases. Pan et al. used plasma-targeted metabolomics approach with the help of GC-MS coupled with LC-MS/MS and quantified 19 metabolites. δ-aminobutyric acid (GABA), kynurenine, tyramine and dopamine provide the difference between MDD patients and healthy controls. These metabolites which were involved in GABAergic, serotonergic and catecholaminergic pathways, were found to be altered [49]. Zheng et al. involved 72 depressive patients while 54 healthy people. In this study, NMR based metabolomics approach was used with least squares-support vector machine (LS-SVM). 20 metabolites such as pyruvate, adipic acid, α-glucose, β-glucose, lactate, poly-UFA, lipids, leucine, isoleucine, tyrosine, valine, alanine, glutamine, glutamate, histidine were affected. Liu et al. studied the therapeutic response of Chinese traditional medicine Xiaoyaosan by ^{1}H NMR metabolomics. The group recruited 16 depressed as well as healthy patients. The levels of lactate, glutamate and trimethylamine oxide increased while those of valine, leucine, choline, alanine, glycine, citrate, glucose and lipids decreased in the plasma samples. After Xiaoyaosan treatment, the levels of alanine, glutamine, lactate, glucose, choline and trimethylamine oxide returned to the normal [50].

4.6. Diabetes

Diabetes Mellitus (DM) is common disease in elderly population. Many biomarkers of type 2 diabetes such as glycated haemoglobin, triglycerides, HDL cholesterol, and inflammatory markers are known. These were not able to understand the complexity of type 2 diabetes. Metabolomics approach may help to identify the novel biomarkers. Urine samples were collected from the patients of type 2 diabetes mellitus. The levels of creatinine, acetoacetate and dimethylamine increased while those of succinate, hippurate, lactate, citrate and 2-ketoglutarate decreased. Floegel et al. used serum targeted metabolomics approach. This group quantified 163 metabolites by flow injection analysis tandem mass spectrometry. The levels of hexose, diacyl-phosphatidylcholines (C32:1, C36:1, C40:5 and C38:3) and phenylalanine increased and of sphingomyelin (C16:1), acyl-alkyl-phosphatidylcholines (C40:6, C34:3, C44:4, C42:5) and lysophosphatidylcholine (C18:2) decreased [42]. Lo et al. collected plasma samples from 486 elders of age more than 65 years for untargeted and targeted metabolomics. The research also differentiated lipid disorder (LD) from diabetes mellitus (DM). Acyl-alkyl phosphatedylcholine (C34:3, C44:3 and C36:3) can predict the progression of DM. The concentration of alanine, branched amino acids, glutamate and α-aminoadipic acid increased in LD patients [51, 52].

4.7. Inborn Errors of Metabolism

This is a genetic disorder caused due to malfunctioning in different metabolisms such as carbohydrate, amino acid, mitochondrial, organic acid and pyrimidine. Here, the toxic substances hinder the particular pathway of metabolism. The NMR studies of the urine collected from the Maple syrup urine disease (MSUD) showed alteration in the number of metabolites including lactate, leucine, 3-methyl-2-oxo-*n*-valerate, 3-hydroxybutyrate and 2-oxo-isocaproate. This approach can help to study the patients affected with MSUD and phenylketonuria (PKU). Proton NMR was used to diagnose the inborn errors of lipid metabolism resulting in disorders such as Smith-Lemli-Optiz syndrome (SLOS), refsum, sitosterolemia and cerebrotendinous xanthomatosis (CTX) using blood plasma or serum [53].

4.8. Sclerosis

Sclerosis is a chronic and multifactorial disease affecting the central nervous system. More than 2.3 million people are suffering from multiple sclerosis. The biomarkers of Amyotrophic lateral sclerosis (ALS) have not been identified. In ALS, glutamate excitotoxicity, creatinine, energy metabolism and oxidative stress pathways are altered. Multiple sclerosis has been studied on chronic mice model. 100 metabolites out of 324 were altered which were related to membrane stability, inflammation and mitochondrial function pathways [54].

The above research shows that metabolomics can help in detection of the early onset of the diseases such as diabetes, depression, dementia, arthritis in the elderly population. In this way, proper care and medical facilities can be provided to the elderly at the right time of the disease progression.

5. Metabolomics as Ageing Biomarker

Metabolomics as a technique to identify ageing biomarkers [55-57] involves identification and quantification of individual metabolites between diseased and control groups which helps in determining the molecules which are different in both the groups. Research in being carried out for past many year to identify metabolic biomarkers in the area of neurodegenerative diseases such as Alzheimer's & Parkinson's disease [58]. Biomarkers have been identified and studied for various other ageing diseases such as cardiovascular disease [59], diabetes [60], coronary heart disease [61], atherosclerosis [62] which can not only predict the present situation but also the future events related to a particular ageing disease. Multiple studies on humans & model systems have been carried out to understand the relation between metabolome changes with age which suggests that metabolic quantification & metabolomics studies are more important biologically to ageing phenotype, morbidities and mortality if better reproducibility and replication can be addressed [63]. Hence, metabolomics alone can serve as an integrative technique for sensitivity and specificity of biomarker prediction. Apart from biomarkers, various cellular networks, how the pathways are getting affected and their correlation also plays an important role in ageing research which is an important aspect of metabolomics [57-59].

This helps in better insight and understanding of biological pathways that affects ageing, age-related diseases and longevity.

6. 'OMICS': INTEGRATED APPROACH AS POTENTIAL SOLUTION IN AGEING RESEARCH

The complete understanding of the biology of ageing and ageing-related diseases requires a framework/model that integrates multiple omics approaches as each 'omics' technique reveals unique information about genetic, biological and biochemical pathways that affect ageing. A comprehensive platform that integrates not only metabolomics and proteomics lying between genotype and phenotype but also proteome, transcriptome, epigenome etc which influence the phenotypes will give a global understanding of ageing and will help in developing targeted lifespan extending interventions. Computational and predictive modelling is being used to develop models which integrates all these modalities and helps in predicting the ageing process at a system level [64, 65].

CONCLUSION

This chapter deals with various ageing problems and diseases with prime focus on role of metabolomics in ageing research. Ageing is a complex process which involves cross correlation between various molecules, cells, organelles, pathways, networks etc and it is required to get a holistic understanding of inter dependence of various cells, pathways & networks, to globally understand the ageing process. Metabolomics gives a wider view by linking all other omics (genomics, proteomics and transcriptomics). Hence, it can help to develop better understanding of the human physiology. As it has been discussed, metabolomics can help to predict and validate the markers, predict the efficacy and toxicity of a drug without administration, identifying new pathways which are altered in the presence of a stimulus (heat, cold, stress, depression etc.), personalised medicine, validation of the beneficial effects of the herbal medicines and many more applications for the elderly as well as other sections of the population. These applications require the development in the database of the human metabolome. The metabolomic approach should be amalgamated with the bioanalytical tools in such a way that the present studies can be combined with the future researches to give a holistic view. This requires the contribution from all (clinicians, researchers and informaticians) to derive the maximum benefit from the study by clinicians. There are some limitations which are needed to be addressed such as sampling of lipids (volume less than 50μL), identification of all the biological molecules present in the particular time point, variation in results due to external stimuli such as diet, physical activities, lifestyle, sample storage and preparation and different analysis methods. These limitations can be outdone by optimising the protocol and using different analytical tools such as LC-MS, NMR, MALDI to draw the results. Metabolomics is the fast growing omics and has a great potential in ageing research if metabolic heterogeneity of individuals and longitudinal studies with replication are taken into consideration.

REFERENCES

[1] Sivaraju et al. 2017. *Caring for our elders: Early responses. India Ageing Report – 2017.* United nation population fund. (Sivaraju et al. 2017)

[2] Jayalakshmi, S., Chakrabarti, S., and Gupta, Nivedita. 2011. *Situation Analysis of the Elderly in India*, Ministry of Statistics & Programme Implementation, Government of India. (Jayalakshmi et al. 2011).

[3] *Changing Cultural Ethos & Impact of Technology* 2018, Elder abuse in India. Study conducted by Ipsos Research Private Limited.

[4] *World Population Prospects: The 2017 Revision.* United Nations, Department of Economic and Social Affairs, Population Division (2017). Online Demographic Profiles.

[5] Jaul, Efraim., and Barron, Jeremy. 2017. "Age-Related Diseases and Clinical and Public Health implications for the 85 Years Old and

Over Population." *Frontiers in Public Health* 5:335. (Jaul 2017, 335).

[6] Mane, Abhay B. 2016. "Ageing in India: Some Social Challenges to Elderly Care." *Journal of Gerontology & Geriatric Research* 5:e136. (Mane 2016, 136)

[7] Rose Michael R., et al. 2012. "What is aging?" *Frontiers in Genetics* 3:134. (Rose 2012, 134)

[8] Bürkle, Alexander., et al. 2015. "MARK-AGE biomarkers of ageing." *Mechanisms of Ageing and Development* 151: 2–12. (Bürkle 2015, 2)

[9] Tkatch, Rifky., et al. 2016 "Population health management for older adults: Review of interventions for promoting successful aging across the health continuum." *Gerontology and Geriatric Medicine* 2: 1-13. (Tkatch 2016, 1)

[10] Kumar, Shailendra., Pradhan, Manas Ranjan., and Singh, Abhishek Kumar. 2017. "Chronic Diseases and their association with disability among the elderly in India." *Social Science Spectrum* 3:22-37. (Kumar 2017, 22).

[11] Yeolekar, ME. 2005 "Elderly in India — Needs and Issues." *Journal of the association of physicians of India*. 53: 843-844. (Yeolekar 2005, 843).

[12] Phillip, Jude M et al. 2015 "The Mechanobiology of Aging." *Annual Review of Biomedical Engineering*. 17: 113-141. (Phillip et al. 2015, 113).

[13] Hasin, Yehudit., Seldin, Marcus., and Lusis, Aldons. 2017. "Multi-omics approaches to disease." *Genome biology* 18:83-98. (Hasin 2017, 83).

[14] Trivedi, Drupad K., Hollywood, Katherine A., and Goodacre, Royston. 2017. "Metabolomics for the masses: The future of metabolomics in a personalized world." *New horizons in translational medicine* 3:294-305. (Trivedi 2017, 294).

[15] Oliver, Stephen G., et al. 1998. "Systematic functional analysis of the yeast genome." *Trends in biotechnology* 16:373-78. (Oliver 1998, 373)

[16] Dettmer, K., Aranov, P. A., Hammock, B. D. 2007 Mass spectrometry based metabolomics. *Mass Spectrom. Rev.*, *26*: 51-78. (Dettmer 2007, 51)

[17] Ryan, D. and Robards, K. 2006 Metabolomics: the greatest omics of them all? *Analytical Chemistry*. 78: 7954-7958. (Ryan 2006, 7954)

[18] Gobey, J et al. 2005 Corr, J. Characterization and performance of MALDI on a triple quadrupole mass spectrometer for analysis and quantification of small molecules. *Analytical Chemistry* 77: 5643-5654. (Gobey 2005, 5643)

[19] Soga, T et al. 2003 Quantitative metabolome analysis using capillary electrophoresis mass spectrometry. *Journal of Proteome Research* 2: 488-494. (Soga 2003, 488)

[20] Christian, W. K. 2004 Chiral separation techniques: A practical approach. *Journal of Chromatography A* 1044: 131-144. (Christian 2004, 131)

[21] Ellis, D. I et al. 2007 Metabolic fingerprinting as a diagnostic tool. *Pharmacogenomics* 8: 1243-1266. (Ellis et al. 2007, 1243)

[22] Allwood, J.W et al. 2006 Metabolic approaches reveal that phosphatidic and phosphatidyl glycerol phospholipids are major discriminatory metabolites in responses by *Brachypodium distachyon* to challenge by *Magnaporthe grisea*. *Plant Journal* 46: 351–368. (Allwood et al. 2006, 351)

[23] Fraser, P. D. et al. 2007 Metabolite profiling of plant carotenoids using the matrix assisted laser desorption ionization time-of-flight mass spectrometry. *Plant Journal* 49: 552-564. (Fraser et al. 2007, 552)

[24] Reo, N. V. 2002 NMR-based metabolomics. *Drug Chemistry Toxicology* 25: 375-382. (Reo 2002, 375)

[25] Can Xu et al. 2017 ^{1}H NMR-Based Metabolomics Study of the Toxicological Effects in Rats Induced by "Renqing Mangjue" Pill, a Traditional Tibetan Medicine. *Frontier in pharmachology* 8:602. (Can et al. 2017, 602)

[26] Pollen K. Yeung. 2018 Metabolomics and Biomarkers for Drug Discovery. *Metabolites* 8:11. (Pollen 2018, 11)

[27] Balashova, Elena et al. 2018 A Metabolomics Approach to Pharmacotherapy Personalization. Journal of Personalized medicine 8:1-15. (Balashova et al. 2018, 1)

[28] Johnson, Caroline H., Ivanisevic, Julijana., and Siuzdak, Gary. 2016 "Metabolomics: beyond biomarkers and towards mechanisms." *Nature reviews Molecular cell biology* 17:451.

[29] (Johnson 2016, 451) Emwas, Abdul Hamid. M., Salek, Reza. M., Griffin, Julian. L., and Merzaban, Jasmeen. 2013. "NMR-based metabolomics in human disease diagnosis: applications, limitations, and recommendations." *Metabolomics* 9:1048–72. (Emwas 2013, 1048)

[30] Kohler, Isabelle., et al. 2017. "Integrating clinical metabolomics-based biomarker discovery and clinical pharmacology to enable precision medicine." *European Journal of Pharmaceutical Sciences* 109:15–21. (Kohler 2017, 15)

[31] Commisso, Mauro., et al. 2013. "Untargeted metabolomics: an emerging approach to determine the composition of herbal products." *Computational and structural biotechnology journal* 4: 1-7. (Commisso et al. 2013, 1)

[32] Shah, Neel Jayesh., Sureshkumar, Srinivasamurthy., and Shewade, Deepak Gopal. 2015. "Metabolomics: a tool ahead for understanding molecular mechanisms of drugs and diseases." *Indian Journal of Clinical Biochemistry* 30:247-54. (Shah 2015, 247)

[33] Yeung, Pollen K. 2018. "Metabolomics and biomarker for drug discovery". *Metabolites* 8:1-3. (Yeung, 2018, 1)

[34] Fetit, Ahmed E., et al. 2013. "Retinal Biomarker Discovery for Dementia in an Elderly Diabetic Population." Paper presented at the Fetal, Infant and Ophthalmic Medical Image Analysis - International Workshop, FIFI 2017 and 4th International Workshop, OMIA 2017 Held in Conjunction with MICCAI 2017. (Fetit 2013)

[35] Hartmann, Samuel., and Kist, Tarso B Ledur. 2018. "A review of biomarkers of Alzheimer's disease in noninvasive samples" *Biomarkers in Medicine* 12:677-90. (Hartmann 2018, 677)

[36] Liang, Q., et al. 2015. "Metabolomics-based screening of salivary biomarkers for early diagnosis of Alzheimer's disease." *RSC Advances.* 5:96074–79. (Liang 2015, 96074)

[37] Lei, Shulei., and Powers, Robert. 2013. "NMR Metabolomics Analysis of Parkinson's Disease." *Current Metabolomics* 1:191-209. (Lei 2013, 191)

[38] Ahmed, S., et al. 2009. "Metabolic profiling of Parkinson's disease: evidence of biomarker from gene expression analysis and rapid neural network detection." *Journal of Biomedical Science* 16:63. (Ahmed 2009, 63)

[39] Tohgi, H., et al. 1991. "A significant reduction of putative transmitter amino acids in cerebrospinal fluid of patients with Parkinson's disease and spinocerebellar degeneration." *Neuroscience letters* 126:155–58. (Tohgi 1991, 155)

[40] Jiménez-Jiménez, F., et al. 1996. "Neurotransmitter amino acids in cerebrospinal fluid of patients with Parkinson's disease." *Journal of the Neurological Sciences* 141:39–44. (Jiménez-Jiménez 1996, 39)

[41] Mally, J., Szalai, G., and Stone, T.W. 1997. "Changes in the concentration of amino acids in serum and cerebrospinal fluid of patients with Parkinson's disease." *Journal of the Neurological Sciences* 151:159–62. (Mally 1997, 159)

[42] Lin, Wei-Chen., et al. 2018. "Ulcerative Colitis in Elderly People: An Emerging Issue." *International Journal of Gerontology* 1-5. (Lin 2018, 1)

[43] Götz, Vera Nina. 2013 "Crohn's diseasedWhat the medical registrar and acute physician needs to know!." *Journal of Acute Medicine* 3:132-37. (Götz 2013, 132)

[44] Zhang, Ai-hua., et al. 2013. "NMR-based metabolomics coupled with pattern recognition methods in biomarker discovery and disease diagnosis." *Magnetic Resonance in Chemistry* 51:549–556. (Zhang 2013, 549)

[45] Al-Rasheed, Rana., et al. 2018. "Malnutrition in elderly and its relation to depression." *International Journal of Community Medicine and Public Health* 5:2156-60. (Al-Rasheed 2018, 2156)

[46] Guma, Monica., Tiziani, Stefano., and Firestein, Gary S. 2016. "Metabolomics in rheumatic diseases: desperately seeking biomarkers." *Nature Reviews Rheumatology* 12:269. (Guma 2016, 269)

[47] Young, Stephen P., et al. 2013."The impact of inflammation on metabolomic profiles in patients with arthritis." *Arthritis & Rheumatism* 65:2015-23. (Young 2013, 2015)

[48] Kanimozhi, S. and Mohan, A Darbastwar. 2017. "Prevalence of depression in the elderly population of rural Puducherry: a community based cross sectional study." *International Journal of Community Medicine and Public Health* 4:4315-20. (Kanimozhi 2017, 4315)

[49] Pan, Jun-Xi., et al. 2018. "Diagnosis of major depressive disorder based on changes in multiple plasma neurotransmitters: a targeted metabolomics study." *Translational psychiatry* 8:130. (Pan 2018, 130)

[50] Zheng, Hong., et al. 2017. "Predictive diagnosis of major depression using NMR-based metabolomics and least-squares support vector machine." *Clinica Chimica Acta* 464: 223-27. (Zheng 2017, 223)

[51] Floegel, Anna., et al. 2013 "Identification of serum metabolites associated with risk of type 2 diabetes using a targeted metabolomic approach." *Diabetes* 62:639-48. (Floegel 2013, 639)

[52] Lo, Chi-Jen., et al. 2019. "Metabolic Signature Differentiated Diabetes Mellitus from Lipid Disorder in Elderly Taiwanese." *Journal of clinical medicine* 8:13. (Lo 2019, 13)

[53] Oostendorp, Marlies., et al. 2006. "Diagnosing inborn errors of lipid metabolism with proton nuclear magnetic resonance spectroscopy." *Clinical chemistry* 52:1395-405. (Oostendorp 2006, 1395)

[54] Lanznaster, Débora., et al. 2018. "Metabolomics Biomarkers: A Strategy Toward Therapeutics Improvement in ALS." *Frontiers in neurology* 9:1-7. (Lanznaster 2018,1)

[55] Ginneken, Vincent Van., 2017. "Are there any Biomarkers of Aging? Biomarkers of the Brain." *Biomedical journal of Scientific & Technical Research* 1:193-207. (Ginneken 2017,193)

[56] Meilin Lui et al. 2018. "Metabolic Biomarkers of ageing and age-related diseases in Chinese middle-aged and elderly men." *The Journal of Nutrition Health & ageing* 10:1189-1197. (Meilin et al. 2018,1189)

[57] Wagner, Karl-Heinz., et al. 2016. "Biomarkers of Aging: From function to molecular biology." *Nutrients* 8:337-349. (Wagner 2016, 337)

[58] Jeromin, Andreas., Bowser, Robert. 2017. Biomarkers in neurodegenerative diseases. *Neurodegenerative diseases.* 15:491-528. (Jeromin 2017, 491)

[59] Ussher, John R et al. 2016. The Emerging Role of Metabolomics in the Diagnosis and Prognosis of Cardiovascular Disease. *Journal of the American College of Cardiology.* 68:2850-2870. (Ussher et al. 2016, 2850)

[60] Guasch-Ferré, Marta et al. 2016. Metabolomics in Prediabetes and Diabetes: A Systematic Review and Meta-analysis. *Diabetes care.* 39:833-846. (Guasch-Ferré, 2016, 833)

[61] Yiping Li et al. 2017. Investigation of novel metabolites potentially involved in the pathogenesis of coronary heart disease using a UHPLC-QTOF/MS based metabolomics approach. *Scientific reports.* 7:1-8. (Yiping, 2017, 1)

[62] Dang, Vi T. and Werstuck, Geoff H. 2016. Metabolomics-Based Biomarkers of the Pathogenesis of Atherosclerosis. *Biomarkers Journal.* 2:1-6. (Dang 2016, 1)

[63] Makinen VP, Ala-Korpela M. 2016. Metabolomics of aging requires large-scale longitudinal studies with replication. *Proc Natl Acad Sci USA.* 113:E3470. (Makinen 2016 E3470)

[64] Zierer J, et al. 2015. Integration of 'omics' data in aging research: from biomarkers to systems biology. *Aging Cell.* 14:933–944. (Zierer 2015, 933)

[65] Smita S, et al. 2016. Deciphering hallmark processes of aging from interaction networks. *Biochim Biophys Acta.* 1860:2706–2715. (Smita 2016, 2706)

In: Current Challenges and Management … ISBN: 978-1-53617-304-8
Editor: Abhai Kumar

Chapter 8

ADVANCEMENT IN BIOMARKERS DISCOVERY FOR ELDERLY POPULATION

Sania Bajaj[1], MSc, Ajay Kumar Sharma[1], PhD, M. H. Yashavarddhan[2], PhD, Arpana Vibhuti[3], PhD and Sandeep Kumar Shukla[1,*], PhD

[1]Institute of Nuclear Medicine and Allied Sciences, Defence Research Development Organization, Delhi, India
[2]Defence Institute of Physiology and Allied Sciences, Defence Research Development Organization, Delhi, India
[3]Department of Biomedical Engineering, SRM University, Haryana, India

ABSTRACT

Advancement in ageing is not just only a visible phenomenon. It is accompanied by many denaturing changes in the body like decrease in hormone levels, increase in inflammatory cytokines, weakening of immune system, increased oxidative DNA damage etc. These changes

* Corresponding Author's Email: sandeepshukla@inmas.drdo.in.

may trigger or lead to onset of diseases in the elderly population. With global increase in elderly population, characterized with increase in their number of disease cases, it is challenging for the health care sector to provide them effective treatment on time. Pre-diagnostic, diagnostic or/and therapeutic target molecules for these diseases can strengthen medical care for our elderly population. Thus it is imperative to look into biomarkers for better on-time treatment for somatic and chronic diseases. Over last two decades, the advancement in tools and technology and availability of data intensive methods under 'OMICS' platform and medical imaging tools has enabled researchers to analyze large biological samples for novel biomarker discovery. The multi-omics approach, not only develops diagnostic markers but can screen high risk population and also provide personalized medicine in near future. The current chapter covers a detail understanding about systems biology approach with their multi-omics tools and techniques. It also provides update on biomarkers discovered using omics technology and imaging techniques like PET SCAN and MRI for elderly population.

Keywords: diseases, elderly population, biomarker discovery, OMICS, imaging techniques

1. INTRODUCTION

Ageing is defined as a natural and fundamental phenomenon with characteristic accumulation of structural and physical changes in the body over time. It is marked by changes like reduce tissue elasticity; build-up of misfolded proteins and waste products; increase oxidative damage and its accumulation; weakening of immune system and regenerative power of tissues (Burtner et al. 2010). Normal ageing process itself is not a disease but with ageing the elderly population is always at risk of developing a disease which needs immediate treatment. Globally, the ageing population (people above 60 years) is growing dramatically and it is reported to grow approximately 22% of the world population by 2050 (Beard et al. 2016). With this rate of growth in elderly population, the cases of geriatric diseases are expected to increase many folds. Although the common age related issues like hearing loss, visual impairment, decrease in vestibular functions, muscle ageing is managed by current medical care. But a large number of people are always at risk of developing or they suffer from chronic diseases like cardiovascular diseases, osteoarthritis, osteoporosis, dementia, Alzheimer's disease, Parkinson's disease etc. which still needs diagnostic and therapeutic advancement. To meet the immediate requirement for their effective health care, it is important to focus our understanding on natural ageing process as well as on the diseases which worsens with growing age. Therefore, for disease management and for development of preventive and personalized treatments it is important to focus on biomarkers.

Biomarkers are biological indicators which reflect a specific physiological state in an organism. Depending on their function and role in a biological pathway, they can help in disease screening, diagnosing, assessing prognosis, evaluating treatment management, drug efficacy etc. (Strimbu et al. 2010). That is why to discover new biomarkers for a pathway or a class of drugs is crucial for established and upcoming methods which measure biological or pharmacological consequences. Among the many potential candidates for biomarkers, the need is particularly high for those targets which are tightly linked to their pathways and functions. Those candidates which are associated with specific biochemical pathway can help to track drug metabolism. Thus with this goal in mind, researches are exploring 'OMIC' tools and technologies as appropriate research approach for molecular biomarker discovery due to recent advances in this field.

The omics platform proves to be a powerful technology and it provides vast amount of data by examining the major features (genome, transcriptome, proteome) in the path of genetic flow of information. It also integrates the information of individual 'omic' tool for better understanding their relationship with each other. Thus it is an ever expanding and improving technology with time. The noninvasive imaging techniques such as PET-SCAN, MRI and ECG are useful and widely used procedures for diagnosing and monitoring disease progression in elderly population. The ongoing technical advancements in these platforms will enrich our knowledge and help to build a better effective and personalized treatments in near future.

1.1. 'Omics' Approach for Biomarker Discovery in Elderly Population

The word 'Omics' is used to denote the technologies which characterize, quantifies and explore relationships between major biomolecules of the cell. These technologies primarily aim at detection and identification of Genes (Genomics), mRNA (Transcriptomics), Proteins (Proteomics) and Metabolites (Metabolomics) in a specific biological sample. In a way the Omics approach is a holistic view of molecules that make up a cell, tissue or organism. When the data from all these techniques is integrated into each other, an interdisciplinary field of biological studies is formed which is known as systems biology. Systems biology experiments are hypothesis-generating, which acquire and analyze complete data to define a hypothesis which can be further tested (Horgan et al. 2011). Overall this strategy has many applications and also potential to develop new approaches that can be predictive, preventive and personalized in the near future.

Today the 'Omics' technology not only helps to understand the normal physiological processes but are also applied in disease conditions. They play a role in disease screening, diagnosis and prognosis, thereby helping to understand disease etiology (Hasin et al. 2017). With potential to investigate multiple biomolecules under different pathophysiological conditions at once, these strategies are major step towards biomarker discovery.

2. The 'OMICS' Technology

The omics strategy is equipped with powerful technologies of genomics, transcriptomics, proteomics and metabolomics (Figure 2.1); that helps in better understanding of major biomolecules individually and their relationships with each another. Thus the technologies and their tools are further described as follows:

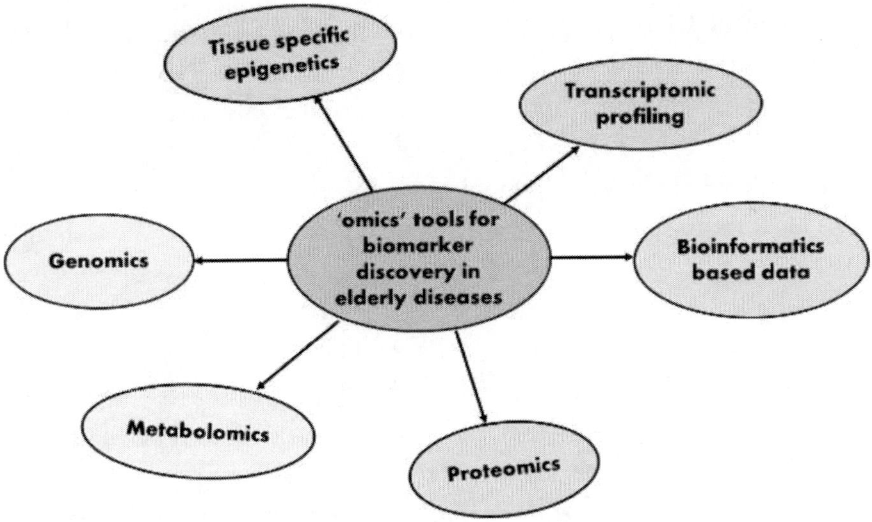

Figure 2.1. Various 'omic' tools used for biomarker discovery in elderly population.

2.1. Genomics

The study of genetic information on DNA, which ultimately holds the fate of a cell is called Genomics. It is systemic study of organism's whole genome. The genome is total DNA of a cell or an organism (Manzoni et al. 2016). Decoding the DNA is one step to understand the complex mechanism which keeps the organism alive and functional. The Human Genome Project (HGP) was launched in 1990 to fulfil this mammoth objective of decoding the human genome. It was then revealed that human genome contains about 3.2 billion bases and 30,000–40,000 protein-coding genes. Traditionally, these genes were analyzed individually but over the years there has been certain advancement in the tools.

2.1.1. Tools to Study Genomics

2.1.1.1. DNA Microarrays

The main tool to study and analyze expression of many genes in a single reaction is DNA microarray analysis. Microarray is an orderly arrangement of DNA samples on microchips where known and unknown DNA sets are matched according to their bases. The DNA spots on the microchips are known as probes which can be either genomic DNA, complementary DNA (cDNA) or oligonucleotides. These probes are used to determine complementary binding of the unknown sequences which allows analysis for gene expression and also gene discovery (Govindarajan et al. 2012). Different categories for Microarray are as follows:

a) **Microarray Expression Analysis**: For analyzing gene expression in a particular physiological condition (diseased conditions) microarray expression analysis is conducted where the complementary or cDNA obtained from the mRNA of known genes is immobilized. Then, the test samples with genes from both the normal as well as the diseased tissues are made to hybridize with immobilized known genes. The spots with more intensity in the test samples are analyzed as overexpression of a gene for that particular disease condition. This expression pattern (whether over or under) is then compared to the expression pattern of a normal tissue to analyze the gene responsible for a disease.

b) **Microarray for Mutation Analysis:** For analyzing a mutation in genetic code, the experimental setup remains the same except that the genomic DNA (gDNA) is used instead of cDNA. As the genes might differ in different people by just a single nucleotide base therefore, a variation is analyzed in the genome of test samples. The single base variation is called single nucleotide polymorphism or SNP. SNPs occur when a nucleotide is substituted with another nucleotide and it results in functional codon for a different amino acid. Thus, a mutation occurs in genetic code which could lead to formation of a disease or a different phenotype. These mutations can also cause the individual patient to respond to drugs differently (Evans et al. 2003). Thereby, SNP profiling becomes an important area to study for diseases linked genetic determination and also pharmcogenetics. The microarray expression analysis remains an important tool for the detection of SNP's in genetic code.

c) **Array Comparative Genomic Hybridization (aCGH):** Array comparative genomic hybridization (aCGH) was developed by combining microarray technique with comparative genomic hybridization (CGH). CGH is a cytogenetic technique which is used to detect and analyze copy number variations (CNV) in test and reference samples. CNVs are repetitive regions of DNA which causes structural variation in the genome of an individual. These variations can cause increase (duplication) or decrease (deletion) of a few base pairs or a whole gene on chromosomal fragments. More than 40 CNVs are identified which are linked with a disease (Clancy, S. 2008). Thus an omic's tool like aCGH allows the researchers to screen the entire genome for these variations/ imbalances with higher resolution than the tradition method (resolution of approx. 5-10 Mb) for clinical applications. For this experimental setup, genomic DNA is extracted from the test sample and reference sample (control). The extracted DNA from two different samples is then labeled with two different colored fluorophores respectively. The denatured and labelled DNA from test and reference samples are then mixed together and applied to the microarray. In the traditional method of CGH, the mixture of DNAs is made to competitively hybridize to metaphase chromosomes. But, in the microarray technique the array slides are made of probes which are immobilized small amount of DNA representing areas of interest. As these probes are several magnitudes smaller than metaphase chromosomes, thereby the resolution of aCGH increases several times over traditional CGH. After digital imaging the relative fluorescence intensities of the labelled DNA probes is quantified. Then, a fluorescence ratio of test and reference hybridization signals is determined at different regions of genome. If there is an altered ratio between the intensities of test and reference sample for a particular probe, then that area indicates either a loss or gain in that region of DNA in the test sample.

2.1.1.2. Next Generation Sequencing (NGS)

Next generation sequencing is a high throughput, ultra-deep sequencing technology which can analyze large number of tissues simultaneously. The ability of this technology to sequence a million nucleotides in a run with high sensitivity than traditional methods allows a researcher to sequence large number of genes and targets in less time and at low cost. The basic methodology of NGS includes following major steps:

- *Library preparation*: The target DNA are randomly fragmented and ligated with adaptor sequences which act as tags and reference point to identify and amplify the target sequence.
- *Amplification:* To achieve amplification of individual target sequence, various methods like bridge PCR, emulsion PCR, in situ polonies are used. All these methods result into amplified sequences generated from single sequence separated spatially.
- *Sequencing*: The sequencing universal primers are added to the amplified individual sequences. The primers bind to the adapter regions right next to the unknown region of interest to be sequenced. Sequencing is performed by enzyme method which can either be a polymerase or a ligase, followed by imaging based data acquisitions.

The advantage of simultaneously sequencing millions of nucleotides from the same or different sources reduces the cost and time of experiments. It results in a large number of data that can be applied to a variety of objectives. This becomes especially useful in the process of drug discovery.

The tools and technologies of genomics have thus allowed researchers to understand not only the fundamental aspects of growth and development, but also the genetic causes of functional abnormalities in the human body.

2.2. Transcriptomics

Although the genetic code is a primary feature to the complex mechanism, it alone does not specify everything that happens within the organism. In a cell, the basic follow of information starts with 'DNA' getting transcribed or copied into another biomolecule called 'RNA'. And a complete set of RNAs produced by the DNA at a specific time in a cell or organism is called its transcriptome. Thus, transcriptomic is expression profiling of active genes which produce RNA in a tissue or cell at a particular time. But the transcribed code i.e., RNA, post transcription does not always resemble the genetic code due to the phenomenon like splicing which are part of RNA maturation pathway (Zhao et al. 2017). Post transcription process produces different species of RNA elements like messenger RNA (which gets translated to protein products), transfer RNA(which help in translation process), ribosomal RNA (essential constituents of ribosomes or the protein factories), small RNA (regulators of all major cellular functions) etc. Therefore, to quantify and analyze transcriptome is essential:

a) To interpret all the species of RNA
b) To determine the transcriptional structure of genes i.e., their start and end sites, their splicing patterns and their post transcriptional modifications.
c) To understand changes in expression of each transcript elements during different physiological conditions.

Also as RNA is a transient intermediary biomolecule between the genomic DNA code and the protein products of those genes, so transcriptomics can incorporate information from genomic, proteomic and metabolomics studies. Hence, the comparison of transcriptomes makes it possible to identify genes that are differentially expressed in individual cell populations, or in response to different treatments.

2.2.1. Tools to Study Transcriptomics

2.2.1. Microarray Technology

This traditional method has been extensively used to study the transcriptome for certain circumstances. In this experimental set up, the short nucleotide oligomers are immobilized on solid surface as probes. Prior knowledge of genome or an EST library of the organism of interest should be known for formation of probe. Then the isolated fragmented transcripts are fluorescently labelled and then hybridized with the probes. The transcript abundance for a particular probe is measured as its the fluorescent intensity at that particular probe location (Lowe et al. 2017). The microarray for transcriptomic is broadly categorized as:

1. **Spotted low density arrays:** The arrays of this category has cDNA probe in the range of picolitres which is higher than high density arrays. Therefore, they have a comparative lower resolution than the high density array. Like the basic methodology of microarray, this set up requires different fluorophores for test and reference samples. The relative abundance of transcripts is calculated as the fluorescence intensity ratio.
2. **High density short probe arrays:** The array of this category has very short probes of 25-mer length for one particular gene. Thus, the transcripts are quantified and analyzed by hybridizing each sample and detecting the signal individually using single fluorophore.

According to the basic principle of the technique of microarray, it can be used to quantify known or predetermined RNA sequences only, and consequently, cannot uncover new RNA sequences.

2.2.2. RNA Sequencing (RNA-Seq)

It is a high through put method for determination of RNA transcripts present in a specific physiological condition. This method indirectly measures the expression of gene in that particular tissue or condition etc.

by sequencing its direct product i.e., RNA via transcript cDNAs. RNA seq, not only maps the transcripts but also measures the transcript abundance by quantifying it directly by counting the transcripts (Wang et al. 2009). The researchers not only validate previously annotated data by sequencing, but also disclose the function of previously unnoted genes.

Its methodology is based on deep sequencing technology therefore this technique has itself improved with development of DNA sequencing methods. The technique has advanced in terms of higher accuracy rate, increased throughput and increased read length. The number of reads produced in every single sample is a very important parameter for the sensitivity and accuracy of RNA-Seq experiment, where number of reads depicts the coverage of sequencing experiment. The RNA-Seq methodology has been rapidly adopted and overtook microarrays as the dominant transcriptomic technique.

The basic experimental setup for sequencing the RNA includes fragmenting the sample. Either the RNA transcripts are directly fragmented or these are first converted to cDNA via reverse transcriptase enzyme and then cDNA is fragmented. These fragments are then amplified via polymerase chain reaction (PCR) to construct libraries. Then these fragments can be sequenced by:

a) Single end sequencing: It is a rapid and economic method of sequencing the transcript along one single direction. It is a method of choice for only determination of expression profile of genes in a particular condition.
b) Paired end sequencing: It allows the researcher to sequence the transcript from both ends of the fragment. With requirement of same amount of sample as single end sequencing, it produces high quality data which can be confidently aligned together. The method detects genomic rearrangement, repetitive sequences and novel transcripts. It also produces twice the number of reads than the single end sequencing method.

2.2.2.1. Advantages of RNA-Seq

a) The method is not limited to known genomic sequences like the hybridization method.
b) It produces very low background signals as transcript mapping is an unambiguous method.
c) It provides deeper information like sequences variations, splicing junctions etc.
d) It is highly sensitive method for quantification than microarray experiments.
e) It shows high levels of accuracy and reproducibility.

Transcriptomic analysis has assisted the study of how gene expression changes and thereby it has been helped in the understanding the development and diseases in humans. The increasing transcriptomics data reveals many mRNA and noncoding RNAs as biomarker in certain diseases (Zhang, C. 2009).

2.3. Proteomics

Proteins are ultimate product in the basic flow of information. This third component after genome and transcriptome is responsible for almost every task within the cell. They are most diverse entities among biomolecules. A complete set of proteins in a cell at a particular time can be referred to as the cell's proteome. The study of protein composition, its structure and function and its interaction with other protcins within a cell is known as proteomics. The proteome is not a static entity and its expression changes from time to time in response to different environmental stimuli. As a result, it is a dynamic reflection of both the gene and the environment. Therefore, the study of proteome helps:

a) To understand the structural and functional properties of proteins,
b) To map their relationship to each other and their interaction other biomolecules,
c) To relate and understand as how they contribute to life processes.

A single gene can encode multiple protein variants which further can undergo several post translational modifications like phosphorylation, methylation, glycosylation etc. to further produce unique proteins according to the requirement (Duan et al. 2015). Thus proteomics tools are powerful techniques to identify specific protein as diagnostic and therapeutic targets and it has till has largely contributed to biomarker studies related to human diseases. As proteomics focuses on the ultimate functional molecule in the cell rather than its genetic code, its studies and analytical tools can take us further towards precision medicine.

2.3.1. Tools to Study Proteomics

Based on their specific functions the technologies can be categorized as follows:

2.3.1.1. Protein Profiling and Analyses Tools

Enzyme Linked Immunosorbent Assay (ELISA)

This method is highly sensitive immunoassay which is commonly used as an analytical tool world over. The technique is based on interaction of antibodies with their specific antigens only.Henceit helps in detection of specific antigens in a particular sample. In its experimental setup either the antigen or antibody are immobilized over a solid surface of wells in a plate. The test sample is processed to contain enzyme conjugated antibodies which are then added to the wells. The enzyme activity is detected and measured which is directly proportional to the quantity of antigen or antibody in the test sample. Thus the technique detects and quantifies molecule of interest which makes it a popular cost effective diagnostic tool of proteomics (Aslam et al. 2017).

Western Blotting

This method is a dominant tool used to detect a known protein in the test sample. It utilizes gel based electrophoresis to separate a complex mixture of proteins into bands of specific molecular weight which are then transferred over a nitrocellulose or polyvinylidene difluoride (PVDF) membrane. Post transfer, the target antigen is detected by its enzyme linked antibody. The enzyme activity is detected and measured which is directly proportional to the quantity of antigen in the test sample. This method not only detects and quantifies target proteins but also confirms the molecular weight of protein. Western blot is usually used as a confirmative test over ELISA in disease diagnostics as it is less likely to give false positive results (Kurien and Scofield 2006).

Protein Microarrays

Microarrays are high throughput technological tool to analyze multiple assays over a glass slide. The data from genomic microarray does not always correlate with the protein expression thus protein microarrays were developed to overcome this limitation. These microarrays are protein spotted chips where immobilized protein can be antigen, antibody, affibodies or full length proteins. These are categorized into analytical protein microarray, functional protein microarray and reverse-phase protein microarray. Analytical protein microarray utilizes a capture antibody which binds to the protein of interest in the test sample and is detected and measured by binding reporter linked to secondary antibody. This tool is used for expression profiling of known proteins. Whereas functional protein microarray contains full form of protein as probes on the solid surface. This tools allows to analyze various interactions like protein-protein, protein-DNA, protein-ligand, protein-RNA, protein-Drug to characterize functions of proteins. And as the name suggest, the reverse phase protein microarray employs opposite format of basic protein microarray technique. Here the sample of interest or the test sample is lysed and arrayed onto the solid support along with reference protein spots. The antibody against target protein of interest is then made to probe with the sample over the slide and the fluorescent signals are detected and measured. This protein microarray tool helps in detection of dysregulation or any alteration in protein for a particular disease (Sutandy et al. 2013). Therefore, protein microarrays are highly sensitive and high throughput technology to understand various aspects of proteome and useful tool in understanding disease biology.

2.3.1.2. Protein Quantification Tools

These tools are required for high throughput technology to separate the complex mixtures of proteins and quantify their differential expression under different physiological condition to identify probable protein biomarkers. These can be categorized as Gel based and Gel-free methods.

Gel-Based Methods

Polyacrylamide based gel electrophoresis has always been a popular technique in proteomics. But combining the basic technique with other tools to achieve high resolution, quantification and identification made these techniques as standard methodological procedures in proteomics. These are further described as follows:

Two Dimensional Gel Electrophoresis (2DE): Since the introduction of this method by O'Farrell and Klose in 1975, it has seen several modifications in its technology and has advanced ever since. It has also been called as the workhorse for proteomic techniques due to its vast usage for detection and analyses of differential expression of proteins (Abdallah et al. 2012). It is a method of choice to study post translational modifications, separation of large number of proteins, visually analyzing the changes in protein expression, identifying new proteins and for biomarkers detection.

This technique combines tools for separation of proteins on the bases of charge (Isoelectric focusing), mass (SDS-PAGE) and further identification of protein via mass spectrometric methods. For the first phase of separation of proteins by iso electric focusing (IEF), the processed samples are loaded on IEF strips of specific length and with gradient pH. The protein resolve according to their net charge at different pH values. For the second phase, the resolved IEF strips are loaded onto SDS-polyacrylamide gels and separation based on molecular weight is performed. The proteins are visualized as spots with appropriate detection method like silver staining, coomassie dye, florescent Sypro Ruby, lava purple, flamingo etc. Sensitivity of 2DE technique is largely dependent on its choice of staining method. Florescent dyes are more sensitive than silver staining methods or coomassie blue whereas PTMs like phosphorylation are visualized using Pro-Q diamond and glycosylation by Pro-Q Emerald dyes. Post resolving the proteins, a gel map is obtained for specific sample (Abdallah et al. 2012; Gygi et al. 2000). The maps obtained are further compared and analyzed using bioinformatics tools like PD Quest by BioRad technologies, Progenesis by Nonlinear Dynamics etc. These softwares generally provide image alignment and spot matching, background adjustments and noise removal, normalization, spot detection and quantification and statistical analysis for differential expression analysis (Klein et al. 2004). After the spot of interest are selected, they are cut out of the gels and fragmented by endopeptidase like trypsin and then concentrated processed further to be identified by mass spectrometric methods.

Although 2DE is a popular, high resolution proteome separation method but this technique suffers from limitations like reproducibility, low detection of proteins with high acidic/basic nature, very high molecular weight or high hydrophobicity.

Two Dimensional Differential Gel Electrophoresis (DIGE): This protein labelling method is an advancement over 2DE method by resolving its limitation of protein expression ratio errors due to gel-to-gel variation. The variation is overcome by loading the test and reference sample onto the same gel, but labelling them with differently resolvable fluorescent CyDyes (Cy2, Cy3 and Cy5 dyes) prior to electrophoresis. These dyes very sensitive and increases the protein detection levels to sub-picomolar levels. Therefore, reduces the need to use large quantity of test samples which also sometime become a limitation in conventional 2DE method. The software used to analysis of DIGE data are DeCyder 2D by GE healthcare, proteome weaver by BioRad technologies etc. This technique lowers the variability and increases the statistical power of the tool (Berth et al. 2007).

One-Dimensional Gel Electrophoresis (1DE): 1DE or the SDS PAGE is very popular method to determine the molecular weight and to assess the protein purity. The test sample are solubilized in SDS detergent and run onto a SDS polyacrylamide with a reference lane of proteins with predetermined molecular weight. This technique is part of western blotting for immunodetection. Now-a-days, it is also coupled with liquid chromatography (LC) prior to identification by MS/MS analysis and is called 1DE-LC approach (Vasilj et al. 2012). This proteomics approach is technically simpler than 2DE and has proved to be better than other fractionation methods like IEF etc. on the parameter of higher proteome coverage and superior performance. It is an efficient method as it can capture and identify those proteins which are otherwise not accessible in 2DE. In this method, after protein separation on SDS-PAGE the lane containing protein bands are directly cut out of the gel and excised into tiny pieces for in-gel digestion. After protein digestion the peptides are fractionated onto LC before final analysis by MS/MS or LC-MS.

Gel-Free Methods

The advancement in the ionization methods to fragmentize the biomolecules into gas phase without their decomposition fueled the development of gel free techniques for differential proteomics. The improvements have made these gel free methods more rapid, sensitive and convenient to use.

Isotope-Coded Affinity Tags (ICATs): ICATs was introduced by Aebersold and co-workers to improve and simplify proteomic analyses. This technique chemically tags the sample which is to be assessed quantitatively. These chemical tags are formed of three elements- a reactive group for tagging cysteine amino acid side chains, an isotopically coded linker with light or heavy isotopes, and a biotin tag for affinity purification (Abdallah et al. 2012). The labelled samples are then pooled and enzymatically cleaved and subjected to affinity chromatography for purification of tagged peptides. The purified samples are then analyzed by LC/MS. The analyzed MS data reflects the relative abundance in the form of ratio of heavy and light forms of similar peptides which are derived from similar proteins. Therefore, a true comparison between expression profiles of any proteome at different physiological state can be measured.

Isotope –Coded Protein Labelling (ICPL): In this technique, the chemical tags are formed of stable isotope derivative which tags free amino groups of intact proteins. Therefore, as compared to ICATs, this method provides high sequence coverage and thus more information on protein isoforms and PTMs. The labelled samples are pooled and digested before subjecting to MS analysis. As peptides of similar sequences are tagged with heavy and light form, they appear as doublets in MS spectra. So a relative abundance of parent protein is determined from the ratios of ion intensities of these doublets (Abdallah et al. 2012; Kellermann, Josef 2008).

Isobaric Tags for Relative and Absolute Quantification (ITRAQ): This technique utilizes chemical isobaric tags which are designed to covalently bind to N-terminus and lysine side chain of peptides. These isobaric tag consists of a reporter group, a neutral balance portion, and a peptide reactive group to give an overall mass of 145.Thus samples with independent reagents of same mass (145) give rise to different reporter ions and ratio of these ions is analyzed in mass spectra for relative quantification of peptides (Abdallah et al. 2012; Wiese et al. 2007). It has certain advantages over the above mentioned techniques like up to 4 or 8 samples can be quantified together. And it has increased analytical precision and accuracy.

Stable Isotopic Labelling with Amino Acids in Cell Culture (SILAC): SILAC is a technique that labels the proteins metabolically for MS based quantitative proteomics. The two cell culture populations are made to grow upon two different mediums containing normal and heavy stable isotopes of specific amino acids such as lysine and arginine. As these two isotopically labeled amino acids are basically chemically identical, their integration into the proteins does not interfere with normal cell growth. But it makes proteins/peptides distinguishable by mass and the technique develops an ideal method for mass spectrometric analysis (Gonneaud et al. 2016). As the samples can be combined and protein is extracted and processed for MS analyses, this methodology reduces vial to vial variation.

2.3.1.3 Protein Sequencing Analysis Tool

Mass Spectrometry

Mass Spectrometry (MS) is now the primary method for protein identification. It is a very reliable and sensitive technique to analyze peptides and protein identification. In general, the MS process comprise of three main steps.

a) Ionization: The protein sample to be analyzed must be transformed togas-phase ions. The commonly used ionization methods are matrix-assisted laser desorption ionization (MALDI), surface enhanced laser desorption/Ionization (SELDI) and electrospray ionization (ESI).
b) Separation of ions: The molecular ion formed during ionization gets fragmented into more ions which are then separated according to their mass to charge (m/z) ratio in a mass analyzer. These separated ions are detected in proportion of their abundance and a mass spectrum of the molecule is produced. The mass spectrum is a plot of ion abundance versus mass to charge ratio.
c) Analysis and identification: The peptides are analyzed by the instrument with high mass accuracy. The analyzed peptide mass data is then compared with predicted mass values from theoretical protein digestion in databases to generate a protein sequences. This method is called Mass fingerprinting or Peptide mass mapping. The spectrum data generated from MS/MS analysis of individual peptide is also used for more accurate identification results. This peptide spectrum data is compared with all hypothetical peptides of the appropriate molecular mass. When greater number of peptide matches to sequences of a single protein, each peptide match can be linked to a protein match and the greater the number of peptides being matched to any one protein and the greater the sequence coverage, the greater the probability of a correct identification (Baldwin et al. 2004).

Thus proteomics is a complex technique which requires maximum tools to understand the biological dynamics of protein. But it provides utmost results as proteins are functional entities of the living organism.

2.4. Metabolomics

Metabolites are low molecular weight (>1500Da), organic or inorganic chemicals which are either a result of a metabolic process or they are part of a metabolic pathway. A metabolome can be defined as a set of all these metabolites present in a biological system i.e., a cell, tissue, organ or any other biological fluid. These metabolites can be required for growth and development of organism thus some metabolites are also absorbed into the system from diet and other exogenous sources. Thus metabolomics becomes an important part of systems biology approach where it qualitatively and quantitatively measures the metabolome a biological sample at a specific point of time. Metabolome comprises of a large network biochemical interactions occurring in an organism which results in its ultimate phenotype under a specific physiological condition. Therefore, metabolomics becomes an important bridge in our understanding between other omics platforms and molecular physiology which is largely influenced by the environment (Barchet, Genoa 2013).

There are currently two leading approaches to study metabolomics: Nuclear Magnetic Resonance (NMR) spectroscopy and Mass spectroscopy.

2.4.1. NMR Spectroscopy

It is a powerful analytical chemistry technique which can determine the molecular structure of the samples from its spectral libraries formed on the basis of magnetic properties of specific nuclei like ^{1}H, ^{13}C etc. The NMR spectroscopy data is based on resonance frequency and spin relaxation of metabolite samples. This technique requires less amount of sample with no preceding sample purification. It is in fact a fast, reproducible method which is also non-destructive, non-invasive and detects hydrophilic as well as lipophilic metabolites (Kruk et al. 2017).

2.4.2. Mass Spectrometry

This is highly sensitive technique which can detect in femtomolar to attamole concentration of samples. The technique can be coupled with tools like gas chromatography or liquid chromatography to produce high resolution accurate mass results for metabolite identification and quantification.

2.4.3. Bioinformatics Tools

The data obtained from metabolomics tools is a complex form which has to be analyzed using tools like chemometric and pattern recognition (PR) analysis methods. Further the available databases for metabolites like METLIN, HMDB, GMD and MassBank are used to match and identify the metabolites obtained in the target samples. To generate and understand the metabolic pathways software like mummichog and metabolite set enrichment analysis (MSEA) are available (Gardinassi et al. 2017).

Therefore, metabolomics is used for biomarkers discovery for drug monitoring, analysis of biochemical pathways, disease diagnosis etc.

3. Medical Non-Invasive Tools

3.1. Positron-Emission Tomography (PET- SCAN)

A pet scan is imaging based medical procedure to detect metabolic activity within the tissue or organ of interest. It helps to evaluate the anatomy, functionality and biochemical properties of the tissue and organs. The technique is based on introduction of a radionuclide into the body and then detection of gamma rays by a large scanner. The rays are created during emission of positron due to breakdown of radionuclide. The computer analyze the data collected from the emission of rays and uses it to create an image. Thus an image with bright coloured regions is created indicating more radionuclide and high metabolic activity in that specific region.

The radionuclide used for PET SCAN technology is an isotope with short half-life attached to a tracer molecule which is naturally used within the body to carry metabolic process. Various isotopes such as fluorine-18 (~110 min), oxygen-15 (~2.2 min), nitrogen-13 (~10 min), carbon-11 (~20 min), are available to be used to scanning purposes. The most common radionuclide for PET SCAN is fluorodeoxyglucose (FDG) which is a glucose analogue with fluorine-18 as glucose metabolism is used by diagnostically important parts of the body. This radiotracer based scanning technology is although expensive but is successful in distinguishing patients suffering from Alzheimer's and Parkinson's disease from healthy cohort (Morbelli and Bauckneht 2018).

3.2. Magnetic Resonance Imaging (MRI-SCAN)

It is another non-invasive imaging technique used to study the anatomical details of an organ. The technique is commonly used for diagnostic study of soft tissue like muscles, tendons, ligaments, brain and spinal cord. As the technique employs a large magnet, patients with pacemaker, metallic valves or clips or metallic prosthetics are not advised for a MRI Scan.

The images are obtained by using body's own magnetic properties. The hydrogen nucleus or proton is present in abundance in the body due to water and fat content. Naturally, these protons spin on their axis and are aligned randomly in the body. The MRI machine contains large powerful magnets and under their influence of magnetic field, these protons align themselves in specific direction. Then a pulse of radio wave frequency current is passed through the body, which deflects the proton from the alignment and excites the nuclei. When this pulse is stopped, the hydrogen nuclei realigns (relaxed state) with the original magnetic field generated by the machine. The detectors placed in the machine detects the amount of energy emitted by the hydrogen nuclei during its time to come back to relaxed state. The amount of energy released and time taken for each nuclei to realign differs according to its chemical nature (the molecule it is a part of) and environment (cells or tissue). Finally, the cross-sectional images are obtained from the received signals. These images are analyzed by specialist to confirm disease related changes in the organs. The application of this technique has been recently linked to biomarker discovery in Parkinson's disease patients.

3.3. Electrocardiogram (ECG)

An ECG is device to detect and plot electric signals from heart into a graphical representation. It is very useful and standard procedure which is non-invasive, cost effective and gives quick results. The equipment is designed to record the occurrence and strength of electrical signal which generates with each heartbeat. When the heart muscle depolarizes, impulses are generated and they travel in the form of electrical waves towards the skin. The ECG electrodes are very sensitive wet sensors to pick up these weak signals. A normal heart beat generates a graph with typical wave pattern on ECG. Any abnormality in this wave pattern is evaluated as indicator of heart related issue. Thus an ECG data analyses reveals a general heart health with clues about its structural abnormalities. With recent advancement in the technology the ECG devices have become more portable and can record ECG for hours or days (Maršánová et al. 2017). The availability of large data from a noninvasive low cost device has prompted researches to use various parameters to understand the data for cardiovascular disease related biomarker discovery.

4. Omics Research in Biomarker Discovery for Elderly Population

Normal ageing is complex molecular phenomenon which affects body's tissue and organ. In general, it is seen as physical and physiological changes in the body over a period of time (Cire, 2016). Therefore, the scientific community has made important efforts to understand biological ageing and establish its markers so that age-related diseases could be prevented. Omics technologies have empowered researchers and contributed to understand ageing in a better way. Techniques like transcriptomic profiling, microarray approach, 2DE, tissue specific epigenomics, metabolomics etc. were applied to target new molecules for biomarker studies in ageing condition (Figure 4.1). Most of the research is centered toward the normal ageing process and few chronic conditions like Parkinson's disease, cardiovascular disease, Alzheimer's, osteoarthritis, dementia etc.

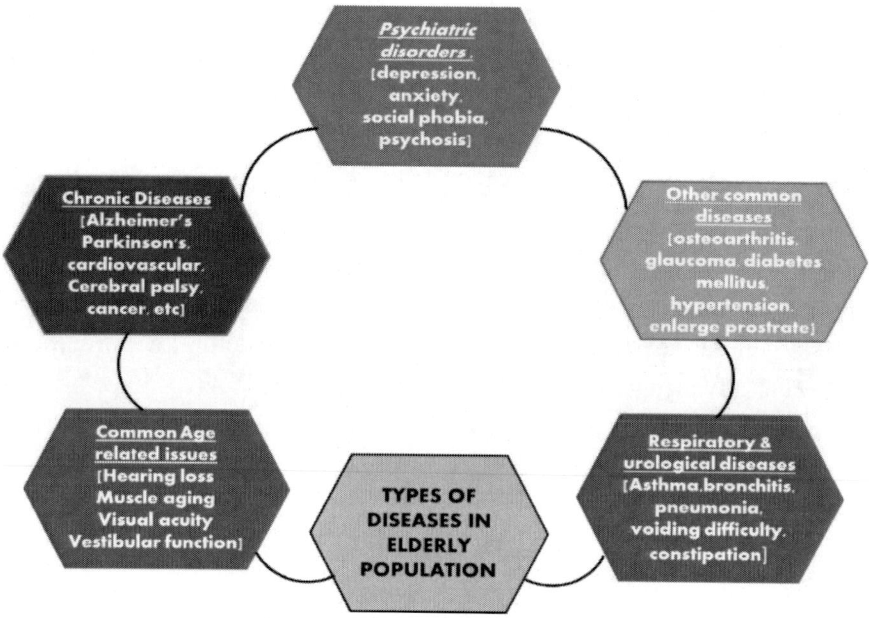

Figure 4.1. Diseases and disorders in elderly population.

4.1. Normal Ageing

Large scale project collaborations like MARK-AGE, conducted on 3200 subjects, were aimed at identifying a set of biomarkers which would measure biological age better than any marker in isolation (Bürkle et al. 2015). Although the project used vast types of technologies to accomplish their objectives but omics techniques like 2DE and LC-MS approach, DNA microarray, miRNA microarray, metabalomics played major roles. According to their published reports they were successful in identifying and validating proteins like transferrin, complement C3b and transthyretin which quantitatively differ in plasma of different age groups (Bürkle et al. 2015). Another group confirms the acidic shift of transferrin protein on

2DE gels in older males (Dunston et al. 2012). Another protein apolipoprotein J/Clusterin (ApoJ/CLU) was studied by MARK-AGE researchers as valuable biomarker for ageing as it is reported to increase in patients with diabetes mellitus, heart diseases and myocardial infarction. The same group reports decreased genetic levels of DNMT1and DNMT3B with increasing age (Capri et al. 2015). Impairment in proteome functioning and reduction in methionine sulfoxide reductase (Msr) activity is reported during ageing and replicative senescence respectively. ApoE and antioxidant proteins was observed to differentially express in the plasma of 10 Japanese supercentenarians compared with 10 young people (Miura et al. 2011). A study on human muscles reports six biological pathways common to several organs such as kidney, muscle and brain ageing via transcriptional profiling (Zahn et al. 2006). They also report the mitochondrial electron transport chain pathway decreases with increasing age in three different species (human, mice and primates). Another study conducted by transcriptional profiling of human skeleton muscle reports hormonal imbalance and mitochondrial dysfunctions along with decreased expression of calcium binding protein EFEMP1and sarcomeric protein MYOZ2 as hallmarks of muscle ageing (Mamoshina et al. 2018). All these reports ascertain the usefulness of systems biology approach in identifying ageing related biomarkers.

4.2. Parkinson's Disease

Patients suffering from this progressive nervous system disorder are increasing each year. The disease is characterized by loss the nigral dopaminergic neurons and accumulation of proteinaceous deposits in the brain. A late stage Parkinson's disease (PD) patient suffers from chewing and swallowing problems, constipation, bladder complications, sleep disorders, tremors, speech changes, depression and emotional problems. There is no cure for Parkinson disease therefore the patient is largely dependent on medicines and surgeries just to improve the symptoms. Advanced techniques have led to identification of genetic markers like alpha-synuclein, parkin, DJ1, PINK1 and LRRK2 for early detection of disease (Caudle et al. 2009). The use of quantitative western blotting and Luminex assay confirms the decrease in DJ1 protein in cerebrospinal fluid (CNF) samples (Emamzadeh et al. 2009). The protein further decreases in late stage PD patients. Recent advancement in biomarker studies has revealed changes in expression levels of alpha-synuclein in blood plasma of PD patients suggesting a better sample source than CNF (Foulds et al. 2011). On the other hand, studies conducted with newly developed technique called Real time quacking induced conversion (RT-QuIC) provided a novel method for detection of abnormal CNF alpha synuclein with 95% sensitivity and 100% specificity (Groveman et al. 2018). In fact, the technique has been further improved to shorten the procedural time and to increase its diagnostic accuracy.

A metabolomics profiling study identified uric acid and glutathione molecule as potential biomarkers for the disease. The study reported significant reduction in concentration of uric acid but increased expression of glutathione in patients with Parkinson's disease (Havelund et al. 2017). The increase glutathione expression probably reflects a response to oxidative damage. Nrf2, which regulates glutathione synthesis, has been identified as promising therapeutic target in PD patients (Deshmukh et al. 2017). It is reported to increase the antioxidant response element (ARE) pathway and several cytoprotective genes. The researchers report and emphasize that by further activating Nrf2/ARE pathway, the nigral dopaminergic neurons can be protected in the diseased subjects (Tufekci et al. 2011).

Accumulation of protease resistant misfolded proteins and aggregated proteins is common phenomenon in neuropathological disorders (Ciechanover et al. 2015). The components of proteolytic pathways and macroautophagy, which are essential to remove misfolded proteins, gets downregulated with age (Ciechanover et al. 2015). Thus even in a healthy individual, it is difficult to clear these cytotoxic misfolded proteins with increasing age. It is known that the activity and components of these pathways further decreases in PD patients. Therefore, to increase proteolytic pathways in PD patients is a good therapeutic strategy for controlling the disease.

Very recent popularization of transcriptomic technique of next generation sequencing (NGS) has been used by researchers to identify microRNA (miRNA) based biomarker for PD. miRNAs are small non-coding RNA molecules which regulate targeted gene expression. A large number of miRNAs are brain specific and can cross the blood brain barrier. Thus these are available in various biological fluids in circulation as well as in exosomes. The study revealed that by combining PD specific miRNAs with PD hallmark protein a new panel comprising of miR-10b-5p, miR-151a-3p, miR-22-3p and α-syn is formed. The analysis of this model revealed that early stage PD patients should have low α-syn protein levels and, low miR-22-3p expression levels in the CSF, and high expression levels of miR-10b-5p and miR-151a-3p. This model showed high predictive value with 97% sensitivity and 90% specificity (dos Santos et al. 2017).

MRI based data analyses of iron content in brain of PD patients has been investigated for biomarker potential to distinguish between a healthy and diseased patient by several researchers (Zhang et al. 2010; He et al. 2015; Guan 2018). It has been suggested that accumulation of iron during disease progression has a strong correlation with nigral neuron degeneration. Although the role of region specific iron accumulation in Parkinson's disease is not yet fully understood, but researchers stress on region specific iron quantification by MRI as potential biomarker for PD (Guan et al.2017).

4.3. Alzheimer's Disease

Alzheimer's disease (AD) is an irreversible, progressive neurodegenerative disorder which slowly destroys memory and thinking skills. It is major cause of dementia in elderly population. Globally, approximately 44 million people are estimated to be living with Alzheimer's disease and only one in four people with the disease get diagnosed. It is an incurable disease characterized by the formation and accumulation of β-amyloid plaques and neurofibrillary tangles in the brain. There are three internationally established biomarkers called amyloid beta ($A\beta_{42}$) protein, total tau (t-tau) protein and phospho-tau protein. Their expression levels are checked in cerebrospinal fluid for diagnosis and progression of Alzheimer's disease (Sharma and Singh 2016). The Amyloid beta ($A\beta_{42}$) protein significantly decreases whereas total tau protein significantly increases in CSF obtained from AD patients. Presence of phosphorylated tau-181 protein is definite marker for neuronal dysfunction. Some studies also suggest, the ratio of CSF $A\beta_{42}$ to t-tau as more sensitive and specific biomarker for distinguishing AD patients from healthy individuals (Huynh et al. 2017). A clinically significant correlation between plasma β-amyloid concentrations and cerebral β-amyloidosis is reported by several researchers as an effective biomarker which is measured by mass spectrometry (Hye et al. 2006; Lashley et al. 2018; Garrido et al. 2019). All biomarkers can be analyzed in CSF with ELISA or with mass spectrometry methods (Sharma and singh 2016). Pet scan imaging is also used to distinguish a healthy brain subjects from AD pathological subjects. Various radiotracers like 8F-florbetapir, 18F-flutemetamol and 18F-florbetaben (Morbelli and Bauckneht 2018) are used to visualize β-amyloid plagues, 18F-AV1451 to visualize tau inclusions in vivo in patients (Schöll et al. 2016). Neurogranin (Ng) a post synaptic protein is reported to increase in AD (Hellwig et al. 2015; Kester et al. 2015) but not in other neurodegenerative disorders. Increase in CSF-Ng is also correlated with reduce glucose metabolism in brain which leads to the tissue atrophy with advancement in disease (Wellington et al. 2016).

CSF sampling requires lumber puncturing the patient which is very painful and very difficult in elderly people. Therefore, circulatory biomarkers were looked into using OMICs techniques and tools. Thus studies conducted in blood from AD patients using a microarray chip and NGS identified a number of miRNAs when compared to controls. Some miRNAs like hsa-miR-34a, hsa-miR-1285-5p, hsa-miR-81b, hsa-miR-107, hsa-miR-103a-3p, hsa-miR-26b-Sp, hsa-miR-26a-Sp, and hsa-let-7f had decreased expression while hsa-miR-151a-3p, brain-mir-161, hsa-let-7d-

3p, brain-miR-112, and hsa-miR-5010-3p had elevated expression in AD patients (Schipper et al. 2007; Huynh et al. 2017). Another study emphasized on miRNA-34c as a biomarker with high diagnostic accuracy than other miRNA. miRNA-34c was found to be highly elevated in the plasma (0.29 versus 0.1) and peripheral blood mononuclear cells (0.08 versus 0.07) of AD patients compared to healthy controls (Bhatnagar et al. 2014).

A very recent study, aimed to provide molecular understanding of pathophysiology of AD reported regional protein expression patterns in human brain using spatial proteomics analysis. The study correlated expression of 4835 proteins in six regions of human brain with Alzheimer's disease progression. The four key regulatory genes which regulated the expression pattern of these were identified as syntaxin binding protein 1 (STXBP1); collapsin response-mediator protein 1 (CRMP1); actin-related protein 10 homologue (ACTR10); and amphiphysin (AMPH). The genes are related neurotransmitter release, development of nervous tissue and hippocampal ageing respectively. AMPH has been stated as candidate risk gene for AD (Xu et al. 2019). Therefore, this data holds high significance with respect to therapeutic point of view.

4.4. Cardiac Diseases

With ever increasing cases of hypertension, number of people entering their geriatric age with the risk of developing a cardiac disease has significantly increased. Till date, cardiac troponin is the only established marker linked with development of cardiovascular disease (CVD) due to its high tissue specificity and sensitivity (Creemers et al. 2012). Whereas non tissue specific marker like myeloperoxidase, copeptin, and growth differentiation factor 15 help in risk assessment of the disease and its development (Tijsen et al. 2018). Therefore, rapidly developing techniques like proteomics (plasma, blood vessels, plasma membrane and mitochondria) and combination all the 'omics' tools like 2DE, ICAT,

LC/MS/MS, microarrays are used for detection of new biomarkers for CVD development. Various proteins, microRNAs, noncoding RNAs (Viereck et al. 2017), SNPs are suggested as candidate biomarkers by researchers. A genomic study conducted with serum and urine samples from hypertensive individuals identified an association between LDL cholesterol (a common risk factor for CVD) and SNPs (rs599839) on 10kb gene locus in chromosome 1p13.3 (Wallace et al. 2008). Another genomic study has identified gene UGT1A1 (major gene controlling serum bilirubin concentrations) to control risk for development of CVD. The reports stated that individuals homozygous for UGT1A1*28 have a significantly lower risk of developing CVD than carriers of the wild-type alleles (Lin et al. 2010).

Other studies reported miRNAs as candidate biomarker for Coronary Artery Disease. miR-133a, miR-208a, miR-126, miR-17, miR-92a, miR-155, miR-145; hsa-miR-140-3p, hsa-miR-182, hsa-miR-92a and hsa-miR-92b; and miR-135a, miR-147 was identified as circulating miRNAs in plasma, whole blood and peripheral blood mononuclear cells (PBMCs) respectively which were associated and differentially expressed in the diseased patients (Fichtlscherer et al. 2010; Taurino et al. 2010; Hoekstra et al. 2010). Another study reports miR-423-5p as most strongly related to the clinical diagnosis of heart failure (Olson et al. 2014).

Studies based on ECG data analysis also relates specific parameters such as ischemic, rhythm, and conduction abnormalities with CVD mortality.

4.5. Osteoarthritis (OA)

Osteoarthritis is a joint disease which is leading cause of large discomfort and disability among elderly population. It is defined as progressive disease characterized with imbalance between degradative and repair process and concomitant inflammation by the doctors. Therefore, there is continuing research to establish the biomarkers for OA. Till date studies have reported inflammatory biomarkers, biochemical biomarkers,

biomarkers from immune system, trascriptomic and metabalomic biomarkers (Daghestani et al. 2016). Urinary C-terminal telopeptides of type II collagen (uCTX-II); serum cartilage oligomeric matrix protein (COMP) and serum hyaluronan are largely studied and commercially available prognostic biomarker for OA (Huang et al. 2018). Several proteomic studies conducted with plasma and serum of affected patients, established proteins like lipoproteins, von Willebrand factor, tetranectin, clusterin, hemopexin, alpha-1 acid glycoprotein-2, fibulin peptides as novel candidate biomarkers for OA (Attur et al. 2013). Further using proteomic and transcriptomic analysis researcher identified complement system and IL-1β as significant candidates for disease progression from synovial fluid and peripheral blood leucocytes respectively (Wang et al. 2011; Panina et al. 2017). Myeloperoxidase (MPO), and chlorinated peptides were another immune system related biomarkers identified in a study conducted in synovial fluid from 30 patients for potential diagnostic markers for early detection of OA (Steinbeck et al. 2007). A serum based metabalomic study concluded Serum branched chain aminoacid to histidine ratio as novel biomarker for knee osteoarthritis (Zhai et al. 2010).

CONCLUSION

As the age advances in human, it grows a large risk of developing a range of diseases such as cardiovascular, neurodegenerative, muscular, metabolic syndromes, etc. Thus it raises the possibility that if a target approach is applied to understand the biology of ageing process, it can delay the onset of many diseases, which otherwise decreases the quality of life in elderly as well as can become a reason for their morbidity. To generate an understanding of molecular events and target molecules which participate in age related diseases, system biology approach proves to be very helpful. The approach includes the in-depth knowledge from genomics, transcriptomics and proteomics data and interlinking it with interdisplinary field of metabolomics. These are ever expanding and improving technologies with time. These approaches utilize various techniques with can be modified or combined with one another to fulfil the larger aim of experiment.

The field of 'omics' technologies have proved to be very fruitful in terms of establishing biomarkers for diseases of elderly population. Every new biomarker candidate discovery increases the likelihood that it will be efficacious, leading us to a better, effective and personalized treatments in near future.

REFERENCES

Abdallah, C., Dumas-Gaudot, E., Renaut, J., & Sergeant, K. (2012). Gel-based and gel-free quantitative proteomics approaches at a glance. *International journal of plant genomics*, 2012.

Aslam, B., Basit, M., Nisar, M. A., Khurshid, M., &Rasool, M. H. (2017). Proteomics: technologies and their applications. *Journal of chromatographic science*, 55(2), 182-196.

Attur, M., Krasnokutsky-Samuels, S., Samuels, J., & Abramson, S. B. (2013). *Prognostic biomarkers in osteoarthritis*. Current opinion in rheumatology, 25(1), 136.

Baldwin, M. A. (2004). Protein identification by mass spectrometry: issues to be considered. Molecular & Cellular Proteomics, 3(1), 1-9.

Barchet, G. (2007). A brief overview of metabolomics: What it means, how it is measured, and its utilization. *The Science Creative Quarterly*, 8, 1-3.

Beard, J. R., Officer, A., De Carvalho, I. A., Sadana, R., Pot, A. M., Michel, J. P., Lloyd-Sherlock, P., Epping-Jordan, J.E., Peeters, G.G., Mahanani, W.R. &Thiyagarajan, J. A. (2016). The World report on ageing and health: a policy framework for healthy ageing. *The Lancet*, 387(10033), 2145-2154.

Berth, M., Moser, F. M., Kolbe, M., & Bernhardt, J. (2007). *The state of the art in the analysis of two-dimensional gel electrophoresis images.* Applied microbiology and biotechnology, 76(6), 1223-1243.

Bhatnagar, S., Chertkow, H., Schipper, H. M., Shetty, V., Yuan, Z., Jones, T., Jenkins, S. & Wang, E. (2014). *Increased microRNA-34c abundance in Alzheimer's disease circulating blood plasma*. Frontiers in molecular neuroscience, 7, 2.

Bürkle, A., Moreno-Villanueva, M., Bernhard, J., Blasco, M., Zondag, G., Hoeijmakers, J. H., Toussaint, O., Grubeck-Loebenstein, B., Mocchegiani, E., Collino, S. &Gonos, E. S. (2015). *MARK-AGE biomarkers of ageing*. Mechanisms of ageing and development, 151, 2-12.

Burtner, C. R., & Kennedy, B. K. (2010). *Progeria syndromes and ageing: what is the connection?* Nature reviews Molecular cell biology, 11(8), 567.

Capri, M., Moreno-Villanueva, M., Cevenini, E., Hervonen, A., & Hurme, M. (2015). *MARK-AGE population: from the human model to new insights*.

Caudle, W. M., Bammler, T. K., Lin, Y., Pan, S., & Zhang, J. (2010). *Using 'omics' to define pathogenesis and biomarkers of Parkinson's disease*. Expert review of neurotherapeutics, 10(6), 925-942.

Ciechanover, A., & Kwon, Y. T. (2015). *Degradation of misfolded proteins in neurodegenerative diseases: therapeutic targets and strategies*. Experimental & molecular medicine, 47(3), e147.

Cheng, Z., Yin, J., Yuan, H., Jin, C., Zhang, F., Wang, Z., Liu, X., Wu, Y., Wang, T. & Xiao, S. (2018). *Blood-derived plasma protein biomarkers for Alzheimer's disease in Han Chinese*. Frontiers in aging neuroscience, 10.

Clancy, S. (2008). *Copy number variation*. Nature Education1, no. 1: 95.

Creemers, E. E., Tijsen, A. J., & Pinto, Y. M. (2012). *Circulating microRNAs: novel biomarkers and extracellular communicators in cardiovascular disease?* Circulation research, 110(3), 483-495.

Daghestani, H. N., & Kraus, V. B. (2015). *Inflammatory biomarkers in osteoarthritis*. Osteoarthritis and cartilage, 23(11), 1890-1896.

Deshmukh, P., Unni, S., Krishnappa, G., & Padmanabhan, B. (2017). *The Keap1–Nrf2 pathway: promising therapeutic target to counteract*

ROS-mediated damage in cancers and neurodegenerative diseases. Biophysical reviews, 9(1), 41-56.

Dos Santos, M. C. T., Barreto-Sanz, M. A., Correia, B. R. S., Bell, R., Widnall, C., Perez, L. T., ... & Maetzler, W. (2018). miRNA-based signatures in cerebrospinal fluid as potential diagnostic tools for early stage Parkinson's disease. Oncotarget, 9(25), 17455.

Duan, G., & Walther, D. (2015). *The roles of post-translational modifications in the context of protein interaction networks.* PLoS computational biology, 11(2), e1004049.

Dunston, C. R., Choudhury, K., & Griffiths, H. R. (2012). *Terminal galactose residues on transferrin are increased in midlife adults compared to young adults.* Proteomics, 12(21), 3147-3153.

Emamzadeh, F. N., &Surguchov, A. (2018). *Parkinson's disease: biomarkers, treatment, and risk factors.* Frontiers in neuroscience, 12, 612.

Evans, W. E., & McLeod, H. L. (2003). *Pharmacogenomics—drug disposition, drug targets, and side effects.* New England journal of medicine, 348(6), 538-549.

Fichtlscherer, S., De Rosa, S., Fox, H., Schwietz, T., Fischer, A., Liebetrau, C., Weber, M., Hamm, C.W., Röxe, T., Müller-Ardogan, M. &Bonauer, A. (2010). *Circulating microRNAs in patients with coronary artery disease.* Circulation research, 107(5), 677-684.

Foulds, P. G., Mitchell, J. D., Parker, A., Turner, R., Green, G., Diggle, P., Hasegawa, M., Taylor, M., Mann, D. &Allsop, D. (2011). Phosphorylated α-synuclein can be detected in blood plasma and is potentially a useful biomarker for Parkinson's disease. *The FASEB Journal,* 25(12), 4127-4137.

Gardinassi, L. G., Xia, J., Safo, S. E., & Li, S. (2017). *Bioinformatics tools for the interpretation of metabolomics data.* Current Pharmacology Reports, 3(6), 374-383.

Garrido-García, A., de Andrés, R., Jiménez-Pompa, A., Soriano, P., Sanz-Fuentes, D., Martínez-Blanco, E., &Díez-Guerra, F. J. (2019). *Neurogranin Expression Is Regulated by Synaptic Activity and*

Promotes Synaptogenesis in Cultured Hippocampal Neurons. Molecular neurobiology, 1-17.

Gonneaud, A., Turgeon, N., Boisvert, F. M., Boudreau, F., &Asselin, C. (2015). *Loss of histone deacetylase Hdac1 disrupts metabolic processes in intestinal epithelial cells.* FEBS letters, 589(19PartB), 2776-2783.

Govindarajan, R., Jeyapradha D., Karunakaran K., and Murugesan P. (2012). *Microarray and its applications. Journal of pharmacy & bioallied sciences.* Suppl 2 S310.

Groveman, B. R., Orrù, C. D., Hughson, A. G., Raymond, L. D., Zanusso, G., Ghetti, B., Campbell, K.J., Safar, J., Galasko, D. & Caughey, B. (2018). *Rapid and ultra-sensitive quantitation of disease-associated α-synuclein seeds in brain and cerebrospinal fluid by αSyn RT-QuIC.* Actaneuropathologica communications, 6(1), 7..

Guan, X., Xuan, M., Gu, Q., Huang, P., Liu, C., Wang, N., ... & Zhang, M. (2017). *Regionally progressive accumulation of iron in Parkinson's disease as measured by quantitative susceptibility mapping.* NMR in Biomedicine, 30(4).

Guan, X., Xu, X., & Zhang, M. (2017). *Region-specific iron measured by MRI as a biomarker for Parkinson's disease.* Neuroscience bulletin, 33(5), 561-567.

Gygi, S. P., Corthals, G. L., Zhang, Y., Rochon, Y., &Aebersold, R. (2000). *Evaluation of two-dimensional gel electrophoresis-basedproteome analysis technology.* Proceedings of the National Academy of Sciences, 97(17), 9390-9395.

Hasin, Y., Seldin, M., &Lusis, A. (2017). *Multi-omics approaches to disease.* Genome biology, 18(1), 83.

Havelund, J. F., Heegaard, N. H., Færgeman, N. J., &Gramsbergen, J. B. (2017). *Biomarker research in Parkinson's disease using metabolite profiling. Metabolites*, 7(3), 42.

He, N., Ling, H., Ding, B., Huang, J., Zhang, Y., Zhang, Z., Z., Liu, C., Chen, K. & Yan, F. (2015). *Region-specific disturbed iron distribution in early idiopathic Parkinson's disease measured by quantitative susceptibility mapping*. Human brain mapping, 36(11), 4407-4420.

Hellwig, K., Kvartsberg, H., Portelius, E., Andreasson, U., Oberstein, T. J., Lewczuk, P., Blennow, K., Kornhuber, J., Maler, J.M., Zetterberg, H. & Spitzer, P. (2015). *Neurogranin and YKL-40: independent markers of synaptic degeneration and neuro-inflammation in Alzheimer's disease.* Alzheimer's research & therapy, 7(1), 74.

Hoekstra, M., van der Lans, C. A., Halvorsen, B., Gullestad, L., Kuiper, J., Aukrust, P., van Berkel, T.J. & Biessen, E. A. (2010). *The peripheral blood mononuclear cell microRNA signature of coronary artery disease.* Biochemical and biophysical research communications, 394(3), 792-797.

Horgan, R. P., & Kenny, L. C. (2011). *'Omic'technologies: genomics, transcriptomics, proteomics and metabolomics.* The Obstetrician &Gynaecologist, 13(3), 189-195.

Huang, M., Zhao, J., Huang, Y., Dai, L., & Zhang, X. (2018). *Meta-analysis of urinary C-terminal telopeptide of type II collagen as a biomarker in osteoarthritis diagnosis.* Journal of orthopaedic translation, 13, 50-57.

Huynh, R. A., & Mohan, C. (2017). *Alzheimer's disease: biomarkers in the genome, blood, and cerebrospinal fluid.* Frontiers in neurology, 8, 102.

Hye, A., Lynham, S., Thambisetty, M., Causevic, M., Campbell, J., Byers, H. L., Hooper, C., Rijsdijk, F., Tabrizi, S.J., Banner, S. & Shaw, C. E. (2006). *Proteome-based plasma biomarkers for Alzheimer's disease*. Brain, 129(11), 3042-3050.

Kellermann, J. (2008). ICPL—isotope-coded protein label. In 2D PAGE: Sample Preparation and Fractionation (pp. 113-123). Humana Press.

Kester, M. I., Teunissen, C. E., Crimmins, D. L., Herries, E. M., Ladenson, J. H., Scheltens, P., van der Flier, W.M., Morris, J.C., Holtzman, D.M. & Fagan, A. M. (2015). *Neurogranin as a cerebrospinal fluid biomarker for synaptic loss in symptomatic Alzheimer disease.* JAMA neurology, 72(11), 1275-1280.

Klein, E., Klein, J. B., &Thongboonkerd, V. (2004). *Two-dimensional gel electrophoresis: a fundamental tool for expression proteomics studies. Proteomics in Nephrology*. Vol. 141, 25-39. Karger Publishers.

Kruk, J., Doskocz, M., Jodłowska, E., Zacharzewska, A., Łakomiec, J., Czaja, K., &Kujawski, J. (2017). *NMR techniques in metabolomic studies: A quick overview on examples of utilization*. Applied magnetic resonance, 48(1), 1-21.

Kurien, B. T., & Scofield, R. H. (2006). *Western blotting*. Methods, 38(4), 283-293.

Lashley, T., Schott, J. M., Weston, P., Murray, C. E., Wellington, H., Keshavan, A., Foti, S.C., Foiani, M., Toombs, J., Rohrer, J.D. &Heslegrave, A. (2018). *Molecular biomarkers of Alzheimer's disease: progress and prospects*. Disease models & mechanisms, 11(5), dmm031781.

Levy, K., Kilgour, L., &Berridge, C. (2018). *Regulating privacy in public/private space: the case of nursing home monitoring Laws*. Elder LJ, 26, 323.

Lin, J. P., Vitek, L., & Schwertner, H. A. (2010). *Serum bilirubin and genes controlling bilirubin concentrations as biomarkers for cardiovascular disease*. Clinical chemistry, 56(10), 1535-1543.

Lowe, R., Shirley, N., Bleackley, M., Dolan, S., &Shafee, T. (2017). *Transcriptomics technologies*. PLoS computational biology, 13(5), e1005457.

Mamoshina, P., Volosnikova, M., Ozerov, I. V., Putin, E., Skibina, E., Cortese, F., &Zhavoronkov, A. (2018). *Machine learning on human muscle transcriptomic data for biomarker discovery and tissue-specific drug target identification*. Frontiers in genetics, 9, 242.

Manzoni, C., Kia, D. A., Vandrovcova, J., Hardy, J., Wood, N. W., Lewis, P. A., & Ferrari, R. (2016). *Genome, transcriptome and proteome: the rise of omics data and their integration in biomedical sciences*. Briefings in bioinformatics, 19(2), 286-302.

Maršánová, L., Ronzhina, M., Smíšek, R., Vítek, M., Němcová, A., Smital, L., & Nováková, M. (2017). *ECG features and methods for automatic classification of ventricular premature and ischemic heartbeats: A comprehensive experimental study*. Scientific reports, 7(1), 11239.

Miura, Y., Sato, Y., Arai, Y., Abe, Y., Takayama, M., Toda, T., Hirose, N. & Endo, T. (2011). *Proteomic analysis of plasma proteins in Japanese semisuper centenarians*. Experimental gerontology, 46(1), 81-85.

Morbelli, S., & Bauckneht, M. (2018). Amyloid PET imaging: standardization and integration with other Alzheimer's disease biomarkers. In Biomarkers for Alzheimer 's disease Drug Development (pp. 203-212). *Humana Press*, New York, NY.

Olson, E. N. (2014). MicroRNAs as therapeutic targets and biomarkers of cardiovascular disease. *Science translational medicine*, 6(239), 239ps3.

Pandey, A., & Mann, M. (2000). *Proteomics to study genes and genomes*. Nature, 405(6788), 837.

Panina, S. B., Krolevets, I. V., Milyutina, N. P., Sagakyants, A. B., Kornienko, I. V., Ananyan, A. A., Zabrodin, M.A., Plotnikov, A. A. & Vnukov, V. V. (2017). *Circulating levels of proinflammatory mediators as potential biomarkers of post-traumatic knee osteoarthritis development*. Journal of Orthopaedics and Traumatology, 18(4), 349-357.

Schipper, H. M., Maes, O. C., Chertkow, H. M., & Wang, E. (2007). *MicroRNA expression in Alzheimer blood mononuclear cells. Gene regulation and systems biology*, 1, GRSB-S361.

Schöll, M., Lockhart, S. N., Schonhaut, D. R., O'Neil, J. P., Janabi, M., Ossenkoppele, R., Baker, S.L., Vogel, J.W., Faria, J., Schwimmer, H.D. & Rabinovici, G. D. (2016). PET imaging of tau deposition in the aging human brain. Neuron, 89(5), 971-982.

Sharma, N., & Singh, A. N. (2016). *Exploring biomarkers for Alzheimer's disease*. Journal of clinical and diagnostic research: JCDR, 10(7), KE01.

Steinbeck, M. J., Nesti, L. J., Sharkey, P. F., &Parvizi, J. (2007). *Myeloperoxidase and chlorinated peptides in osteoarthritis:*

potential biomarkers of the disease. Journal of orthopaedic research, 25(9), 1128-1135.

Strimbu, K., &Tavel, J. A. (2010). *What are biomarkers?* Current Opinion in HIV and AIDS, 5(6), 463.

Sutandy, F. R., Qian, J., Chen, C. S., & Zhu, H. (2013). *Overview of protein microarrays. Current protocols in protein science*, 72(1), 27-1.

Taurino, C., Miller, W. H., McBride, M. W., McClure, J. D., Khanin, R., Moreno, M. U., Dymott, J.A., Delles, C. & Dominiczak, A. F. (2010). Gene expression profiling in whole blood of patients with coronary artery disease. Clinical science, 119(8), 335-343.

Tijsen, A. J., Creemers, E. E., Moerland, P. D., de Windt, L. J., van der Wal, A. C., Kok, W. E., & Pinto, Y. M. (2010). MiR423-5p as a circulating biomarker for heart failure. Circulation research, 106(6), 1035.

Tufekci, K. U., Civi Bayin, E., Genc, S., & Genc, K. (2011). *The Nrf2/ARE pathway: a promising target to counteract mitochondrial dysfunction in Parkinson's disease.* Parkinson's disease, 2011.

Vasilj, A., Gentzel, M., Ueberham, E., Gebhardt, R., & Shevchenko, A. (2012). *Tissue proteomics by one-dimensional gel electrophoresis combined with label-free protein quantification*. Journal of proteome research, 11(7), 3680-3689.

Viereck, J., &Thum, T. (2017). *Circulating noncoding RNAs as biomarkers of cardiovascular disease and injury*. Circulation Research, 120(2), 381-399.

Wallace, C., Newhouse, S. J., Braund, P., Zhang, F., Tobin, M., Falchi, M., Ahmadi, K., Dobson, R.J., Marçano, A.C.B., Hajat, C. & Burton, P. (2008). *Genome-wide association study identifies genes for biomarkers of cardiovascular disease: serum urate and dyslipidemia.* The American Journal of Human Genetics, 82(1), 139-149.

Wang, Q., Rozelle, A. L., Lepus, C. M., Scanzello, C. R., Song, J. J., Larsen, D. M., ... & Hwang, I. (2011). *Identification of a central role for complement in osteoarthritis. Nature medicine*, 17(12), 1674.

Wang, Z., Gerstein, M., & Snyder, M. (2009). *RNA-Seq: a revolutionary tool for transcriptomics.* Nature reviews genetics, 10(1), 57.

Wellington, H., Paterson, R. W., Portelius, E., Törnqvist, U., Magdalinou, N., Fox, N. C., Blennow, K., Schott, J.M. & Zetterberg, H. (2016). *Increased CSF neurogranin concentration is specific to Alzheimer disease.* Neurology, 86(9), 829-835.

Wiese, S., Reidegeld, K. A., Meyer, H. E., &Warscheid, B. (2007). *Protein labeling by iTRAQ: a new tool for quantitative mass spectrometry in proteome research.* Proteomics, 7(3), 340-350.

Xu, J., Patassini, S., Rustogi, N., Riba-Garcia, I., Hale, B. D., Phillips, A. M., Waldvogel, H., Haines, R., Bradbury, P., Stevens, A. & Faull, R. L. (2019). *Regional protein expression in human Alzheimer's brain correlates with disease severity*. Communications biology, 2(1), 43.

Zahn, J. M., Sonu, R., Vogel, H., Crane, E., Mazan-Mamczarz, K., Rabkin, R., Davis, R.W., Becker, K.G., Owen, A.B. & Kim, S. K. (2006). *Transcriptional profiling of aging in human muscle reveals a common aging signature*. PLoS genetics, 2(7), e115.

Zhai, G., Wang-Sattler, R., & Hart, D. J. (2010). *Serum branched-chain amino acid to histidine.*

Zhang, C. (2009). *Novel functions for small RNA molecules.* Current opinion in molecular therapeutics, 11(6), 641.

Zhang, J., Zhang, Y., Wang, J., Cai, P., Luo, C., Qian, Z., Dai, Y. & Feng, H. (2010). *Characterizing iron deposition in Parkinson's disease using susceptibility-weighted imaging: an in vivo MR study*. Brain research, 1330, 124-130.

Zhao, B. S., Roundtree, I. A., & He, C. (2017). *Post-transcriptional gene regulation by mRNA modifications*. Nature reviews Molecular cell biology, 18(1), 31.

In: Current Challenges and Management … ISBN: 978-1-53617-304-8
Editor: Abhai Kumar

Chapter 9

The Role of Natural Polyphenols on Neurodegenerative Disorders

***Shambhoo Sharan Tripathi*[1], *Mallika Chatterjee*[2] *and Abhishek Kumar Singh*[2,*]**

[1]Department of Biochemistry, Faculty of Science, University of Allahabad, Allahabad, India

[2]Amity Institute of Neuropsychology and Neurosciences, Amity University Uttar Pradesh, Noida, India

Abstract

Neurodegenerative disorders are related to neuronal cell death and are one of the many global challenges. It affects the quality of life of human beings. There are different kinds of identified neurodegenerative diseases which are caused by either genetic or environmental factors. These factors induce different signaling pathway(s) which affect cell renewal as well as the cell death process. Several plant-derived polyphenols with neuroprotective capacities have been discovered. In this chapter we have collected information regarding neurodegeneration, types of neurodegenerative disorders, signaling pathways involved in

* Corresponding Author's Email: aksingh20@amity.edu.

pathogenesis of neurodegeneration, and plant-derived polyphenols that have potential as therapeutic interventions against neurodegenerative disorders.

Keywords: polyphenols, neurodegenerative disorders, oxidative stress, neuroprotection, mTOR/AMPK signaling

1. Introduction

Neurodegenerative diseases are related to a chronic collapse and disappearance of the neuronal cells. These diseases consist of a wide range of pathological symptoms that affect the central nervous system (CNS) and have a broad impact on the human population. Continuous aggregation of misfolded proteins is one of the major reasons that have been identified for these diseases. The protein clump overload in neuronal cells interferes with signal transduction of neurotransmitters through synaptic regions. Other cellular transporters also face the same problem. Moreover, another mechanism of neurodegeneration is the free radical mediated molecular damage of the cellular and mitochondrial membranes, which affects the membrane integrity of the cells. Both mechanisms are involved in the loss of neuronal cell function and eventual death (Pavlin et al. 2016).

Most of the neurodegenerative diseases are progressive, incurable, predominantly of idiopathic origin and eventually lethal disorders of the central nervous system (CNS). Parkinson's disease (PD) and Alzheimer's disease (AD) are two most prominent types of neurodegenerative disorders (Xie et al. 2014). There are also several other neurodegenerative disorders but their incidence are lower than PD and AD (Kumar et al., 2016; Rasool et al., 2014). Environmental and genetic factors are also known to initiate the onset and pathogenesis of neurodegenerative diseases. From last few years, several genes mutations have been identified that are connected with neurodegenerative disorders. But exact mechanisms of pathogenesis in most of these disorders are still not clear.

2. Types of Neurodegeneration

2.1. Alzheimer's Disease

Alzheimer disease (AD) is one of the most common neurodegenerative disorders, affecting approximately 28 to 38 million people around the world (Katsnelson et al. 2016, Bagli et al. 2016). The typical pathological symptoms of the disease start with mild memory loss and successive changes in cognitive behavior (Bagli et al. 2016). Clinically, AD is characterized by neuronal loss and neuropathologic lesions in the brain (Smith and Mallucci 2016). AD is a multifactorial disease and the pathophysiology of AD is not clearly known. Moreover, approximately 70% familial AD patients carry the mutant gene from their parents. Hypertension, depression and head injuries are also reasons for AD. The initiation of disease is associated with aggregation of amyloid-beta plaques and neurofibrillary tangles of hyper-phosphorylated tau-protein in the neuronal cells (Diack et al. 2016). AD can be diagnosed by the history of the illness, blood test and cognitive testing with medical imaging. There are no proper medicines or supplements available to reduce the risk associated with AD.

2.2. Parkinson's Disease

Parkinson's disease (PD) is the second most common neurodegenerative disorder, related to memory loss and the progressive destruction of motor control (Bagli et al. 2016). Voluntary motor function destruction is associated with the different signs and symptoms including akinesia, bradykinesia, hypokinesia, postural instability, rigidity, stooped posture, and tremor at rest. These signs and symptoms are used in diagnosis and prognosis of PD (Smith and Mallucci 2016, Navone et al. 2015). These symptoms are due to the pathological changes in brain like the progressive loss of neurons in the substantia nigra pars compacta. These neurons are connected with signal transduction of dopamine to other neurons. Neuronal degeneration leads to disruption of the neuronal circuitry in the basal ganglia and motor cortical areas. Mechanism of neuronal loss includes deposition of α-synuclein also known as Lewy body inclusions (Diack et al. 2016, Rohowetz et al. 2018, Douglas and Dillin 2010). Finally, abnormalities in movement- the major manifestations of PD, affect the individual's behaviour as well as quality of life (Smith and Mallucci 2016).

2.3. Huntington's Disease

Huntington's disease (HD) is another neurodegenerative disease which is characterized by the dominant inherited repeat of CAG trinucleotide in the huntingtin gene present on chromosome 4 (Wexler et al. 2016, Wild and Tabrizi 2017, Telenius et al. 1994). The prevalence of HD in western populations is 10-13 individuals per 100 000 (Bates et al. 2015). The characteristics of HD are cognitive, motor and psychiatric disturbance. Mutation in huntingtin gene produces toxic mutant protein which leads to disruption of protein homeostasis, transcription and mitochondrial function and finally neuronal death. The pathological lesions are visualized in the striatum and cortex region with the progression of disease. Till date there are no disease treatments, therefore management of disease symptom is the form of treatment that is given to these individuals (McColgan and Tabrizi 2017).

3. Causes and Symptoms

The main reason of neurodegenerative disorders such as AD, PD, and HD are the deposition of anomalous protein isoforms which synthesized inside neuronal cells. The exact mechanism of disease progression is not clear, consequently development of early therapeutic intervention is challenging. Amongst these disorders, the transmissible spongiform encephalopathies (TSEs) or prion diseases are very unique, which can transmit from one to other individuals (Diack et al. 2016).

A gross scheme of neurodegeneration on the molecular level is based on two pathways. Firstly, reactive species oxidize heavy atom ions, which enhance the interaction of alpha-synuclein, thus promoting its folding to the beta form and giving rise to insoluble amyloid plaques (Gaggelli et al. 2006, Zecca et al. 2004, Singh et al. 2014). The latter prevents the function of vesicular transport leading to gradual neuronal death (Pahnke et al. 2014). In the second pathway, free radical species, -OH in particular, react with the methylene groups of the apolar part of the lipid bilayer of either the cell or mitochondria, resulting in membrane leakage followed by dyshomeostasis, loss of resting potential and neuronal death (Cordeiro 2014). Unlike all other CNS relevant biogenic amines, dopamine and noradrenaline are capable of a non-enzymatic auto-oxidative reaction, which produces hydrogen peroxide. This reaction is not limited to the mitochondrial membrane where scavenging enzymes, such as catalase, are located (Bottelbergs et al. 2010). On the other hand, dopamine and its metabolites, such as dopamine-o-quinone, dopaminechrome, 5, 6-dihydroxyindole and indo-5, 6-quinone, also interact directly with alpha-synuclein and reversibly inhibit plaque formation. The current analysis can be employed in developing strategies for the prevention and treatment of neurodegeneration, and, hopefully, aid in the building of an overall kinetic molecular model of neurodegeneration itself (Pavlin et al. 2016).

4. Molecular Mechanism and Signalling

4.1. mTOR Signalling in Neurodegeneration

The mammalian target of rapamycin (mTOR) signalling pathway is one of the important pathways that regulate cellular senescence, aging and age-associated disorders. mTOR possess serine/threonine kinase activity and essential components of protein complexes: mTORC1 and mTORC2, which are different in their upstream and downstream signaling (Jung et al.

2010). Growing evidence emphasizes that interruption in mTOR signalling pathway in the brain affects glucose metabolism, mitochondrial function, energy production, cell proliferation and autophagy (Jung et al. 2010, Godoy et al. 2014, Finley and Haigis 2009). mTOR signalling pathway is an important player in the pathogenesis of AD. From last few years, mTOR signalling pathway has been comprehensively studied in human AD brain and animal model of AD indicating an anomalous upregulation (Oddo 2012, Pei and Hugon 2008). Post-mortem analysis of human AD brains demonstrates that the phosphorylation of mTOR at Ser-2448 and Ser-2481 as well as its downstream signalling cascade, p70S6K and eIF4E, are significantly higher in the region of the hippocampus and in other brain areas (Griffin et al. 2005, Li et al. 2005, Sun et al. 2014). Moreover, there are correlations between the increased activity of mTOR and Braak stages and/or disease severity of AD patients. Additionally, it has been seen that, at early stages of development of AD, over activation of mTOR signaling (Tramutola et al. 2015) is observed in the inferior parietal lobule (IPL) of mild cognitively impaired (MCI) subjects. On the other hand, phosphoinositide-3 kinase (PI3-K/Akt)-acting upstream of the mTOR signalling cascade, is diminished in AD brains (Martin et al. 2001, Wei et al. 2002). Aberrant activation and abnormal sub-cellular level of PI3-K has been reported in cortical neurons and hippocampal region of the brain (Kwak et al. 2010, O' Neill 2013, Pei et al. 2003, Sonoda et al. 2010). In PD, mTOR protein is over-expressed in the temporal cortex of patients due to the accumulation of α-synuclein (Crews et al. 2010). Moreover, α-synuclein accumulation inhibits autophagy perhaps via inducing mTOR signalling. Conversely, mTOR inhibitors, such as rapamycin, have the ability to restore the elevated activity of mTOR that have been induced by the accumulation of α-synuclein (Gao et al. 2015).

4.2. AMPK Dysregulation

Adenosine monophosphate-activated protein kinase (AMPK) is a sensor for cellular metabolism and is an evolutionarily conserved protein.

It is present in immune cells and an essential regulator of inflammatory responses (Carroll et al. 2013, Galic et al. 2011). AMPK negatively regulates nuclear factor-kB and toll-like receptor. Dysregulation of AMPK plays an important role in neurodegenerative diseases, for instance in AD, multiple sclerosis, HD, and PD etc. Moreover, AMPK activator has a neuroprotective role. However, clinically available and well tolerated pharmacological activators, such as metformin, resveratrol, and GPA have not been in clinical use till date for neurodegenerative diseases in human patients (Peixoto et al. 2017).

The pathogenesis of major neurodegenerative diseases for example Alzheimer's disease (AD) and Parkinson's disease (PD) is multifactorial and not very clear. Accumulating evidence proposes that oxidative stress is one of reasons for these illnesses. Although AD and PD have different signs and symptoms, in both illnesses oxidative stress contributes to neuronal damage. Glutamate is an important neurotransmitter and is related to calcium homeostasis and mitochondrial function (Cassano et al. 2016). Human genetics studies have shown that disease-causing rare mutations and risk-associated common alleles overlap in different neurodegenerative disorders. Shared pathological mechanisms include defective protein quality-control and degradation pathways, dysfunctional mitochondrial homeostasis, stress granules, and maladaptive innate immune responses. Research efforts have started to bear fruit, as shown by recent treatment successes and an encouraging therapeutic outlook (Gan et al. 2018).

5. Oxidative Stress and Neurodegeneration

Brain has limited levels of antioxidants as compared to other organs and which is therefore less able to ameliorate reactive oxygen and nitrogen species (ROS/RNS) production (Cobb and Cole 2015). Redox imbalance is consequence of reduction of the antioxidant capacity, and leads to activation of alternating pathways that generally do not work in normal conditions.

Oxidative stress has a significant role in a variety of diseases including neurodegenerative disorders. Optimum iron concentration is essential for the activity a large number of proteins and enzymes, but elevated level of iron could also be toxic. Excess of iron produces oxidative stress, predominantly in brain, where antioxidant systems are comparatively low. In the brain, iron accumulation in particular area is linked with pathogenesis of neurodegenerative diseases such as Parkinson's disease, Alzheimer's disease, and Huntington's chorea etc. Mostly Fe^{++} ion is a part of catalyst of Fenton reaction that generates a large number of free radicals like hydroxyl radicals (OH). It has been proved in clinical studies that patients with neurodegenerative disorders exhibit dramatic accumulation of iron in brain as well as increase in reactive oxygen species (Carocci et al. 2018).

6. Apoptosis

Apoptosis in the cells is characterized by phenotypical changes such as shrinking of the cell, membrane blebbing, compartmentalization, chromatin condensation, and DNA fragmentation. Apoptosis in neuronal cells was first reported in a cell based model of PD that had been induced by neurotoxin MPP+ (Dipasquale et al. 1991). Apoptosis has also been shown to be predominant in the substantia nigra (SN) region of post-mortem brains of PD patients (Mochizuki et al. 1996, Anglade et al. 1997, Tompkins et al. 1997). But these findings could not be reproduced by the other researchers (Kosel et al. 1997, Banati et al. 1998, Wullner et al. 1999). TUNEL staining of post-mortem tissue has subsequently confirmed the incidence of apoptosis in PD pathology (Tatton et al. 1998, Tatton 2000) and also activation of caspase-3, caspase-8, and caspase-9 in nigrostriatal dopaminergic neurons (Hartmann et al. 2000, Tatton 2000) and increased activities of caspase-1 and caspase-3 in SN (Mogi et al. 2000). Additionally, in case of AD pathogenesis, a lysosomal protease cathepsin D strongly expressed in the brain plays a vital role in the regulation of apoptosis (Malik et al. 2011). Moreover, constant production of hydroxyl radicals through Fenton chemistry fails to react iron, leading to apoptosis via inducing the nuclear factor kappa-B (NF-kB) signalling pathway (Chen et al. 2012) in many neurodegenerative diseases like AD (Kell 2010). Although many *in vivo* and *in vitro* data are in favour of involvement of apoptosis in neurodegenerative processes, there is considerable evidence that other complex events may also contribute to neuronal cell death with possible repair mechanisms, the elucidation of which may prove useful for future prevention and therapy of neurodegenerative disorders (Jellinger 2001).

7. Therapeutic Interventions

Neurodegenerative diseases (NDs) such as Parkinson's disease (PD), Alzheimer's disease (AD), Huntington's disease (HD), and amyotrophic lateral sclerosis (ALS) are major health concerns throughout the world. Till date, there are no effective therapies available. Since most of the disorders are age associated, therefore, an approach of delaying pathogenesis and providing patients symptomatic reliefs have been adopted so far. Mitochondria of the cell not only regulate the energy production process but are also involved in programmed cell death and mitochondrial dysfunctions have therefore been causally linked to the above-listed neurodegenerative disorders. Therefore, study of the mechanism of mitochondrial dysfunction may be important for therapeutic intervention. Mitochondrial dysfunction and associated loss of mitochondrial membrane potential lead to bioenergetic function collapse and eventual neuronal cell death. This can be seen in ischaemic reperfusion injury and also in a number of other diseases. Disturbance in mitochondrial homeostasis causes impaired mitochondrial biogenesis and mitophagy. This impairment in mitochondrial homeostasis is emerging as an important aspect of various neurodegenerative and neuromuscular disorders (Corona and Duchen 2015).

Targeting glutamate metabolism might be the potential therapeutic intervention for the treatment of neurodegenerative disorders. Glutamate acts as a neurotransmitter and metabolite for neurons. Glutamate dehydrogenase (GDH) catalyzes the conversion of glutamate to α-ketoglutarate and the latter serves as a TCA cycle intermediate. There is correlation of GDH dysregulated activity with neurological disorders. On the basis of different studies, it has been concluded that the administration of allosteric modulators of GDH in GDH deficient mice improves the energy metabolism and delays the early onset of Alzheimer's disease, Parkinson's disease, spinocerebellar atrophy and temporal lobe epilepsy. Thus modulation GDH activity in energy crisis situation might be a good approach for the therapy of neurodegenerative diseases (Kim and Baik 2019).

8. Therapeutic Intervention Involving Polyphenols

Plant-derived polyphenolic compounds are able to efficiently reduce oxidative stress generated in neurodegenerative diseases (Solayman et al. 2017). Dietary antioxidants, particularly flavonoids, are being identified as a therapeutic strategy to restrict or delay the pathogenesis of neurological and age-related disorders. Generally, the pharmacological target of natural flavonoids is extracellular signal-regulated kinases (ERK) that act as a therapeutic agent. Depending upon the chemical structure, flavonoids are categorized into different subgroups including anthocyanins, flavones, flavanones, flavan-3-ols, flavonols, and isoflavones. Evidence from different studies revealed that many of the flavonoids collected from different kind of plants or dietary fruits as well as herbal sources reduce oxidative stress in several neurodegenerative disorders. The polyphenolic natural products are generally extracted from medicinal plants, act as antioxidants, and have been recognized as a safe and non-toxic in nature (Farzaei et al. 2018).

Table 1. Natural Product Inhibitor, *in vivo* Efficacy: Animal Studies and Clinical Trials

Natural Product	**Targeted-Protein/Animal Model/Human Trial**	**Effects**	**Reference**
In vivo Animal studies			
Curcumin	Aβ/Tg2576 mouse	Low and high doses of curcumin significantly lowered oxidized proteins and proinflammatory cytokine IL-1β With low-dose but not high-dose, soluble and insoluble Aβ, plaque burden, and the astrocytic marker GFAP were significantly reduced	(Lim et al. 2001)
Epigallocatechin gallate (EGCG)	α-synuclein/N-methyl-4-phenyl-1,2,3,6-tetrahydropyridine-and 6-hydroxydopamine-induced neurodegenerative C57-BL mice	EGCG prevented the accumulation of iron and α-synuclein in the substantia nigra pars compacta.	(Mandel et al. 2004)
Ferulic acid	Aβ/APP/PS1 mouse	Decreased in brain parenchymal and cerebral vascular β-amyloid deposits as well as Aβ oligomer abundance Reversed transgene-associated behavioral deficits including hyperactivity, object recognition, spatial working, and reference memory	(Mori et al. 2013)
Hopeahainol A	Aβ/APP/PS1 mouse	Protected against mitochondrial dysfunction and suppressed oxidative stress. Rescued synaptic dysfunction and memory impairment.	(Zhu et al. 2013)

Table 1. (Continued)

Natural Product	Targeted-Protein/Animal Model/Human Trial	Effects	Reference
Myricetin	Aβ/Tg2576 mouse	Aβ plaque depositions in mice brains significantly decreased TBS-soluble, A11-positive oligomers in the mice brain significantly reduced	(Hamaguchi et al. 2009)
Oleuropein	Aβ/TgCRND8 mouse	Ameliorated memory dysfunction Enhanced autophagic response	(Grossi et al. 2014)
Scyllo-inositol	Amyloid β peptide (Aβ)/TgCRND8 mouse	Inhibit Aβ high-molecular –weight oligomers in the brain Ameliorate several AD-link phenotypes: Impaired cognition, Altered synaptic physiology, Cerebral Aβ pathology, Accelerated mortality	(McLaurin et al. 2006)
Quercetin	Aβ/C. elegan CL2006	Decreased the amount of aggregated proteins in solution and also paralysis in CL2006. Increased proteasomal activity and the flow of proteins through the macroautophagy pathway	(Regitz et al. 2014)
Resveratrol	Aβ/Tg19959 mouse	Reduced plaques in medial cortex, striatum, and hypothalamus. Brain glutathione reduced and brain cysteine increased Neither resveratrol nor its conjugated metabolites were detectable in brain	(Karuppagounder et al. 2009)
Resveratrol	Aβ/APP/PS1 mouse	Long-term treatment significantly prevented memory loss. Reduced the amyloid burden in the brain.	(Solberg et al. 2014)
Rifampicin	Tau609 mouse	Reduced accumulation of Aβ oligomers, tau hyperphosphorylation, synapse loss, and microglial activation improved memory.	(Umeda et al. 2016)

Natural Product	Targeted-Protein/Animal Model/ Human Trial	Effects	Reference
Rosmarinic acid	Aβ/Tg2576 mouse	Aβ plaque depositions in mice brains significantly decreased TBS-soluble Aβ monomers was increased TBS-soluble, A11-positive oligomers in the mice brain significantly reduced.	(Hamaguchi et al. 2009)
Rutin	Aβ/APP/PS1 mouse	Reduced oligomeric Aβ level, increased glutathione/glutathione disulfide ratio Attenuated memory deficits. Reduced microgliosis and astrocytosis, and inflammatory IL-1β and IL-6 levels in brain.	(Xu et al. 2014)

Clinical Studies

Curcumin	Aβ and tau; Clinical trial	No changes in the AD Assessment Scale-cognitive Subscale, Aβ40 and Aβ42 levels in plasma, levels of Aβ42 and total and phosphorylated tau in cerebrospinal fluid (CSF) Suggested limited bioavailability: levels of native curcumin were undetectable in the CSF	(Ringman et al. 2012)
EGCG/Green Tea/Green Tea Extract	Transthyretin/Clinical trial	No increase of left ventricular (LV) wall thickness and LV myocardial mass was observed. Suggested an inhibitory effect of GT/GTE on the progression of cardiac amyloidosis.	(Kristen et al. 2012)

Polyphenolic compounds have exhibited neuroprotective attributes in various research experiments (Table 1). These protective outcomes can be described by the antioxidant capacity of polyphenols. Moreover, their roles in cellular defense and interactions with neurotoxic proteins have also been confirmed. In the case of Alzheimer's disease, it has been explained in recent research that polyphenols inhibit the aggregation of toxic beta-amyloid protein through direct interaction. Green tea derived polyphenol like epigallocatechin-3-gallate (EGCG) and the phytoalexin resveratrol are good examples (Smid et al. 2012). Presently, plant-derived alkaloids are predominantly used as therapeutic drugs for Alzheimer's disease in which galantamine and rivastigmine are used for protection of the cholinergic system. However, as the alkaloids hold the most critical place of the phytochemical spectrum, and they are usually connected with side effects (Wightman 2017).

Although flavonoids have various pharmacological functions,, human and animals are not able to synthesize them. Nonetheless, they are known to be produced in approximately all types of plants and have demonstrated exceptional impact on human health.

Concluding Remarks and Perspectives

The growing incidence of neurodegenerative diseases is a global health burden. There is an utmost requirement of effective therapeutic interventions. A number of polyphenols have been characterized for their neuroprotective roles. Each and every existing polyphenols has different molecular targets, in the future they can be used as combinatorial therapies for the treatment of neurodegenerative disorders. In this regard, more research is required to screen the neuroprotective activities of plant derived polyphenols. Moreover, we do not have good diagnostic and prognostic markers for the neurodegenerative disorders, therefore, we should also think about in this direction as well.

Acknowledgments

D. S. Kothari Post-Doctoral Fellowship scheme of University Grant Commission (UGC), New Delhi, India, is acknowledged for providing financial support (F.4-2/2006 (BSR)/BL/17-18/0381) to SST.

References

Anglade, P., et al. 1997. Apoptosis and autophagy in nigral neurons of patients with Parkinson's disease. *Histol Histopathol,* 12(1), 25-31.

Bagli, E., et al. 2016. Natural Compounds and Neuroprotection: Mechanisms of Action and Novel Delivery Systems. *In Vivo,* 30(5), 535-547.

Banati, R. B., Daniel, S. E. and Blunt, S. B. 1998. Glial pathology but absence of apoptotic nigral neurons in long-standing Parkinson's disease. *Mov Disord,* 13(2), 221-227.

Bates, G. P., et al. 2015. Huntington disease. *Nat Rev Dis Primers,* 1, 15005.

Bottelbergs, A., et al. 2010. Axonal integrity in the absence of functional peroxisomes from projection neurons and astrocytes. *Glia,* 58(13), 1532-1543.

Carocci, A., et al. 2018. Oxidative stress and neurodegeneration: the involvement of iron. *Biometals,* 31(5), 715-735.

Carroll, K. C., Viollet, B. and Suttles, J. 2013. AMPKalpha1 deficiency amplifies proinflammatory myeloid APC activity and CD40 signaling. *J Leukoc Biol,* 94(6), 1113-1121.

Cassano, T., et al. 2016. Glutamate and Mitochondria: Two Prominent Players in the Oxidative Stress-Induced Neurodegeneration. *Curr Alzheimer Res,* 13(2), 185-197.

Chen, C. H., et al. 2012. Increased NF-kappaB signalling up-regulates BACE1 expression and its therapeutic potential in Alzheimer's disease. *Int J Neuropsychopharmacol,* 15(1), 77-90.

Cobb, C. A. and Cole, M. P. 2015. Oxidative and nitrative stress in neurodegeneration. *Neurobiol Dis,* 84, 4-21.

Cordeiro, R. M. 2014. Reactive oxygen species at phospholipid bilayers: distribution, mobility and permeation. *Biochim Biophys Acta,* 1838(1 Pt B), 438-444.

Corona, J. C. and Duchen, M. R. 2015. Impaired mitochondrial homeostasis and neurodegeneration: towards new therapeutic targets? *J Bioenerg Biomembr,* 47(1-2), 89-99.

Crews, L., et al. 2010. Selective molecular alterations in the autophagy pathway in patients with Lewy body disease and in models of alpha-synucleinopathy. *PLoS One,* 5(2), e9313.

Diack, A. B., et al. 2016. Insights into Mechanisms of Chronic Neurodegeneration. *Int J Mol Sci,* 17(1).

Dipasquale, B., Marini, A. M. and Youle, R. J. 1991. Apoptosis and DNA degradation induced by 1-methyl-4-phenylpyridinium in neurons. *Biochem Biophys Res Commun,* 181(3), 1442-1448.

Douglas, P. M. and Dillin, A. 2010. Protein homeostasis and aging in neurodegeneration. *J Cell Biol,* 190(5), 719-729.

Farzaei, M. H., et al. 2018. Targeting ERK signaling pathway by polyphenols as novel therapeutic strategy for neurodegeneration. *Food Chem Toxicol,* 120, 183-195.

Finley, L. W. and Haigis, M. C. 2009. The coordination of nuclear and mitochondrial communication during aging and calorie restriction. *Ageing Res Rev,* 8(3), 173-188.

Gaggelli, E., et al. 2006. Copper homeostasis and neurodegenerative disorders (Alzheimer's, prion, and Parkinson's diseases and amyotrophic lateral sclerosis). *Chem Rev,* 106(6), 1995-2044.

Galic, S., et al. 2011. Hematopoietic AMPK beta1 reduces mouse adipose tissue macrophage inflammation and insulin resistance in obesity. *J Clin Invest,* 121(12), 4903-4915.

Gan, L., et al. 2018. Converging pathways in neurodegeneration, from genetics to mechanisms. *Nat Neurosci,* 21(10), 1300-1309.

Gao, S., et al. 2015. Alpha-synuclein overexpression negatively regulates insulin receptor substrate 1 by activating mTORC1/S6K1 signaling. *Int J Biochem Cell Biol,* 64, 25-33.

Godoy, J. A., et al. 2014. Signaling pathway cross talk in Alzheimer's disease. *Cell Commun Signal,* 12, 23.

Griffin, R. J., et al. 2005. Activation of Akt/PKB, increased phosphorylation of Akt substrates and loss and altered distribution of Akt and PTEN are features of Alzheimer's disease pathology. *J Neurochem,* 93(1), 105-117.

Grossi, C., et al. 2014. Employing Alzheimer disease animal models for translational research: focus on dietary components. *Neurodegener Dis,* 13(2-3), 131-134.

Hamaguchi, T., et al. 2009. Phenolic compounds prevent Alzheimer's pathology through different effects on the amyloid-beta aggregation pathway. *Am J Pathol,* 175(6), 2557-2565.

Hartmann, A., et al. 2000. Caspase-3: A vulnerability factor and final effector in apoptotic death of dopaminergic neurons in Parkinson's disease. *Proc NatlAcadSci USA,* 97(6), 2875-2880.

Jellinger, K. A. 2001. Cell death mechanisms in neurodegeneration. *J Cell Mol Med,* 5(1), 1-17.

Jung, C. H., et al. 2010. mTOR regulation of autophagy. *FEBS Lett,* 584(7), 1287-1295.

Karuppagounder, S. S., et al. 2009. Dietary supplementation with resveratrol reduces plaque pathology in a transgenic model of Alzheimer's disease. *Neurochem Int,* 54(2), 111-118.

Katsnelson, A., De Strooper, B. and Zoghbi, H. Y. 2016. Neurodegeneration: From cellular concepts to clinical applications. *Sci Transl Med,* 8(364), 364ps318.

Kell, D. B. 2010. Towards a unifying, systems biology understanding of large-scale cellular death and destruction caused by poorly liganded iron: Parkinson's, Huntington's, Alzheimer's, prions, bactericides, chemical toxicology and others as examples. *Arch Toxicol,* 84(11), 825-889.

Kim, A. Y. and Baik, E. J. 2019. Glutamate Dehydrogenase as a Neuroprotective Target Against Neurodegeneration. *Neurochem Res,* 44(1), 147-153.

Kosel, S., et al. 1997. On the question of apoptosis in the parkinsonian substantia nigra. *Acta Neuropathol,* 93(2), 105-108.

Kristen, A. V., et al. 2012. Green tea halts progression of cardiac transthyretin amyloidosis: an observational report. *Clin Res Cardiol,* 101(10), 805-813.

Kwak, Y. D., et al. 2010. NO signaling and S-nitrosylation regulate PTEN inhibition in neurodegeneration. *Mol Neurodegener,* 5, 49.

Li, X., et al. 2005. Levels of mTOR and its downstream targets 4E-BP1, eEF2, and eEF2 kinase in relationships with tau in Alzheimer's disease brain. *FEBS J,* 272(16), 4211-4220.

Lim, G. P., et al. 2001. The curry spice curcumin reduces oxidative damage and amyloid pathology in an Alzheimer transgenic mouse. *J Neurosci,* 21(21), 8370-8377.

Malik, M., et al. 2011. A novel approach for characterization of cathepsin D protease and its effect on tau and beta-amyloid proteins. *Neurochem Res,* 36(5), 754-760.

Mandel, S., et al. 2004. Cell signaling pathways in the neuroprotective actions of the green tea polyphenol (-)-epigallocatechin-3-gallate: implications for neurodegenerative diseases. *J Neurochem,* 88(6), 1555-1569.

Martin, D., et al. 2001. Effect of the Alzheimer amyloid fragment Abeta (25-35) on Akt/PKB kinase and survival of PC12 cells. *J Neurochem,* 78(5), 1000-1008.

McColgan, P. and Tabrizi, S. J. 2017. Huntington's disease: a clinical review. *Eur J Neurol,* 25(1), 24-34.

McLaurin, J., et al. 2006. Cyclohexanehexol inhibitors of Abeta aggregation prevent and reverse Alzheimer phenotype in a mouse model. *Nat Med,* 12(7), 801-808.

Mochizuki, H., et al. 1996. Histochemical detection of apoptosis in Parkinson's disease. *J Neurol Sci,* 137(2), 120-123.

Mogi, M., et al. 2000. Caspase activities and tumor necrosis factor receptor R1 (p55) level are elevated in the substantia nigra from parkinsonian brain. *J Neural Transm (Vienna),* 107(3), 335-341.

Mori, T., et al. 2013. Ferulic acid is a nutraceutical beta-secretase modulator that improves behavioral impairment and alzheimer-like pathology in transgenic mice. *PLoS One,* 8(2), e55774.

Navone, F., Genevini, P. and Borgese, N. 2015. Autophagy and Neurodegeneration: Insights from a Cultured Cell Model of ALS. *Cells,* 4(3), 354-386.

Oddo, S. 2012. The role of mTOR signaling in Alzheimer disease. *Front Biosci (Schol Ed),* 4, 941-952.

O'Neill, C. 2013. PI3-kinase/Akt/mTOR signaling: impaired on/off switches in aging, cognitive decline and Alzheimer's disease. *Exp Gerontol,* 48(7), 647-653.

Pahnke, J., Langer, O. and Krohn, M. 2014. Alzheimer's and ABC transporters--new opportunities for diagnostics and treatment. *Neurobiol Dis,* 72 Pt A, 54-60.

Pavlin, M., et al. 2016. The Chemistry of Neurodegeneration: Kinetic Data and Their Implications. *Mol Neurobiol,* 53(5), 3400-3415.

Pei, J. J. and Hugon, J. 2008. mTOR-dependent signalling in Alzheimer's disease. *J Cell Mol Med,* 12(6B), 2525-2532.

Pei, J. J., et al. 2003. Role of protein kinase B in Alzheimer's neurofibrillary pathology. *Acta Neuropathol,* 105(4), 381-392.

Peixoto, C. A., et al. 2017. AMPK activation: Role in the signaling pathways of neuroinflammation and neurodegeneration. *Exp Neurol,* 298(Pt A), 31-41.

Regitz, C., Dussling, L. M. and Wenzel, U. 2014. Amyloid-beta (Abeta (1)(-)(4)(2))-induced paralysis in Caenorhabditis elegans is inhibited by the polyphenol quercetin through activation of protein degradation pathways. *Mol Nutr Food Res,* 58(10), 1931-1940.

Ringman, J. M., et al. 2012. Oral curcumin for Alzheimer's disease: tolerability and efficacy in a 24-week randomized, double blind, placebo-controlled study. *Alzheimers Res Ther,* 4(5), 43.

Rohowetz, L. J., Kraus, J. G. and Koulen, P. 2018. Reactive Oxygen Species-Mediated Damage of Retinal Neurons: Drug Development Targets for Therapies of Chronic Neurodegeneration of the Retina. *Int J Mol Sci,* 19(11).

Singh, N., et al. 2014. Iron in neurodegenerative disorders of protein misfolding: a case of prion disorders and Parkinson's disease. *Antioxid Redox Signal,* 21(3), 471-484.

Smid, S. D., Maag, J. L. and Musgrave, I. F. 2012. Dietary polyphenol-derived protection against neurotoxic beta-amyloid protein: from molecular to clinical. *Food Funct,* 3(12), 1242-1250.

Smith, H. L. and Mallucci, G. R. 2016. The unfolded protein response: mechanisms and therapy of neurodegeneration. *Brain,* 139(Pt 8), 2113-2121.

Solayman, M., et al. 2017. Natural Products Combating Neuro-degeneration: Parkinson 's disease. *Curr Drug Metab,* 18(1), 50-61.

Solberg, N. O., et al. 2014. Optical and SPION-enhanced MR imaging shows that trans-stilbene inhibitors of NF-kappaB concomitantly lower Alzheimer's disease plaque formation and microglial activation in AbetaPP/PS-1 transgenic mouse brain. *J Alzheimers Dis,* 40(1), 191-212.

Sonoda, Y., et al. 2010. Accumulation of tumor-suppressor PTEN in Alzheimer neurofibrillary tangles. *Neurosci Lett,* 471(1), 20-24.

Sun, Y. X., et al. 2014. Differential activation of mTOR complex 1 signaling in human brain with mild to severe Alzheimer's disease. *J Alzheimers Dis,* 38(2), 437-444.

Tatton, N. A. 2000. Increased caspase 3 and Bax immunoreactivity accompany nuclear GAPDH translocation and neuronal apoptosis in Parkinson's disease. *Exp Neurol,* 166(1), 29-43.

Tatton, N. A., et al. 1998. A fluorescent double-labeling method to detect and confirm apoptotic nuclei in Parkinson's disease. *Ann Neurol,* 44(3 Suppl 1), S142-148.

Telenius, H., et al. 1994. Somatic and gonadal mosaicism of the Huntington disease gene CAG repeat in brain and sperm. *Nat Genet,* 6(4), 409-414.

Tompkins, M. M., et al. 1997. Apoptotic-like changes in Lewy-body-associated disorders and normal aging in substantia nigral neurons. *Am J Pathol,* 150(1), 119-131.

Tramutola, A., et al. 2015. Alteration of mTOR signaling occurs early in the progression of Alzheimer disease (AD): analysis of brain from subjects with pre-clinical AD, amnestic mild cognitive impairment and late-stage AD. *J Neurochem,* 133(5), 739-749.

Umeda, T., et al. 2016. Rifampicin is a candidate preventive medicine against amyloid-beta and tau oligomers. *Brain,* 139(Pt 5), 1568-1586.

Wei, W., et al. 2002. Abeta 17-42 in Alzheimer's disease activates JNK and caspase-8 leading to neuronal apoptosis. *Brain,* 125(Pt 9), 2036-2043.

Wexler, A., Wild, E. J. and Tabrizi, S. J. 2016. George Huntington: a legacy of inquiry, empathy and hope. *Brain,* 139(Pt 8), 2326-2333.

Wightman, E. L. 2017. Potential benefits of phytochemicals against Alzheimer's disease. *Proc Nutr Soc,* 76(2), 106-112.

Wild, E. J. and Tabrizi, S. J. 2017. Therapies targeting DNA and RNA in Huntington's disease. *Lancet Neurol,* 16(10), 837-847.

Wullner, U., et al. 1999. Cell death and apoptosis regulating proteins in Parkinson's disease--a cautionary note. *Acta Neuropathol,* 97(4), 408-412.

Xie, A., et al. 2014. Shared mechanisms ofneurodegeneration in Alzheimer's disease and Parkinson's disease. *Biomed Res Int,* 2014, 648740.

Xu, P. X., et al. 2014. Rutin improves spatial memory in Alzheimer's disease transgenic mice by reducing Abeta oligomer level and attenuating oxidative stress and neuroinflammation. *Behav Brain Res,* 264, 173-180.

Zecca, L., et al. 2004. Iron, brain ageing and neurodegenerative disorders. *Nat Rev Neurosci,* 5(11), 863-873.

Zhu, X., et al. 2013. Hopeahainol A attenuates memory deficits by targeting beta-amyloid in APP/PS1 transgenic mice. *Aging Cell,* 12(1), 85-92.

In: Current Challenges and Management … ISBN: 978-1-53617-304-8
Editor: Abhai Kumar

Chapter 10

ROLE OF DIET AND NUTRITION IN BRAIN HEALTH

Kanishka Singh**, *MD (AM)
Department of Home Science (Foods & Nutrition), Meerut College,
Chaudhary Charan Singh University, India

ABSTRACT

The role of nutrition and diet for human body has been in prime importance and very well-known since the time of human existence. As we age the need to have balanced well-planned diet and nutrition according to age increases, particularly during old age. In older ages lack of nutrients leads to neurotoxicity, oxidative stress, amyloid-beta toxicity, etc. and thus older people tend to be affected by impaired brain functioning and decreased cognition and learning leading to brain disorders and diseases like AD, PD, dementia, depression, anxiety, epilepsy, etc. Among all serotonin is one of the prime concern of studies for older population, as its level decreases with age and it is thought to be responsible for mood and behavioral responses, cannot cross BBB unlike tryptophan. Besides serotonin, another nutrient of study concerns is tyrosine as it has an important role in pain-relieving and works greatly

* Corresponding Author's Email: kanishkasingh2@gmail.com.

regulates stress and metabolism. And like serotonin its stores and levels also depletes as we ages. This chapter discusses about brain health, all major nutrients, their role in brain physiology and different types of diets to improve brain functioning and treating brain diseases in older population.

Keywords: nutrition, brain functioning, brain health, serotonin, tyrosine, omega-3 fatty acid, cholesterol, vitamin B12, DASH diet, MIND diet

1. INTRODUCTION

The major purpose of this chapter is to bring in light the role of foods, nutrition and diet in brain health and how geriatric nutrition is an important aspect of one's life. This chapter aims to guide the readers with different aspects of nutrition and applied physiology i.e., diseases and brain health in older people across the globe. This fact is well known from ages that the knowledge of food and its nutrition is highly important because what one chooses to eat & drink greatly influences the physical, mental and emotional nutritional status, overall health and quality of life. In the past, food was known and understood for its abilities in providing energy (carbohydrates & fats), and body building (proteins), but the upcoming researches around the globe and continuously bringing out more specific and molecular functions of food, and thus continuous remolding and development of the role of diet in brain health is taking place with the base of previously known facts and existing knowledge.

It is a known fact that the population is aging globally. Thc global population aged 60 years or over is numbered 962 million in 2017, which is more than twice as large as in 1980, worldwide, and it is expected to grow double again by 2050, and is projected to reach nearly 2.1 billion(UN, World Population Aging- Highlights 2017).

According to a recent UN report (2017), the greying of the population is much rapid in developing countries than in developed countries, with over two-third of the world's older population being contributed by the former itself.

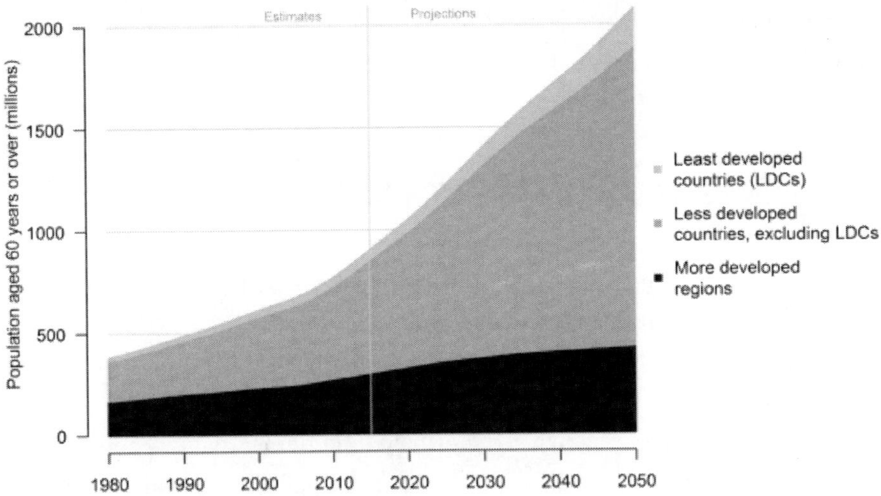

Data source: United Nations (2017), World Population Prospects-the 2017 revision.

Figure 1. Number of population aged 60 years and above.

The greying of the population worldwide, especially in developing regions, is because of many factors like economic growth, continuous enhancement and availability of affordable health and medical care, improved and enhanced control of diseases, improved lifestyles, better nutrition, improved water and sanitation facilities, increased number of small and nuclear families, increasing immigration rates, etc. All these factors have relatively reduced the size of the younger population in comparison to the older one. It was estimated in 2014, that the U.S. population of 65 years and above will be larger than the population under 18 years of age by 2056 (Colby and Ortman, 2014). The studies have shown that women live longer than men all-over the world. Another recent report throws up an interesting fact that "While the female advantage exists everywhere, the cross-country differences are large. In Russia, women live 10 years longer than men, while in Bhutan the difference is less than half a year" (ourworldindata.org). So on an average the life expectancy of women is more in comparison to men globally. The greying of the population has a socio-economic impact depending upon the proportion of that population which is healthy and able-bodied. This trend is now proliferating and the diseases that were once considered as the part of an old age package, like joint pain, ischemic stroke, Type 2 diabetes, COPD, osteoarthritis, etc. are now considered as lifestyle diseases and factors.

2. Ageing as a Science

- **Gerontology:** The word was coined by llya llyich Mechnikov in 1903. Gerontology is the scientific study of normal aging, including social, cultural, psychological, cognitive and biological aspects of aging.
- **Geriatrics:** Geriatrics or Geriatric medicine, is a specialty that focuses on the healthcare of the elderly people. Its main focus and objective is to promote health among older people by preventing and treating diseases, disorders and inabilities among them.

The changes that cause and influence ageing are complex. Let us focus on majorly two kinds of ageing-

- **Primary Ageing:** "It is a gradual and inevitable process of bodily deterioration that begins early in life and continues through the years, irrespective of what people do to stave it off."
- **Secondary Ageing:** "It consists of the results of disease, abuse and disabuse- factors that are often avoidable and within people's control." (Diane E. Papalia, Human Development)

3. Nutrition in Older Adults

For all individuals of all ages physical, mental and social health is very important, they are interrelated and forms the basic strand for life. Among these three mental health holds a very important and crucial place as the other two health are highly dependent on mental well-being When it comes to old age and, aging the aspect of nutrition in brain health or mental health becomes even more important as nutrition is one of the essential determining factors in the age of 60 years and above. The reason why some older adults experiences good physical and mental functioning in old age too, while some have a very weak and poor health and they need some or the other support to meet up their regular and basic requirements is because of the changes that are associated with ageing which are actually neither linear nor they are constant.

Besides the shifts in social roles and the needs to be in close relationships, etc. old age frequently involves biological changes and, changes in their nutritional and dietary requirements. Thus, in older adults, the role and importance of nutritional and dietary care is not merely confined to the therapeutic nutrition in any specialized condition or disease or any disorder, rather it has much broader spectrum and sense, and is also associated with great focus on healthy lifestyle and prevention of diseases and other disorders and illnesses during this age. Now-a-days all round the world older people in comparison of their age are more concerned with nutrition & dietary information and are also very willing to make changes and adopt healthier food behaviors for better, maintained and healthier lives with help and support in improving self-care.

3.1. As a Preventive Aspect of Treatment, Nutritional and Dietary Care is Majorly of Three Types

- **Primary Prevention**, in which health promotion and disease prevention are in the main focus areas of treatment mode and are combined with physical activities & balanced and healthy dietary behaviours.
- **Secondary Prevention,** in which reduction of health risk and deceleration of nutrition related chronic diseases to maintain the strength & mobility (i.e., functionality) & quality of life.
- **Tertiary Prevention,** in which the main concern is on the case-care management and discharge panning. This is due to the issues of chewing and digestive problems, modified diets and their follow ups and limitations in patient's functional abilities.

Krause's Food and the nutrition care process- L.K. Mahan & J.L. Raymond)

4. Brain

Brain is the command center for all the activities performed by the human body majorly. Human brain is the largest brain in relation to its body size among all the vertebrates. It weighs around 1300-1400 gm i.e., 3 pounds, and about 15 cms in length. Comparatively, men have 100gms larger brain than women in normal. In women, parts of frontal lobe & limbic cortex are bigger in comparison to men. These parts are associated with problem solving and regulations of emotions. While, in men parietal cortex and amygdala, and their areas are associated with perception of space and social & sexual behaviors. The size of the brain can be associated with some diseases like Alzheimer's disease, in which the patient's hippocampus (majorly in older adults) tends to be smaller, and it is associated with memory (www.verywellmind.com). Like the whole human body, human brain also ages, i.e., its size reduces due to shrinkage, speed slows down, it becomes lesser adaptable to changes. It thus becomes more vulnerable to diseases like Parkinson's due to increased susceptibility to oxidative changes. An individual's lifestyle plays a major role in defining the brain health, and it can be well done during young age so that in late adulthood good sharp memory and good brain health can be achieved and maintained. Though good nutrition and balanced diet is important in all ages, but due to lot many factors in later adulthood geriatric nutrition becomes highly important.

5. Brain Health

According to latest WHO report mental health problems are one of the leading cause of poor health and disorders all over the world, it is because every individual experiences mental health issues in some or the other stage of their lives. Approximately 450 million people worldwide are currently suffering from poor brain and mental health, which makes one in four people to suffer from one or the other mental/neurological issues (www.who.int). It becomes very essential to understand and make the difference in decline in brain health which is related with age and impairment due to special conditions like dementia in brain health. On an average, it can be seen that there is a decline of 5-10% in human brain weight between 20 to 90 years of ages (Galvin JE, Sadowsky, 2012). Thus, mental or brain health issues are also often related to behavioral problems and disorders like inattention, hyperactivity, impulsivity, criminal activity, drug abuse, defiant behavior, ADHD, ODD, conduct disorder, etc. There are several factors which affects the brain health includes genetic factor, stress, nutrition and diet, physical activity level, drugs and other factors associated with environment (So Young Lim et al., 2016). Among all these above factors nutritional and dietary factor plays an important role as it ameliorate the signs, symptoms and progression of mental diseases and disorders to much extent.

6. Nutrition in Brain Health

Human brain is highly metabolically active organ and consumes approx. 20% of total calories per day required by the body which accounts about 400-500 calories/day for a man and 350-400 calories/day for a woman. The soul fuel for brain is the glucose, and human brain consumes approx. 120gm glucose/day. This is similar to an energy input of approx. 420 Kcal which makes approx. 60% of the total glucose utilization by the whole body at the resting stage. This is mainly because the human brain has to synthesize neurotransmitters and their receptors for impulse transmissions, for which brain needs to maintain the Na^+-K^+ membrane potential pump to transmit impulses. As fatty acids are bound to albumin protein in the plasma and are unable to cross Blood Brain Barrier (BBB) they are unable to give energy and serve as fuel to human brain. However during the condition such as starvation the ketone bodies which are produced by the liver acts as fuel to some extent for the brain (Biochemistry- Jeremy M. Berg et al.).

Brain health is closely related to heart health, thus the foods which are good for heart heath are good for brain health too, as heart patients often experiences mental health problems in later life. There are five basic nutrients required by the human body i.e., carbohydrates, proteins, fats, vitamins and minerals. Among all the nutrients we eat in our diets, the nutrients which plays major roles in brain health and have highly beneficial effects on brain health includes- Omega-3 fatty acids, phospholipids, folate, niacin, cholesterol, vitamin B6, vitamin B12 and vitamin D. While on the contrary, those which have highly negative & detoriating brain health effects includes- saturated fats, trans fats (found in partially hydrogenated oils), simple sugars, processed foods, excess salt consumption, refined grain flours, and alcohol consumption. Different foods are linked with our behavior from centuries, and it is a well-known fact that different foods have their effects on the behavior and cognitive performance of human brain. Cognition or thinking is the prime brain functioning on which diet and nutrition has its greatest effects. Infancy to early childhood are the stages when neural connectivity is greatest and thus it is considered as the neural developmental stage too. The direct effects of diet and nutrition on individual's cognition can thus be seen during neural developmental stage and then again during the latter adulthood i.e., during ageing.

During ageing various mental health issues can be observed and experienced, among which some common neurological and neurodegenerative diseases (NDD) are- depression, schizophrenia, epilepsy, dementia, Alzheimer's disease, Parkinsonism, bipolar disorders or manic depressive disorder, anxiety disorders, obsessive compulsive disorder, eating disorders, etc. They basically starts as during ageing the breakdown of synapse and atrophy of brain (shrinkage) takes place. The lack of nutrients develops neurotoxicity as the brain ages. Poor or under nutrition of brain leads to neural degeneration and results in death of neurons in an uncontrolled manner, mitochondrial dysfunction, oxidative stress and amyloid-beta toxicity (www.myvmc.com). So the dietary and nutritional factors affect brain functioning processes ranging from regulation of pathways of neurotransmitters, to fluidity of membrane, synaptic transmissions, and signal transduction pathways.

Here we will discuss about some important nutrients that play an important role in brain health of older population, both in terms of promoting good brain health and as well as those that have their negative brain health impacts.

Nutrients that are beneficial and promote brain health are discussed below:-

6.1. Lipids

Human brain is composed of 60% of fat. Thus proper and right fats are essential to develop and maintain cell membrane of the brain. The neuroplasticity depends on the health of the neuron and which ultimate is dependent on the amount of right fat consumed. (Rewire your brain). The lipids are of three types simple, compound and derived. Among them compound lipids are further sub-classified as phospholipids, glycolipids and lipoproteins, while derived lipids are sub-classified into fatty acids and cholesterol.

Out of the several forms of lipids which are consumed in the dietary form, PUFA (Poly Unsaturated Fatty Acids) (omega 3, omega 6) and cholesterol plays the major role in neural activities. The omega 3 which is considered as the most important neural nutritional component is of three types- ALA (Alpha-linolenic acid), EPA (eicosapentaenoic acid) and DHA (docosahexaenoic acid). While omega 6 fatty acids are mainly of following types- LA (linoleic acid), gamma-linoleic acid and ARA (arachidonic acid), among which linolenic acid and ARA are considered as most important. LA and ALA actually compete for same desaturation enzymes and elongation thus more dietary LA leads to lesser conversion of ALA into long chain omega 3 PUFA. Long chain PUFA are closely linked and associated with the development and functioning of serotonergic, dopaminergic and noradrenergic like pathways i.e., monoaminergic systems. ALA and LA are the essential fatty acids and among which ALA can be further converted into EPA and DHA, which takes place primarily in liver, in very lesser quantities, due to which there arises the need to intake them from the dietary sources.

Fatty acids which are most abundant and, accounting for approx. $1/5^{th}$ of the brain's dry weight are DHA (20%) and ARA (15%) (Bentsen, Havard. 2017). In comparison to other body tissues, the brain tissues (synaptic membrane) has higher concentration of DHA. The concentration of DHA varies with diet and as an individual ages this concentration lowers down. The major omega 3 fatty acid for brain is DHA alone which accounts about 10-15% of the total fatty acids. The women have higher biosynthesis efficiency of EPA and DHA in comparison to men. (Dietary lipids for healthy brain functioning, Claude Leray). The dosage of adequate intake (AI) for DHA can vary according to the condition and may normally ranges from 0.5 gm/day – 1 gm/day in older adults. The AI for ALA in older adults is 1.6gm/day (men) and 1.1gm/day (women), while AI of LA ranges from 14gm/day (men) and 11gm/day (women) (lpi.oregonstate.edu).

Table 1. Adequate intake of nutrient dosage issued by different organizations/institutes

Organizations/ Institutes	Nutrient + Dosage
EFSA	LA (4% of total energy), ALA (0.5% of total energy), EPA + DHA (250mg/day)
WHO	omega 6 FA (6-11% of energy), omega 3 FA (0.5-2% of energy), EPA + DHA (0.250-2 gm/day)
ISSFAL	LA (2% of energy), ALA (0.7% of energy), EPA + DHA (500 mg/day)
AHA	EPA + DHA, for people without documented CHD (500 mg/day), with documented CHD (1gm/day), who need to lower serum triglycerides (2-4gm/day)

Date source: lpi.oregonstate.edu

EFSA: European Food Safety Authority

WHO: World Health Organization

ISSFAL: The International Society for the study of Fatty Acids and Lipids

AHA: American Heart Association

Studies have shown that with the long term dietary interventions and modifications the brain's lipid concentration can be changed or altered which directly affects and influences the mood and emotional behaviour of an individual. The deficiency of lipids, particularly omega 3 fatty acids, leads to the induction of depression and anxiety in an individual. Thus general enhancement in the dietary lipids (mainly omega 3) acts as an antidepressant. It is also found in several researches worldwide that omega 3 prevents memory loss and greatly helps in treating dementia in older adults, and also has a great link between AD (Alzheimer's disease) and omega 3 in the diet. It is due to ageing that older population suffering from AD have lower omega 3 levels in brain. Increased dietary omega 3 levels decreases the stroke incidences that are associated with increased AD, and also prevents cognitive decline in AD patients (Hooper, C. et al., 2018). Cholesterol being one of the major nutrient in brain plays a major role in neural development and activities with sphingolipids, particularly in myelin form. Human brain is said to be the most cholesterol-rich organ, and contains about 25% of the total body's cholesterol. The major process which derives cholesterol in the body is de-nova synthesis.

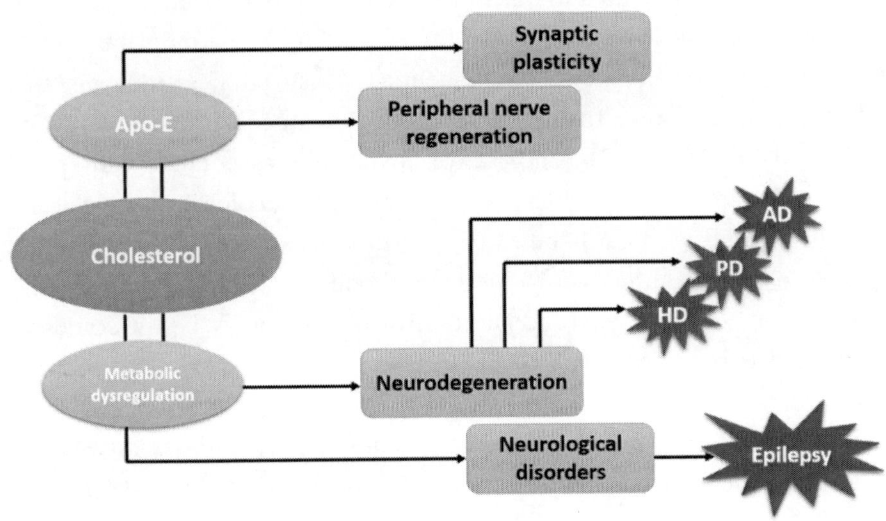

Figure 2. Role of cholesterol in brain health and its disorders.

The deficiency of cholesterol in the brain leads to diseases like AD and PD (Parkinsonism disease). As many pathways are regulated by the cholesterol it plays major role in brain health and thus also in nerve regeneration. It plays an important nutritional role in PNI (peripheral nerve injury) as it has a crucial role in nerve regeneration in both, CNS and PNS. Neural cell death is caused by increased high levels of cholesterol in membrane leading to Aβ (β-amyloid) incorporation in membrane and enhancement of cytosolic calcium levels. High dietary cholesterol levels enhances Aβ peptide levels (which starts neurodegeneration and synaptic dysfunction). Low LDL cholesterol dietary levels are said to regulate AD. In PD, which is another leading NDD in older people, α-synuclein accumulation and lewy bodies formation, and their main pathological characteristics are highly stimulated by high lipid levels. Thus, high cholesterol and oxysterol levels can be said to be the main contributors in AD and PD. Studies have also shown the links of reduced LDL cholesterol with increased epilepsy risks, as 3-hydroxy-3-methylglutarly-CoA reductase and proprote in convertase subtilisin kexin 9 genes cause mutation leading to deficiency of LDL cholesterol. However, there is unavailability of much data in this reference (Hussain, Ghulam et al. 2019).

In dementia, however, there are mixed findings regarding the role of cholesterol in development of dementia. Most studies indicate that cholesterol plays a protective role in cognitive decline. It is also revealed in researches that high LDL cholesterol levels are associated with good cognitive health among older adults. As high cholesterol levels are invariably linked with cardiac health, so it becomes important to maintain good cholesterol health during young adulthood too. Simply stated, during young age one should keep the cholesterol levels low. When it comes to linkage between omega 3 and dementia, there is evidence of consumption of omega 3 has a positive role in improving dementia. Dietary interventions of omega 3 in the early stages of dementia improves the condition while in later stages it is not founf effective. (www.alzheimer s.org.uk)

6.2. Proteins

Proteins is the building block of human body. As we age the body's protein stores starts depleting leading to increased requirement for protein in older ages. After lipids, proteins plays the major role in neural health and are essential for the cognitive development and health of elderly. Proteins plays a significant role in maintaining the heart-and-brain balance. The pronouncing role of dietary protein in brain's health is that they are essential for the production of signaling chemicals like serotonin, which are the chemical messengers and transmit signals/impulses for neural communication. Among CNS and PNS, the AA (amino acids) such as tryptophan, tyrosine, histadine and arginine are essentially required, mainly by CNS, for the production and synthesis of neuromodulators and neurotransmitters (Davin Wahl et al. 2016).Tryptophan is responsible for alertness, depression levels and pain sensitivity in human body. It has been found that tryptophan decreases the pain sensitivity (Lieberman, Harris R. 1999).

Among all, serotonin is one of the prime concern of studies for older population, as its level decreases with age and it is thought to be responsible for mood and behavioral responses, can not cross blood brain barrier like tryptophan. Tryptophan, which is an amino acid and a precursor of serotonin, can easily pass across the barrier through specialized channels. After passing through the barrier this tryptophan gets transformed into 5-HTP (5- hydroxyl-tryptophan) which further gets converted to serotonin leading to the fulfilment of serotonin requirements. The deficiency of serotonin may lead to detrimental decline in the cognitive function in elderly population (Davin Wahl et al. 2016). The dietary protein: carbohydrate ratio has been found significantly affecting the brain's serotonin levels. In this regard, as the carbohydrate increases in comparison to protein, the brain's serotonin levels also increases. Increase in the dietary protein decreases the serotonin levels, and increase in carbohydrate increases the serotonin levels in hypothalamus & cortex, and hypothalamus plays an important role in appetite regulation.

Table 2. Different amino acids in brain, their neurotransmitters/ neuromodulators and their functions in body

Amino Acids	Their neurotransmitters/ Neuromodulators	Neurotransmitter/ neuromodulator function
Tryptophan	Serotonin and Melatonin*	Mood, Pain, Food intake & Arousal
Tyrosine/Phenylalanine	Dopamine	Motor function, Mood, Arousal
	Norepinephrine	Arousal, Attention, Anxiety
	Epinephrine/Adrenaline	Stress regulation, cardiac output (↑es) and BP regulation (↑es), blood glucose regulation (↑es), regulation of circulating free fatty acids (↑es)
Histidine	Histamine	Food intake, Arousal, Thermo-regulation
Arginine	Nitric Oxide (NO)	Arousal, Anxiety, Memory
Threonine	Glycine	Motor function

* Melatonin is secreted by pineal gland is not considered to be a NT (neurotransmitter), but behaviorally is an active tryptophan metabolite.

In protein food, in comparison to tryptophan, tyrosine is found in larger quantities. Besides serotonin, another nutrient of study concern is tyrosine, as it has an important role in pain relieving and works greatly in regulating stress and metabolism. Its requirement increases with ageing while its storage and levels depletes as we ages. (Lieberman, Harris R. 1999). In recent study by Catharine Paddock in Medical News Today on November 8, 2018, it was found that, "Netrin which is a protein seems to play an important role in neural connectivity in brain of an embryo and infant, is now also found strengthening neural synaptic connections in the hippocampus of an adult brain. Thus it can be said that netrin plays the strengthening role learning and memory development in adulthood, as hippocampus is concerned with these two aspects" (www.medicaln ewstoday.com). Though much studies have not been done on elderly population revealing the role of protein in cognitive function in older people, but it has been observed that low dietary protein shows lower verbal memory in late adulthood, whereas high dietary protein is linked with increased non-verbal learning, verbal memory and decreased dementia risk (Moore, Katie et al., 2018). According to Judith Graham in the recently published article in Kaiser Health News on January 17, 2019,

"In most place the most cited standard RDA of protein for elderly is 0.8 gm proteins/kg body weight/day. But in 2013 physicians and many nutrition experts suggested the new RDA of protein for elderly that is 1-1.2 gm protein/kg body weight/day, and this RDA was also accepted by the European Society of Clinical Nutrition and Metabolism." (www.khn.org).

6.3. Carbohydrate

Carbohydrates are the main sources of energy for the body to perform any activity by the body. As stated earlier, of all the organs the human brain consumes the largest part of the total body glucose for energy in performing its activities. The link between carbohydrates and cognitive function in older adults is still quite unclear as much studies are not been done in this regards. We consume two forms of carbohydrates in our daily routine i.e., simple carbohydrates and complex carbohydrates. It has been shown that high dietary carbohydrates and sugars gives rise to MCI (mild cognitive impairment) and dementia in the later life of individuals and are also linked with increased depression risks in older adults (Moore, Katie et al., 2018). It is a well stated fact that dietary carbohydrate levels sparks the insulin levels which cause the rise in the blood glucose levels. The increased insulin levels helps more tryptophan to cross BBB and thus affects the neurotransmitters levels such as for serotonin. (www.dietiti ans.ca). In a published report by Christian Benedict in Eurek Alert-The global source for science news on Feb. 1, 2012, "The insulin level in the brain is found to enhance the memory in humans, but the capacity of insulin to metabolize glucose in the body decreases with ageing. Thus it greatly affects the cognition in elderly population. It was also stated that in a research done in Uppsala University recently, it was found that insulin resistance is linked with smaller size of brain and language skills degradation in older people."

The decline in central insulin concentration and insulin receptor binding ability are linked to decreased central concentration of insulin, which causes degradation of glucose homeostasis in brain. Low insulin receptor activity leads to AD and type 2 diabetes is greatly linked with high increased risk in developing AD. (Baranowska-Bik, Agnieszka and Bik, Wojciech 2017).Obesity and type-2 diabetes are strongly linked with the decline of memory and cognition in ageing individuals, and AD is also referred as "Type-3 diabetes" in reference to older population because to its linkage with insulin resistance and ageing. As the glucose metabolism in older people gets affected so, short-term high levels of glucose can be proved with detrimental effects in them in the longer term. Thus, in older age, carbohydrates which are simple and refined must be avoided, as they provide quick calories for short period, rather they must be replaced with complex dietary carbohydrates. The complex carbohydrates are slower with digestibility in older people and gives lesser calories in comparison to simple carbohydrates in a given period of time. However, they provide more stable supply levels of energy to the body in elderly populance which is far more vital for them, than the higher levels for shorter periods at that stage of age for an individual.

6.4. Vitamins

Vitamins are the essential micro-nutrients required by the human body to perform many metabolic function. As macronutrients, vitamins also play a major role in maintaining the brain health as we age. Vitamins are the organic compounds and are of two types i.e., water soluble and fat soluble. Like amino acids in protein, vitamins also play an important role in the production and activities of neurotransmitters. Human body is not capable of producing most of the vitamins, except vitamin D. Thus, in regards to vitamins it becomes essential to source them from the dietary sources. Vitamins also provide energy to the body, though not themselves directly, but acting as energy source. They support the body by metabolizing energy sources like fats and carbohydrates and utilize their energy efficiently. The oxidative stress during ageing is found to be a major factor for NDD and depression. (Moore, Katie et al., 2018). Among all the vitamins required by the body, vitamin B1 (thiamine), B3 (niacin), B6 (pyridoxine), B9 (folate/folic acid), B12 (cobalamin), C, D, E are highly important for the healthy functioning of the brain in elderly people.

Let us discuss each of the above mentioned vitamins and their functioning in brain health in brief:-

6.4.1. Vitamin B1 (Thiamine)

This sulphur containing vitamin plays its role in energy metabolism by converting carbohydrates, proteins and fats to energy sources in the body. Thiamine plays an important role in brain glucose metabolism. This water soluble vitamin also plays a key role in nerve signaling in the brain functioning. Its deficiency may lead to PD and AD in older adults.

6.4.2. Vitamin B3 (Niacin)

Niacin too is a water soluble vitamin but unlike thiamine, it does not get stored in human body. Niacin is a potent antioxidant for brain. It primarily works in decreasing LDL-C and increasing HDL-C thus preventing heart diseases and, boosting brain health. In the glucose and fat metabolism, niacin acts as a coenzyme for energy-transfer. It prevents neuro degeneration and protects the brain functioning. Niacin deficiency is associated with confusion, memory loss, depression and dementia in older adults. In a published article by UHN Staff iUHN Daily on December 7, 2017, "Dietary niacin prevents AD and age related cognitive decline. It supports in nerve cell growth and acts as an antioxidant for the brain." As stated by Nordqvist Christian in Medical News Today on February 21, 2019, "On one hand niacin is essential for brain health, while on the other hand, its excess reduces glucose tolerance and insulin resistance which can badly affect brain health in older people". According to the NIH (National Institutes of Health) the daily recommended dietary allowance of niacin is 16mg/day for all individuals above 4 years of age".

6.4.3. Vitamin B6 (Pyridoxine)

"According to a publication by Lizzie Streit in Health line on October 1, 2018. This water soluble vitamin plays a big role in mood regulation. Pyridoxine is found to be helpful in the production of serotonin, dopamine and GABA. It is also associated strongly with decreasing blood homocysteine levels. Thus it has a great role in preventing depression and many psychiatric health problems. As during older age blood vitamin levels decrease, it was found that the decreased pyridoxine levels doubled the tendency of depression in older adults. Although the researches are controversial, but pyridoxine has also been found to prevent AD and memory impairment, as it declines the circulating homocysteine levels. The excess of this vitamin i.e., over 100mg/day, can cause nerve damage, pain or even numbness in hands/feet."

6.4.4. Vitamin B9 (Folic Acid/Folate)

Folic acid is the more stable form of folate and is another water soluble vitamin. It mainly functions as coenzyme, and in energy and amino acid metabolisms. This vitamin is essential for brain development and functioning and works in combination with cobalamin i.e., vitamin B12. Long term deficiency of this vitamin leads to brain degeneration. Folic acid plays a huge role in brain health. It acts as coenzyme for the conversion of tryptophan to serotonin and tyrosine to epinephrine and norepinephrine. It also slows down the annihilation of brain's tryptophan therefore enhancing the serotonin function. Folic acid is significantly involved in energy metabolism executing high energy metabolism through formation of high energy compounds. Folate is also found to be involved in the synthesis of an excitatory neurotransmitter i.e., dopamine (www.dietitians.ca). Its deficiency is likely to cause depression, schizophrenia, dementia, AD. Excess levels of folate may mask the deficiency of vitamin B12 and may deteriorate the condition of anemia and cognition in older individuals (Watson, Jessica et al. 2017). The RDA for folate is 400 mcg DFE for both men and women (www.ods.od.nih.gov).

6.4.5. Vitamin B12 (Cobalamin)

Vitamin B12 level in the body is of high concern area in most of the researches related to role of vitamins in brain health. Besides being involved in the metabolism of all cells in the body it is also closely associated with the energy production. Cobalamin plays a major role myelin synthesis, and is thus greatly involved in the nerve impulse conduction. It is also found to have a role in monoamine neurotransmitters synthesis. In a Havard Health blog posted by Patrick J. Skerrett on January 10, 2013, it was acknowledged that "Vitamin B12 deficiency causes severe depression, paranoia, delusions, loss of memory, etc. The neuro-cognitive development and health in elderly is greatly affected by vitamin B12 and folic acid, cognitive degradation and increased homocysteine levels are caused by their deficiencies in elderly (www.dietitians.ca). Declined levels of cobalamin are found to causes mental slowness, confusion, psychosis, stammering, weak limbs and depression (Rewire your Brain, John B. Adren, 2010). Individuals who are vegan in their dietary habits are more prone to cobalamin deficiencies because almost all sources are andiet diets in one or the other way. In a publication by Deane Alban in Be brain Fit on February 7, 2019, it was revealed that "Vitamin B12 deficiency is closely linked with depression, social withdrawal, emotional inexpressiveness, psychiatric disorders, dementia, AD, loss of appetite, brain fog, decline in memory, focus and concentration, anxiety, disorientation, hallucination, schizophrenia, neuropathy, brain damage, and brain atrophy."

6.4.6. Vitamin C (Citric Acid)

Vitamin C is a known highly potent antioxidant and works with B vitamins as cofactors. High levels of vitamin C are found in brain. It works as a primary antioxidant and also plays a role of free radical scavenger (Rewire your Brain, John B. Adren, 2010). Vitamin C is also known for producing neurotransmitter norepinephrine which acts as a vasoconstrictor and aids during stress (Roth, Ruth A., Nutrition and Diet Therapy 2011). "In a published report by Anna Bolton O'Byrne in Natural Calm on June 16, 2018, it was mentioned that vitamin C is one of the primary ingredients of calm balance as it plays roles in preventing anxiety, depression, and declined memory. It reduces oxidative stress in elderly. It also acts as a neuroprotective nutrient and plays role in myelin production and development of nerve cells. According to Canada Health the RDA for vitamin C is 60-90mg/day is recommended and 2000mg/day as its upper dietary limit". Notwithstanding this, much of the role played by vitamin C in brain functioning in and more studies are the elderly is still unclear.

6.4.7. Vitamin D (Cholecaliferol)

It is the only vitamin that is present in the body in liver as calcidiol and in kidneys as calcitriol. In studies, low serum vitamin D levels are seen associated with AD, dementia, depression and worsening cognition. On the other hand, the higher vitamin D levels are associated with greater brain volumes (Moore, Katie et al., 2018). According to Food and Nutrition Board in The National Academies the RDA's for vitamin D are 600 IU/15 mcg (for 51-70 years male and female) and 800 IU/20 mcg (for > 70 years male and female) (www.ods.od.nih.gov).

6.4.8. Vitamin E

It is a potent antioxidant and is a fat soluble vitamin. It acts as a protective agent for the damage caused by free radicals during ageing. Vitamin E decreases amyloid-beta deposition, reactive oxygen and NO synthesis leading to the prevention of AD and impairment in cognition (So Young Lim et al., 2016). It boosts the immune power in older people and gives protection from many NDDs. In a published report by Cathleen Crichton –Stuart in Medical News Today on May 14, 2018, it was revealed that, "Difficulty in coordination and the muscle weakness caused due to vitamin E deficiencies are the neurological symptoms of central and peripheral degeneration in older adults." Much role of vitamin E in brain health of elderly population, however, is still unclear.

6.5. Minerals

Unlike macronutrients and vitamins, minerals also play a significant role in the brain's health and maintenance. There are several minerals like copper, magnesium, zinc, cobalt, iron, selenium manganese, calcium, phosphorus, potassium, iodine, etc. that play major roles in the metabolism of the human body at different stages of age. But when we start ageing or are in old age, a few specific minerals amongst them play highly influential roles in brain health. There are two kinds of charges according to which minerals are classified i.e., cations (+ve ions) and anions (-ve ions). They acts as electrolytes, and are important in the nerve impulse conduction.

Minerals important for brain health are discussed below:-

6.5.1. Calcium

During ageing, cognitive functions gets significantly affected by the age related decline in the neuro-glial networks of the pre-frontal cortex region of the brain, and the interruption in the glial Ca^{2+} signaling has been associated with declined cognitive function (Sonia Guerra-Gomes et al., 2018). The dysregulation of calcium levels may cause and give rise to detrimental crosstalk in between Fe-Ca finally leading to neural dysfunction and death (Marco Tulio Nunez and Cecilia Hidalgo, 2019). In a published report by Lana Barhum in Medical News Today on May 21, 2018, "The calcium deficiency has no early symptoms, but its deficiency is linked with depression and mood disorders." Elderly people are much prone to calcium loss and its deficiencies thus calcium balance during old age becomes more critical.

6.5.2. Zinc

Zinc is the most abundant intracellular micronutrient, and more than 95% of body zinc being intracellular. Brain contains high levels of zinc in it. Studies showed the association of decreased plasma zinc levels with ageing. The decline in zinc level cause impairment in zinc homeostasis and neurological malfunctioning. Like calcium, zinc has also been found to act as secondary messenger and its increase is likely to result in AD. During ageing the deficiency of zinc is common. It plays an important role in enzymatic and mitochondrial function, cognition and memory loss (Lester Packer et al., 2010). Zinc also plays an important role in reducing oxidative stress and in synthesis, control and release of insulin in the body, thereby affecting the neurological function. Deficiency of zinc is associated with memory loss and mental lethargy. Vegetarian diet are found to be low in zinc in comparison to non-vegetarian diets, thus vegans are more prone to zinc deficiencies and thus require to supplement zinc by other modes.

Body pool of an individual greatly affects the zinc status/level of absorption in the body (similarly to iron). In individuals who are zinc deficient their gut absorbs zinc more readily and efficiently than others. Zinc is absorbed through the small intestine. Proximal intestinal portion is efficient, but the net absorption is done by distal intestinal part. Phytate rich foods support zinc reabsorption through faces, and zinc absorption is also enhanced by dietary proteins. On the other hand, high dietary intakes of Ca, P and Fe hinders and declines zinc absorption in the body. Adequate intake of zinc for adult men (19 years and above) is 11mg and for women (19 years and above) is 8 mg, while the corresponding tolerable upper intake levels is 40 mg for both categories (19 years and above) (ods.od.nih.gov/factsheets/Zinc-HealthProfessional/).

6.5.3. Iron

Iron is the most abundant element on earth and for human body it is essentially required for many physiological activities. In human body iron is found majorly in two forms with protein- one is hemoglobin (haem + globin) in blood and the other is myoglobin (myo + globin) found in muscles. Both both these forms of protein are oxygen-carrying in nature. The bioavailability of iron greatly dependent on the effective electron transfer properties of iron. Thus in many oxidation-reduction reactions in the body iron acts as the co-factor and thus has a role in energy metabolism of the body. Besides electron transport, iron is important for neurotransmitter synthesis and myelin production.

The iron requirements keeps on varying and when the iron stores in the body reaches their maximum levels, further iron absorption in the body declines, while iron absorption peaks to its highest level. Iron absorption is influenced by many factors like- food composition, meal composition, solubility level of the form of dietary iron, intake of vitamin C and animal protein (it increases Fe absorption), phytate, phenols, vegetable protein and calcium (they decreases Fe absorption). According to US Food and Nutrition Board, 2001, the RDA's for iron for adult man is 8 mg (19 years and above) and for woman 18-8 mg (19-50 years, and 51 years and above respectively). During older ages, iron intake is of greater concern because of many reasons. When it comes to brain health in later adulthood, iron plays an important role in anemia, AD, PD, multiple sclerosis, neuroferritinopathy and Friedrich's Ataxia (FA) (Stankiewicz, James et al.). During ageing, the iron gets accumulated in different regions of brain which causes impairment of cognitive function and behaviour. The abnormal metabolism of iron by fenton reaction develops hydroxyl radicals which targets oxidative stress reactions, spoils cellular lipids, protein, structure and functioning of DNA, finally leading to cell death (Jun-Lin Liu et al.).

6.5.4. Magnesium

Magnesium is the fourth most abundant mineral in human body that acts as a co-enzyme in many body processes. It is involved in energy conversion, protein formation, gene maintenance, muscle contraction and relaxation and neural regulation through neurotransmitters. It has a great influential role in improving brain plasticity which greatly improves learning, memory and cognitive abilities in older adults. Magnesium also greatly influences mood changes, and its deficiency is often linked with increased risks of depression, NDD, AD, etc. in older population. Comparatively, older individuals tends to consume lesser magnesium than younger ones, thus, besides dietary intake they need magnesium supplements to meet their daily requirements. No single supplement contains complete DV (Daily Value) of magnesium. So for elderly, it is much required to balance their consumption of magnesium rich foods with its supplements in regular diet. According to "The Food and Nutrition Board of the Institute of Medicine" for older adults (> 50yrs.) adequate intake of magnesium is 3.4gm/day (Adequate Intake) for men and 2.6gm/day (Adequate Intake) for women (lpi.oregonstate.edu).

6.5.5. Sodium

Sodium plays an important role in brain cell signaling. Low sodium level is a major concern in older adults as it is closely associated with hypertension and CVD, which ultimately is associated with cognitive functioning. Low dietary sodium considerably affects the homeostasis maintain ability of an individual and this in turn leads to changes in cognitive functions (Rush, M Toni et al., 2017). In a blog entry by Takahashi, Y. Paul in Mayo Clinic on July 15, 2017, "Hyponatremia (Low blood sodium levels) lead to altered personality, lethargy, confusion, and in severe case can also leads to seizures, coma and can also cause death." Both high and low sodium levels, both, are associated with cognitive decline in elderly. According to WHO 5gm/day salt is the RDA for adults. According to Institute of Medicine's Foods and Nutrition Board 1.3gms Na/day for people of 51-70 years and 1.2gmNa/day for 70+ years of age is recommended.

7. Diet in Brain Health

Diet plays a very important role in developing brain and maintaining brain health. Many researches across the globe have shown that imbalanced, poor or deficient diet (any nutrient in particular) greatly affects the memory and learning in an individual. Healthy diet prevents and reduces the risk of many diseases like depression, AD, PD, PTSD, epilepsy, anxiety, memory loss, declined learning ability, etc. There are different kind of diets which are proven to have great impact on brain health, like- Mediterranean diet, DASH diet and MIND (Mediterranean-DASH Intervention for Neurodegenerative Delay) diet. It is a well-established fact that the contemporary and typical western diet is unhealthy for brain's health as it is high in sugar, salt, excessive calories and carbohydrates. Single kind of food and diet does not work for maintaining good brain health thus there must be the combination of nutrients and food combinations in order to maintain health. Many studies have also claimed that plant based diet is a proven way to enhance and maintain good brain health (Global Council on Brain Health).

7.1. Mediterranean Diet

Mediterranean diet is a traditional diet of the Mediterranean countries. It is also known as an anti-inflammatory diet. This diet focuses on fruits, vegetables, nuts, olive oil, whole grains, steamed and grilled non-veg food items like chicken and sea food, herbs, legumes, dairy products (low fat) and moderate amount of wine. It additionally restricts red meat and sweets consumption. Mediterranean diet has been proven to aid in brain health. It is associated with larger brain volumes and enhanced memory and cognitive function. It is also known to play a high influential role in treating depression, AD, mild cognitive impairment, dementia and other neurological diseases.

Here is a list of food items that are included in mediterranean diet:-

- ***Vegetables and Greens***- Tomato, Onion, Pepper, Eggplant, Cucumber, Green beans, Okra, Zucchini, Garlic, Peas, Potato, Mushrooms, Cauliflower, Broccoli, Carrot, Celery leaves, Spinach, Beets, Cabbage, Romaine Lettuce, Chicory, Dandelion, Beet greens, Amaranth (focus on locally grown and season vegetables).
- ***Dairy products***- Milk, Yogurt, Fresh cheese, fresh mozzarella, Parmesan and other full- fat dairy items (less processessed).
- ***Fats & Oils***- Olive oil (Extra virgin), Almonds, Nuts, Pine nuts, Pistachios, Sesame seeds, Avocado oil, Cashew nut, pumpkin seeds, Sunflower seeds, Hazelnuts, Walnuts, Raisins, etc.
- ***Pulses & Beans***- Lentils, Chickpeas, White beans, Yellow split peas.
- ***Meat, Poultry & Sea foods***-Chicken, Duck, Turkey, Ground beef, Pork, Shrimp, Cod, Anchovies (fresh/canned form), Sardines (fresh/canned form), Tuna, Mackerel, Oysters, Crab, Mussels, Octopus, Red meat can be consumed once in a week in smaller amounts.

- ***Fruits***- Watermelon, Oranges, Tangerines, Lemons, Apples, Pears, Cherries, Cantaloupe, Peaches, Apricots, and Figs (Consume more locally available seasonal citrus fruits)
- ***Breads and Grains***- Whole grain breads/chapaties/tortillas, Buckwheat, Brown rice, Whole oats, Rye, Barley, Paximadi (Barley husk), Pita bread, Pasta, Rice, Egg pasta, Couscous, etc.
- ***Herbs and Spices***- Cumin, Oregano, Parsley, Mint, Basil, Dill, All spice, Cinnamon, Pepper, Sea salt, Thyme, Sage, Mountain tea, Chamomile, Nutmeg, Garlic, etc.
- ***Beverages***- Water (drink as much as u can), red wine (moderate amounts), Tea and Coffee

7.1.1. Do Not Eat Foods

Refined oils, added sugars, sugar sweetened beverages, processed meats, grains, highly preserved and processed foods. Always try to choose the least processed and low preservative option for your diet on a regular basis.

7.2. DASH Diet

DASH diet is a Dietary Approach to Stop Hypertension (DASH). This diet is basically formulated to prevent and fight against hypertension and heart diseases. This diet is prescribed for brain health as hypertension is closely related to the risks of mental health issues like strokes. In Cognitive Vitality, a report written by Yoko Hara on January, 30, 2019 it was mentioned that, "Researches done on DASH diet combined with aerobic exercises had been seem to be proven to have high improvements in cognitive function." "Many researches have proven that high BP increases the risk of AD and dementia for about 50% in older adults of age 60 years or more. Moreover overweight and obesity is directly linked with high BP and poor cardiac health, which is further in turn associated with decreased mental health. Similar to Mediterranean diet, DASH diet also emphasizes on fruits, beans, vegetables, whole grain, fish, poultry, lean meats, and low-fat dairy products. DASH diet involves potassium rich foods and restricts sodium rich foods, preserved foods, added sugars, fatty and red meats, full fat dairy products, and oils like coconut and palm oil (tropical region oils). In DASH diet it is recommended to have 4-5 servings of vegetables, 4-5 servings of fruits, 7-8 servings of whole grains, 2 servings or less of lean meat, poultry and fish, 4-5 servings/week of nuts and seeds, 2-3 servings of fats and oils (www.heartandstroke.ca).

DASH diet advocates the following recommendations:-

- Consumption of lesser processed foods and eating of more natural foods
- Lowering consumption of sodium in any form (if required one must also restrict sodium intake).
- Restricting preserved food items consumption (as most preserved items contains high sodium content).
- Choose alternative modes for food seasoning and flavoring like lime juice, blended seasoning, herbs, etc.
- Restrict addition of table salt after cooking in the meal.
- Avoid sauces, pickles, cured foods, canned foods, soy sauce, items prepared from smoking, etc.
- Avoid eating red meat.
- Restrict consumption of sweetened beverages, added sugars (in any form)
- Increase intake of whole grains (in any cooked forms), poultry, fish, lean meats, and nuts in the diet.
- Eat poultry and fish two times a week.
- Plentiful consumption of calcium, potassium, magnesium and fiber.
- DASH diet restrains the sodium intake between 1500 2300 miligram/day (www.mayoclinic.org)

7.3. MIND Diet

Seeing the level of improvements and deep impacts of Mediterranean and DASH diets scientists have developed a new improved and combined version of these two diets i.e., Mediterranean and DASH diet as named it as "MIND Diet". The term MIND diet stands for "Mediterranean-DASH Intervention for Neurodegenerative Delay". This diet has been proven to treat dementia, AD, heart diseases, BP, diabetes, and declined cognitive function with ageing. MIND diet also focuses on the consumption of whole grain, poultry, low-fat dairy, green leafy vegetables, nuts, berries, beans, fish, non-tropical oils like olive oils and wine (a glass/day).

Recommendations from MIND diet are:-

- 6 servings/week of green leafy veggies
- 1 serving/week of other vegetables
- 5 servings/week of nuts and seeds
- 2 or more servings/week of berries
- Minimum 3 servings/week of beans
- 3 or more servings/day of whole grains (in any cooked form)
- Fish must be consumed once/week
- Chicken/Turkey (i.e., poultry) is recommended 2 times/week
- Olive oil consumption is said to be included as a regular cooking oil
- Wine
- Avoid eating red meat
- Reduce the consumption of butter or margarine up to not more than 1tbsp/day
- Not more than 1 serving of cheese/week
- Avoid pastries and sweets and limit them to max. not more than 5 servings/week
- Restrict fried and fast food and limit it to not more than 1 serving/week.

Table 3. Different nutrients and their regulated brain functions

Nutrients	Their Brain Functions
Carbohydrates	Provides glucose, triggers the release of insulin that helps blood glucose enter the cells. As insulin levels rise, more of the amino acid tryptophan crosses the blood brain barrier that affects levels of neurotransmitters such as serotonin
Fats/Lipids	The lipid concentration of the brain partly reflects the dietary intake. About 35% of the brain/nervous system tissue comprises polyunsaturated fatty acids that include the essential fatty acids, eicosapentaenoic acid (EPA), and docosahexaenoic acid (DHA). EPA and DHA form phospholipids in brain cell membranes and have important roles in signal transduction.
Proteins	Provide amino acids; the precursors of neurotransmitters, and therefore facilitates neurotransmission and neuromodulation. The dietary precursors of serotonin (precursor is tryptophan), dopamine (precursor is phenylalanine), norepinephrine (precursor is tyrosine), and histamine (precursor is histadine) have been the main protein derivatives investigated
Thiamine (Vitamin B1)	Functions as a coenzyme in the synthesis of acetylcholine, γ-aminobutyric acid (GABA), and glutamate, Can mimic action of acetylcholine
Niacin (Vitamin B3)	Nicotinamide adenine dinucleotide (NADH) increases tyrosine hydroxylase activity and dopamine production in pheochromocytoma cells, Involved in synthesis of serotonin (5-HT)
Pyridoxine (Vitamin B6)	Role in the synthesis of many neurotransmitters (e.g., dopamine, serotonin, norepinephrine, epinephrine, histamine, GABA), Deficiency tends to reduce production of serotonin and GABA
Folic Acid (Vitamin B9)	Functions as a cofactor for enzymes that convert tryptophan into serotonin and tyrosine into norepinephrine/noradrenaline, Can heighten serotonin function by slowing destruction of brain tryptophan, Helps form compounds involved in brain energy metabolism, Involved in the synthesis of dopamine
Cobalamin (Vitamin B12)	Involved in the synthesis of monoamine neurotransmitters, Involved in maintaining myelin sheaths for nerve conductance, Functions in folate metabolism
Pantothenic Acid	Changes to coenzyme A that helps convert macronutrients into energy, Production of red blood cells, hormones, and nerve regulators, Needed for the uptake of amino acids and acetylcholine, Is necessary to make vitamin D and works closely with B vitamins such as biotin, niacin, vitamins B1, B2, and B6
Vitamin C	Acts as part of the intracellular antioxidant network, and is an important neuroprotective constituent, Acts as a neuromodulator and enzyme cofactor in noradrenaline and dopamine synthesis
Vitamin A	Retinoids influence hormone pathways (steroid and thyroid hormones) known to cause mood elevation and depression
Vitamin D	1,25-Dihydroxyvitamin D3 affects cholinergic activity in several brain regions and may have a role in the neuroendocrine regulation of certain aspects of anterior pituitary function
Vitamin E	Alpha-tocopherol protects cells from damage by free radicals, May reduce brain amyloid beta peptide accumulation, known to be relevant in Alzheimer's disease
Vitamin K	Involved in the development of the nervous system and affects calcium regulation in the brain through osteocalcin
Choline	Essential roles in structural integrity of cell membranes, cell signaling (precursor to acetylcholine), and nerve impulse transmission, Major source of methyl groups for methylation reactions

Table 3. (Continued)

Nutrients	Their Brain Functions
Calcium	Important intracellular messenger, cofactor for enzymes and release of neurotransmitters
Copper	Modulator of NMDA-receptor activity
Chloride	Negatively charged chloride ions cause influx of sodium ions and reverts the brain cell to its resting state
Chromium	Involved in glucose and lipid homeostasis
Iron	Essential cofactor for the production of ATP, Plays an essential role in hemoglobin for ensuring there is sufficient oxygen in the brain for oxidative metabolism, Functions in the enzyme system involved in the production of serotonin, norepinephrine, epinephrine, and dopamine
Magnesium	Functions as a coenzyme; roles in the metabolism of carbohydrates and fats to produce ATP, and in the synthesis of nucleic acids (DNA and RNA) and proteins, Important for the active transport of ions (such as potassium and calcium) across cell membranes, and for cell signaling
Manganese	deficiency results in lowering the catecholaminergic content of the brain
Phosphate	Helps maintain membrane potential and role in energy metabolism
Potassium	In the brain, potassium channels regulate neuronal signaling. Potassium channels may also regulate cell volume and protect neurons under metabolic stress. Role in energy metabolism
Selenium	Glutathione peroxidase maintains the integrity of the cellular and subcellular membranes. This antioxidative protective system of glutathione peroxidase depends heavily on selenium
Vanadium	Inhibits Na+-K+-ATPase pump activity
Zinc	Roles in protein synthesis, as well as structure and regulation of gene expression, Serves in neurons and glial cells. Certain zinc-enriched regions (e.g., hippocampus) are especially responsive to dietary zinc deprivation, which can cause learning impairment and olfactory dysfunction

Data Source: www.dietitians.ca

CONCLUSION

Diet and nutrition are the vital aspects of one's life and they become more important as an individual ages. Among all forms of health, mental health plays a crucial role as other health aspects are dependent on brain's health and its functioning. As older population undergoes great social and biological changes with passing years, their lifestyle, dietary and nutritional aspects becomes more important for them to stay healthy. Studies have shown that of all the nutrients in diet, amino acids, omega-3 fatty acids, phospholipids, folate, cholesterol, niacin, vitamin B6, 12, vitamin D, vitamin C, phosphorus, zinc, iron, magnesium plays a major role in neural health and brain's physiology, while their metabolism and level declines with age. On the contrary, saturated fats, trans fats, simple sugars, processed foods, excess salt, refined flours, and alcohol negatively affects the brain functioning and declines cognition and thinking. Several studies have shown that with ageing, a well-balanced diet greatly improves cognition and learning, and is highly effective in treating diseases like PD, AD, dementia, depression, anxiety, bipolar disorders, etc. For brain health diets like – Mediterranean diet, DASH diet, MIND diet are highly used as the dietary treatment mode for treating neural diseases and disorders, particularly in old age. Studies have also shown that plant based diet also effectively enhances the brain functioning.

REFERENCES

Adren, John B. (2010). Fueling your brain: Vitamins and Minerals. Rewire your brain. New Jersey: John Wiley and Sons., (Adren, John B., 2010, 101-102).

Arden, John B. (2010). Rewire your brain: Think your way to a better life. New Jersey: John Wiley and Sons., (Arden 2010, 107-116).

Baranowska-Bik, Agnieszka. & Bik, Wojciech. (2017). "Insulin and brain ageing". *Menopause Review.*, *16*(2), 44-46. doi: 10.5114/pm.2017. 68590. (Baranowska-Bik, Agnieszka and Bik, Wojciech 2017, 44-46).

Bentsen, Havard. (2017). "Dietary polyunsaturated fatty acids, brain function and mental health". *Microbial Ecology in Health and Disease*, *28*, 1-4. Doi: 10.1080/16512235.2017.1281916 (Bentsen, Havard 2017, 1-4).

Colby, S. L. & Ortman, J. M. (2014). *The Baby Boom Cohort in the United Stated*: 2012 to 20160.

Galvin, J. E. & Sadowsky, C. H. (2012). Practical guidelines for the recognition and diagnosis of dementia, *J Am Board Fam Med*, *25*, 367, 2012.

Gibney, J. Michael., et al. (2009). "*Introduction to human nutrition*". *Minerals and trace elements.* edited by JJ (Sean) Strain and Kevin D

Cashman. 188-237. Blackwell publishing: John Wiley and Sons. Originally published by The Nutrition Society., Zinc, 2nd edition (Gibney J, Michael et al. 2009, 209-212).

Global council on brain health. (2018). "Brain foods: GCBH recommendations on nourishing your brain health". 1-36. doi:10.264 19/pia.00019.001. (Global council on brain health. 2018, 2-26).

Gomez-Pinilla, Fernando. (2008). "Brain foods: the effects of nutrients on brain function". *Nature Reviews Neuroscience*, *9*, 575-578. doi: 10.1038/nrn2421. (Gomez-Pinilla, Fernando 2008, 572-573).

Hooper, C., et al. (2018). "The relationship of omega 3 polyunsaturated fatty acids in red blood cell membranes with cognitive function and brain structure: A review focused on Alzheimer's disease". *The journal of prevention of Alzheimer's disease.*, *5*, 78-84. doi: 10.14283/ jpad.2017.19 (Hooper, C. et al. 2018, 78-79).

Hussain, Ghulam., et al. (2019). "Role of cholesterol and sphingolipids in brain development and neurological diseases." *Lipids in health and disease.*, *18*, 26-38. Doi: 10.1186/s12944-019-0965-z. (Hussain, Ghulam et al. 2019, 27-33).

Jeremy, M. Berg., John, L. Tymoczko. & Lubert, Stryer. "Biochemistry." The integration of metabolism: Major metabolic pathways and control sites, edited by Susan Moran, 1260-1275. W. H. Freeman and Company., (Jeremy M. Berg, 1253).

Jun-Lin, Liu., et al. (2018). "Iron and Alzheimer's disease: From pathogenesis to therapeutic implications". *Frontiers in neuroscience.*, *12* (632), 1-14. doi:10.3389/fnins.2018.00632. (Jun-Lin Liu et al. 2018, 1-10).

Krikland, E. Anna., et al. (2018). "The role of magnesium in neurological disorders". *Nutrients.*, *10*, 730, 1-23. doi: 10.3390/nu10060730. (Krikland, E. Anna et al. 2018, 1-2).

Marco, Tulio Nunez. & Cecilia, Hidalgo. (2019). "Noxious Iron-Calcium connections in neurodegeneration" *Front. Neurosci.*, *13* (48), 1-18. doi: 10.3389fnins.2019.00048 (Marco Tulio Nunez and Cecilia Hidalgo. 2019, 1-12).

Moore, Katie., et al. (2018). "Diet, nutrition and the ageing brain: current evidences and new directions". Proceedings of the nutrition society. 77:152-163. doi: 10.1017/S0029665117004177. (Moore, Katie et al. 2018, 153-157).

Packer, Lester., et al. (2010). "Micronutrients in brain health". In Animal models of zinc deficiency. Edited by Packer, Lester et al.

Rush, M. Toni., et al. (2017). "Association of dietary sodium intake and cognitive function in older adults". *J Nutr Health Ageing, 21* (3), 276-283. doi: 10.1007/s12603-016-0766-2. (Rush, m. Toni et al. 2017, 276-283).

So Young, Lim., et al. (2016). "Antioxidants". *Nutritional factors affecting mental health.*, *5*(3), 143-152. doi: 10.7762/cnr.2016.5.3.143 (So Young Lim et al. 2016, 146).

So Young, Lim., et al. (2016). "Nutritional factors affecting mental health". *Clinical Nutrition Research*, *5*(3), 143-152. Doi.org/10.7762/cnr.2016.5.3.143 (So Young Lim et al. 2016).

Sonia, Guerra-Gomes., et al. (2018). "The role of astrocytic calcium signaling in the aged prefrontal cortex". *Front. Cell. Neurosci.*, *10*, 1-9. doi: 10.3389/fncel.2018.00379 (Sonia Guerra-Gomes et al. 2018, 1-9).

Stankiewicz, James., et al. (2014). 'Iron in chronic brain disorders: Imaging and neurotherapeautic implications". *Mech Ageing Dev.*, 136-137, (100), 22-28. doi:10.1016/j.mad.2013.11.005. (Stankiewicz, James et al. 2014, 22-26)

The role of nutrition in mental health promotion and prevention. https://www.dietitians.ca/Downloads/Public/Nutrition-and-Mental-Health-1.aspx

Watson, Jessica., et al. (2018). "Consequences of inadequate intakes of vitamin A, Vitamin B12, Vitamin D, Calcium, Iron and Folate in older persons". *Current Geriatrics Report.*, *7*(2), 103-113. doi:10.1007/s13670-018-0241-5. (Watson, Jessica et al., 2018, 106).

Whal, Davin., et al. (2016). "Nutritional Strategies to optimize cognitive function in the ageing brain". *Ageing Res Rev.*, *31*, 80-92. doi:10.1016/j.arr.2016.06.006. (Whal, Davin et al. 2016, 87).

Websites

http://trap.ncirl.ie/1965/1/dionnesmith.pdf.

http://www.census.gov/prod/2014pubs/p25-1141.pdf.accessed December 30,2014.

http://www.un.org/en/development/desa/population/publications/pdf/ageing/WPA2017_Highlights.pdf.

https://2012books.lardbucket.org/books/an-introduction-to-nutrition/index.html.

https://apps.who.int/iris/bitstream/handle/10665/186463/9789240694811_eng.pdf;jsessionid=95E0ECFB937DBB3CB269A6101E54B9CB?sequence=1.

https://bebrainfit.com/vitamin-b12-benefits/.

https://braintest.com/lean-protein-really-protect-brain/.

https://core.ac.uk/download/pdf/84755544.pdf.

https://en.wikipedia.org/wiki/Geriatrics.

https://en.wikipedia.org/wiki/Gerontology.

https://faculty.washington.edu/chudler/facts.html.

https://healthyeating.sfgate.com/much-sodium-should-elderly-consume-5893.html.

https://healthyeating.sfgate.com/potassium-memory-11232.html.

https://khn.org/news/why-older-adults-should-eat-more-protein-and-not-overdo-protein-shakes/.

https://lpi.oregonstate.edu/mic/life-stages/older-adults.

https://lpi.oregonstate.edu/mic/life-stages/older-adults.

https://naturalcalm.ca/vitamin-c-brain-health-mood-anxiety-focus/.

https://ods.od.nih.gov/factsheets/Folate-HealthProfessional/.

https://ods.od.nih.gov/factsheets/Magnesium-HealthProfessional/.

https://ods.od.nih.gov/factsheets/Omega3FattyAcids-HealthProfessional/.

https://ods.od.nih.gov/factsheets/VitaminD-health%20Professional/.

https://ourworldindata.org/why-do-women-live-longer-than-men

https://universityhealthnews.com/daily/memory/b-vitamins-for-memory-niacin-benefits-for-alzheimers-disease/.

https://www.aarp.org/content/dam/aarp/research/survey_statistics/health/2017/brain-health-nutrition.doi.10.26419%252Fres.00187.001.pdf.

https://www.aarp.org/health/brain-health/global-council-on-brain-health/nutrition/.

https://www.afar.org/pdfs/AFAR-Guide-to-Theories-of-Agingsm.pdf

https://www.alzdiscovery.org/cognitive-vitality/blog/exercise-with-dash-diet-improved-cognitive-functions-in-older-adults.

https://www.alzheimers.org.uk/omega-3-and-dementia.

https://www.google.com/search?q=UN+world+older+population+prospects+2017&tbm=isch&tbs=rimg:CTrxdVwwrHEMIjh3qaLzpA041cEaxzLxi9OqhvGvwZfmLeE-0ibMna6O59TSoZngeVu8mzoBmRu7Tw-eoHQLEHiEXioSCXepovOkDTjVEcIU9CPEQzCfKhIJwRrHMvGL06oRPUcXyBNc6S4qEgmG8a_1Bl-Yt4RGY-QH83rr6NioSCT7SJsydro7nEcF_1CejKUSHOKhIJ1NKhmeB5W7wRiHb2Io0s-dMqEgmbOgGZG7tPDxFc0wyymnfV1CoSCZ6gdAsQeIReEZbd-ScYKliS&tbo=u&sa=X&ved=2ahUKEwiw-q7v_PzgAhUE6Y8KHW6kDG0Q9C96BAgBEBg&biw=1366&bih=608&dpr=1#imgrc=RtNO93sJOWRLSM.

https://www.google.com/search?q=UN+world+older+population+prospects+2017&tbm=isch&tbs=rimg:CUbTTvd7CTlkIjhd_19o8S7WBVbbgK2aGDNytnhxevq3sehwS-ha6y3RNFCn1_1S8RCLKu82lzbY63QHU0irZF3a3eNyoSCV3_12jxLtYFVEdaWWdJBXjymKhIJtuArZoYM3K0R8WDYvr5ExSUqEgmeHF6-rex6HBHiQgosjTwczyoSCRL6FrrLdE0UES5lM5BUFsecKhIJKfX9LxEIsq4RlyY8LbVH56MqEgnzaXNtjrdAdRHnyu_1CySIhPSoSCTSKtkXdrd43EQvvN1rdmsQS&tbo=u&sa=X&ved=2ahUKEwiT4uaf_fzgAhXXknAKHf_TA8gQ9C96BAgBEBg&biw=1366&bih=608&dpr=1#imgrc=Aqjz8RsGK0bAGM.

https://www.health.harvard.edu/blog/nutritional-psychiatry-your-brain-on-food-201511168626.

https://www.healthline.com/nutrition/10-proven-magnesium-benefits#section1.

https://www.healthline.com/nutrition/vitamin-b6-benefits.

https://www.heartandstroke.ca/get-healthy/healthy-eating/dash-diet.

https://www.ifnacademy.com/wp-content/uploads/2015/08/Drew-Ramsey-Updated-PPT-version-9.28.17-1.pdf.

https://www.lifeextension.com/Magazine/2016/6/Unique-Magnesium-Compound-Reverses-Brain-Aging/Page-01.

https://www.livescience.com/29365-human-brain.html.

https://www.mayoclinic.org/diseases-conditions/hyponatremia/expert-answers/low-blood-sodium/faq-20058465.

https://www.mayoclinic.org/healthy-lifestyle/nutrition-and-healthy-eating/in-depth/dash-diet/art-20050989.

https://www.medicalnewstoday.com/articles/321800.php.

https://www.medicalnewstoday.com/articles/321865.php.

https://www.medicalnewstoday.com/articles/323623.php.

https://www.myvmc.com/lifestyles/nutrition-and-brain-health/

https://www.un.org/development/desa/publications/world-population-prospects-the-2017-revision.html.

https://www.upi.com/Study-High-cholesterol-linked-to-better-brain-health-after-age-85/5731520279738/.

https://www.verywellhealth.com/age-related-diseases-2223996.

https://www.verywellmind.com/how-big-is-the-brain-2794888.

https://www.who.int/whr/2001/media_centre/press_release/en/.

https://www2.gov.bc.ca/assets/gov/people/seniors/health-safety/pdf/healthy-eating-seniorsbook.pdf.

ABOUT THE EDITOR

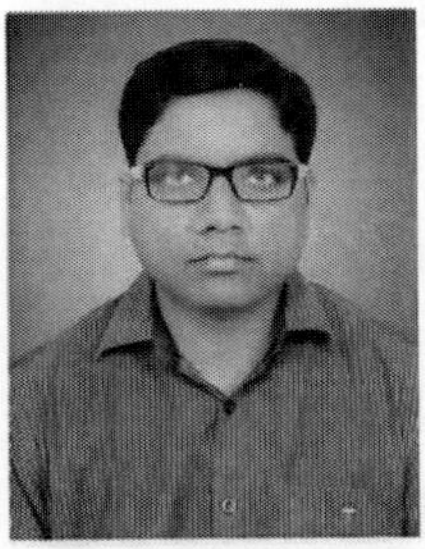

Dr. Abhai Kumar is working as principal research scientist at Department of Science and Technology, Government of India sponsored project at Interdisciplinary School of Life Sciences, and Department of Neurology, Institute of Medical Sciences, Banaras Hindu University, Varanasi, India. He did his masters in Biotechnology from Deen Dayal Upadhyay Gorakhpur University, Gorakhpur, India in 2002 and later his doctoral studies from CSIR-Indian Institute of Toxicology Research, Lucknow, India in 2008 in area of Biotechnology. Dr. Kumar has done his postdoctoral work from prestigious University of Pittsburgh Medical Centre, Pittsburgh, PA, USA. Expertise in Neuroscience research and used sophisticated techniques like plasma proteomics, microarray, mass spectrometry in elucidating disease mechanism and early diagnosis, he is recipient of various awards and international fellowship from Ministry of

Science and Technology, Government of India, New Delhi, University Grants Commission, New Delhi, India and other societies related to Cognitive Neuroscience and Neuroscience research for his outstanding work on early diagnosis of mild cognitive impairment in elderly population. Dr. Kumar has several peer reviewed articles in international and national journal of repute, book chapters, in international acclaimed books on biomarkers, diseases and nutrition. Dr. Kumar is member of various scientific societies and awarded by INSA, New Delhi. He is the recipient of fellowship, research award in International meetings on Cognition and Neurochemistry. Dr. Kumar is Project Director for Ageing Health Services of Chand Foundation, Gorakhpur for delivering mental health management to elderly people in rural and urban settings. The work on AD done by Dr. Kumar has produced international publications and several book chapters for awareness of disease among health care workers and public in general.

INDEX

D

E

G

H

I

M

N

O

P

S

T

V